Best of Five Questions for
MRCP Part 1

This book is dedicated to mother and father – for perseverence.

It is also dedicated to the memory of Dr Steven Feenan, a truly good man.

Commissioning Editor: Ellen Green
Project Development Manager: Janice Urquhart
Project Manager: Frances Affleck
Designer: Erik Bigland
Illustration Manager: Bruce Hogarth
Illustrator: Richard Morris

Best of Five Questions for
MRCP Part 1

Helen Fellows BSc MB BS MRCP
Clinical Fellow, Intensive Care Medicine, Royal Cornwall Hospital, Truro, UK

Simon Noble MB BS MRCP PGCE DipPalMed
Specialist Registrar in Palliative Medicine, Cardiff, UK

Harry Dalton BSc DPhil FRCP DipMedEd
Consultant Physician, Royal Cornwall Hospital, Truro, UK

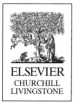

ELSEVIER
CHURCHILL
LIVINGSTONE

EDINBURGH LONDON NEW YORK OXFORD PHILADELPHIA
ST LOUIS SYDNEY TORONTO 2005

ELSEVIER
CHURCHILL
LIVINGSTONE

First published 2005

ISBN 0 443 10020 9

British Library Cataloguing in Publication Data
A catalogue record for this book is available from the British Library

Library of Congress Cataloging in Publication Data
A catalog record for this book is available from the Library of Congress

Notice
Medical knowledge is constantly changing. Standard safety precautions must be followed, but as new research and clinical experience broaden our knowledge, changes in treatment and drug therapy may become necessary or appropriate. Readers are advised to check the most current product information provided by the manufacturer of each drug to be administered to verify the recommended dose, the method and duration of administration, and contraindications. It is the responsibility of the practitioner, relying on experience and knowledge of the patient, to determine dosages and the best treatment for each individual patient. Neither the Publisher nor the authors assume any liability for any injury and/or damage to persons or property arising from this publication.
The Publisher

your source for books,
journals and multimedia
in the health sciences
www.elsevierhealth.com

The
publisher's
policy is to use
**paper manufactured
from sustainable forests**

Printed in China

We have attempted to provide you with 350 examination-style questions on topics that you are likely to encounter in the examination. When choosing the best option from the five possible answers, it is important to understand why the other four options are not correct. Often more than one of the answers is plausible and so be careful to check exactly what the examiners are looking for, by reading the question carefully.

The questions have been arranged in a random fashion – that is, they are not arranged by specialty. This mirrors the way in which you will encounter the questions in the exam. Knowing that some candidates also like to review questions by topic, we have included an appendix of subject categories that lists all the questions that pertain to a specialty.

This book originally arose from the authors' involvement in local SHO teaching programmes. The questions we wrote as part of the teaching were well received and, we are told, pitched at an appropriate level for the exam. There are several classic topics that come up in the exam and on occasion we have included some deliberately difficult questions. This is to illustrate important topics and provide a focus for learning. We have tried to provide expanded answers to the questions, with essential lists and tables where relevant. The examination has become far more clinically relevant and this is reflected in the scope of questions.

We have piloted the questions to several cohorts of MRCP candidates and have enlisted the help of senior colleagues (including college examiners) to review questions on their particular speciality. We are grateful to the following people for their advice and comments during the preparation of this book: Alex Murray, John Barnes, Shaheena Sadiq, Meg Williams, Emma Mason, Nick Reynolds, Tony Mourant, Paul Johnston, Rob Parry, Brendan McLean, Moya O'Doherty. A special thanks goes to Dr Austin Hunt for his help with regards to all things creepy crawly.

HF   2004
SIRN
HRD

Contents

QUESTIONS

Q

1   Answer on p.117.

A 22-year-old lady presents to her GP with facial swelling, most marked in the morning, and shortness of breath. Urinalysis shows protein +++.
Results were as follows:

24-hour urinary protein	4.2 g	
Haemoglobin (Hb)	10.8 g/L	(11.5–16.0 g/L)
Urea	22.8 mmol/L	(2.5–6.5 mmol/L)
Creatinine	374 µmol/L	(70–150 µmol/L)
C_3	0.24 g/L	(0.55–1.2 g/L)
C_4	0.29 g/L	(0.2–0.5 g/L)

Which of the following is the most likely diagnosis?

A. Minimal change nephropathy
B. Systemic lupus erythematosus
C. Rheumatoid arthritis
D. Cryoglobulinaemia
E. Diabetes mellitus

2   Answer on p.118.

A 52-year-old man was admitted after returning from holiday abroad. A diagnosis of pneumonia had been made by his GP; however, he failed to respond to a course of amoxicillin.

On admission he has a dry cough, myalgia and abdominal pain. He is pyrexial at 38°C, heart rate of 110 and respiratory rate of 28. An initial chest X-ray (CXR) shows diffuse bilateral basal opacities. Blood cultures taken at the time show no growth after 48 hours. Whilst in hospital he becomes increasingly confused, his Glasgow Coma Scale (GCS) dropping to 11 and blood test as follows:

Sodium (Na)	118 (135–145 mmol/L)	Hb	14.1 (13–18 g/dL)
Potassium (K)	4.2 (3.5–5.3 mmol/L)	White blood cell count (WCC)	13.2 (4–11 × 10⁹/L)
Urea	9.2 (2.5–6.7 mmol/L)	Neutrophils	10.1 (2–7.5 × 10⁹/L)
Creatinine	180 (50–120 µmol/L)	Lymphocytes	1.0 (1.5–4 × 10⁹/L)

Which of the following is the most likely diagnosis?

A. Churg–Strauss
B. Sarcoidosis
C. *Legionella* pneumonia
D. *Mycoplasma* pneumonia
E. *Pneumocystis carinii* pneumonia

3 Answer on p.119.

A previously fit 79-year-old gentleman is found to have a blood pressure (BP) of 180/90 mmHg on three occasions, 1 month apart. He takes aspirin 75 mg that was started 2 years ago for 'dizzy turns'. Examination is unremarkable, as is the electrocardiogram (ECG) and chest X-ray.
  Which of the following courses of action would you recommend?

A. Monitor BP on a 2-month basis and treat if the diastolic BP is > 100 mmHg
B. Take no further action
C. Oral atenolol
D. Oral angiotensin-converting enzyme (ACE) inhibitor
E. Oral bendrofluazide

4 Answer on p.119.

A 40-year-old female presents with a mole that has changed in appearance. A biopsy diagnoses melanoma with a Breslow's thickness of less than 0.75 mm.
  What is the next course of management?

A. Localized radiotherapy
B. Chemotherapy
C. Excision of remaining mole with a clear margin of skin
D. Excision of mole and draining lymph nodes
E. Interferon

5 Answer on p.120.

An 18-year-old insulin-dependent diabetic is seen in A&E. Over the last 4 days she has suffered from diarrhoea and vomiting, and has cut down on her insulin injections. Her mother has brought her in because she has become drowsy and confused. Her blood results are as follows:

WCC	16.4×10^9/L	$(4–11 \times 10^9$/L)
Hb	$17.8 \times$ g/dL	(12–16 g/dL)
Platelets	597×10^9/L	$(150–400 \times 10^9$/L)
Na	146 mmol/L	(135–145 mmol/L)
K	6.6 mmol/L	(3.5–5 mmol/L)
Urea	8.4 mmol/L	(2.5–6.7 mmol/L)
Creatinine	145 μmol/L	(60–120 μmol/L)
Random glucose	26 mmol/L	(4.5–5.6 mmol/L)

  You are with one nurse in the resuscitation room. What is the first thing you are going to ask her to do?

A. Start an insulin sliding scale
B. Give 1 L of normal saline over 30 minutes
C. Run to the lab with blood gases
D. Draw up 10 mL of 10% calcium gluconate
E. Give 100 mmol bicarbonate intravenously (iv)

6   Answer on p.121.

A 70-year-old man with is admitted with new-onset atrial fibrillation with an apical rate of 120/minute and a BP of 100/70 mmHg. Shortly after admission he develops moderate lower abdominal pain and diarrhoea with dark red blood.
   Which is the most appropriate course of action?

A. Cardioversion
B. Unfractionated heparin
C. Mesenteric angiography
D. Laparotomy
E. Digoxin

7   Answer on p.122.

A patient has the following test results:

VDRL   1:16
TPHA   negative

   Which of the following would be consistent with these results?

A. Primary syphilis
B. Secondary syphilis
C. Tertiary syphilis
D. Systemic lupus erythematosus
E. Previous infection with yaws

8   Answer on p.122.

A 24-year-old man presents to his A&E department with a sudden-onset painful right eye. He is otherwise fit and well. On examination, there is a right-sided ptosis. On lifting the eyelid, the pupil is fixed and dilated and there is diplopia on all eye movements except gaze to the right.
   Which of the following is the most likely diagnosis?

A. Subarachnoid haemorrhage
B. Multiple sclerosis
C. Optic nerve glioma
D. Cavernous sinus thrombosis
E. Posterior communicating artery aneurysm

9 Answer on p.123.

A 65-year-old man presents with erectile problems. He has requested sildenafil but is already on several medicines.
Which of the following drugs contraindicates it being prescribed?

A. Isosorbide mononitrate
B. Atenolol
C. Enalapril
D. Digoxin
E. Simvastatin

10 Answer on p.124.

Which of the following is an absolute contraindication to electroconvulsive therapy (ECT)?

A. Pregnancy
B. Raised intracranial pressure
C. Age > 60 years
D. Presence of cardiac pacemaker
E. Previous stroke

11 Answer on p.124.

A 51-year-old patient with rheumatoid arthritis is admitted with pneumococcal pneumonia. On examination she has splenomegaly and the following blood test results:

Hb	10 g/dL	(12–16 g/dL)
WCC	2.1×10^9/L	(4–11×10^9/L)
Platelets	123×10^9/L	(150–400×10^9/L)

Which of the following HLA haplotypes is the patient most likely to possess?

A. B27
B. DR3
C. DR4
D. DR1
E. DQ2

12 Answer on p.125.

A 60-year-old female has been on long-term treatment for rheumatoid arthritis. She presents with dyspnoea on minimal exertion and a non-productive cough. Oxygen saturation on air is 84% and chest radiograph shows diffuse bilateral interstitial infiltrates. Extensive investigation for an infective cause is negative.

Which of the following drugs is most likely to be responsible?

A. Methotrexate
B. Penicillamine
C. Pednisolone
D. Cyclosporin
E. Hydroxychloroquine

13 Answer on p.126.

A 65-year-old man has the following blood results on admission to hospital:

Na	132 mmol/L	(135–145 mmol/L)
K	8.6 mmol/L	(3.5–5 mmol/L)
Urea	42.4 mmol/L	(2.5–6.7 mmol/L)
Creatinine	1178 µmol/L	(70–150 µmol/L)

The patient appears unwell and the ECG shows tented T waves, absent P waves and widened QRS.

Which of the following therapeutic interventions should be performed first?

A. Immediate haemodialysis
B. Intravenous insulin and dextrose
C. Intravenous calcium gluconate
D. Nebulized salbutamol
E. Oral calcium resonium

14 Answer on p.127.

Which of the following is true regarding troponins?

A. They remain raised for 3 weeks
B. They have equal sensitivity as CK-MB
C. They are a useful indicator of severity of ischaemic heart disease
D. Peak levels occur after 12 hours
E. They can be used to rule out ischaemic heart disease

15
Answer on p.127.

A 42-year old male treated for scabies with malathion becomes re-infected.

Which of the following is the most likely cause for this?

A. Malathion resistance
B. Failure to apply malathion to scalp
C. Not changing underwear daily
D. Failure to wash bedding
E. Failure to apply malathion on three separate occasions

16
Answer on p.128.

A 35-year-old woman with polycystic ovary syndrome presents with anovulatory infertility. She has been on a diet and exercise programme, but cannot get her body mass index below 27 kg/m^2.

Which of the following is the most appropriate treatment for her infertility?

A. Clomiphene
B. Metformin
C. Gonadotrophins
D. Orlistat
E. *In vitro* fertilization

17
Answer on p.129.

The polymerase chain reaction is routinely used in the laboratory diagnosis of which of the following conditions?

A. Down's syndrome
B. Phenylketonuria
C. Cystic fibrosis
D. Di George's syndrome
E. Turner's syndrome

18
Answer on p.130.

A British Army soldier presents on return from exercises in Belize, Central America, with a 3-month-old ulcerating lesion on the upper lip. He is referred for investigation to the ENT Department. Examination reveals widespread nasopharyngeal involvement.

Which of the following is the most likely causative organism?

A. *Dermatobium hominis*
B. *Trypanosoma cruzi*
C. *Leishmania mexicana*
D. *Leishmania braziliensis*
E. *Dracunculus medinensis*

---

19   Answer on p.131.

A weakness of which one of the following would *not* be expected by damage to the radial nerve in the axilla?

A. Elbow extension
B. Elbow flexion in half supination
C. Elbow pronation
D. Wrist extension
E. Finger flexion

---

20   Answer on p.131.

A 56-year-old male presents to his GP with galactorrhoea.
   Which of the following oral medicines could be responsible?

A. Cimetidine
B. Domperidone
C. Spironolactone
D. Bromocriptine
E. Griseofulvin

---

21   Answer on p.133.

The following blood tests were taken at a routine clinic attendance:

Na	138 mmol/L	(135–145 mmol/L)
K	4.0 mmol/L	(3.5–5.0 mmol/L)
Cl	108 mmol/L	(95–106 mmol/L)
Bicarbonate	20 mmol/L	(22–30 mmol/L)
Urea	6.8 mmol/L	(2.5–6.7 mmol/L)
Creatinine	108 µmol/L	(70–150 µmol/L)

Which of the following is the correct value of the anion gap?

A. 8 mmol/L
B. 10 mmol/L
C. 12 mmol/L
D. 14 mmol/L
E. 16 mmol/L

22 Answer on p.133.

A patient has an elective lumbar puncture for investigation of suspected multiple sclerosis.

Which of the following is least likely to contribute to the development of a post-lumbar puncture headache?

A. Multiple attempts at lumbar puncture
B. Angle of needle bevel inserted horizontally
C. Angle of needle bevel inserted vertically
D. Large bore lumbar puncture needle
E. Removal of the lumbar puncture needle without first replacing the introducer stylet

23 Answer on p.134.

A 65-year-old man had a transient ischaemic attack (TIA) 3 months ago. Investigations revealed significant stenosis in the corresponding carotid artery, but he was considered a major anaesthetic risk and not appropriate for surgery. He presents with a further TIA. He is normotensive and in sinus rhythm. He is currently taking aspirin 150 mg for secondary prevention.

What is the next step to prevent further embolic events?

A. Increase aspirin to 300 mg
B. Continue aspirin and start warfarin
C. Continue aspirin and start dipyridamole 200 mg bd
D. Continue aspirin 150 mg and start clopidogrel 75 mg
E. Stop aspirin and start warfarin

24 Answer on p.135.

Concerning adrenal physiology, which of the following hormones is secreted by the zona glomerulosa?

A. Adrenaline
B. Noradrenaline
C. Cortisol
D. Aldosterone
E. Angiotensin II

25 Answer on p.135.

A 26-year-old male is reviewed in outpatients following admission with abdominal pain. At the time he was noted to have a left wrist drop and a blistering photosensitive rash. His test results from the acute admission have now come back and include:

Urinary δ-aminolaevulinic acid	Raised
Urinary porphyrins	Raised
Faecal porphyrins	Raised

What is the most likely diagnosis?

A. Acute intermittent porphyria
B. Variegate porphyria
C. Hereditary coproporphyria
D. Porphyria cutanea tarda
E. Congenital porphyria

26   Answer on p.137.

A 38-year-old male is referred to outpatients with abnormal liver function tests (LFTs), found on a routine medical examination for insurance purposes. He has no risk factors for chronic liver disease but takes an ACE inhibitor for mild hypertension. He drinks 20 units of alcohol per week but has not drunk any alcohol for 3 months. Examination is unremarkable.
Bloods are as follows:

	6 months ago	3 months ago	Now	Normal range
Alanine transaminase (ALT; IU/L)	68	47	72	3–35
Alkaline phosphatase (ALP; IU/L)	100	96	78	3–110
Bilirubin (μmol/L)	4	8	7	3–17

Which of the following is the most likely diagnosis?

A. Chronic hepatitis C
B. Excess alcohol
C. Chronic hepatitis B
D. Non-alcoholic steatohepatitis
E. Drug reaction to ACE inhibitor

27   Answer on p.137.

What is the main advantage of a post-marketing surveillance scheme of a newly released drug?

A. To detect Type A adverse drug events
B. To detect Type B adverse drug events
C. To monitor effectiveness
D. To assess safety of the drug in the patient population
E. To assess patient satisfaction

---

28 Answer on p.138.

A 33-year-old female is seen in the maternity department. She suffers from SLE. Her child was born with profound bradycardia.
Which of the following antibodies is most likely to be present?

A. Anti-Ro
B. Anti-La
C. Anti-Jo
D. Anti-Scl-70
E. Antiphospholipid antibodies

---

29 Answer on p.138.

Which of the following is not associated with Epstein–Barr virus infection?

A. Burkitt's lymphoma
B. Nasopharyngeal carcinoma
C. Oral hairy leukoplakia
D. Hodgkin's lymphoma
E. Kaposi's sarcoma

---

30 Answer on p.140.

A 76-year-old man attends clinic with his wife. She gives a history of transient memory loss and confusion in her husband. She reports being downstairs when he came into the room appearing not to recognize her. Furthermore, he did not know who or where he was. He was able to carry out conversations regarding his surroundings but had impaired memory of past events. His symptoms remained for the rest of the day but awoke the following morning back to normal. His retrograde amnesia was limited to a short period of time prior to coming down stairs. He has a past history of hypertension and migraine. Which of the following diagnoses best suit this clinical picture.

A. Frontal lobe dementia
B. Subdural haematoma affecting right frontal lobe
C. Transient ischaemic attack affecting left temporal lobe
D. Transient global amnesia
E. Migraine with aura

---

31 Answer on p.140.

A 67-year-old man presents with nausea and pain in his right upper quadrant. On examination, he has tender hepatomegaly with an irregular edge. His blood tests are as follows:

Hb	8 g/dL	(11.5–16 g/dL)
WCC	17.8×10^9/L	(4–11×10^9/L)
Platelets	104×10^9/L	(150–400×10^9/L)
Neutrophils	68%	
Normoblasts	8%	
Myeloblasts	8%	
Myelocytes	5%	
Metamyelocytes	5%	
Lymphocytes	15%	

What is the most likely cause of his anaemia?

A. Gaucher's disease
B. Leukaemoid reaction secondary to acute infection
C. Myelosclerosis
D. Malignant infiltration of bone marrow
E. Osteopetrosis

32   Answer on p.141.

A well-designed randomized controlled trial finds that, in cancer patients, using long-term low-molecular-weight heparin (LMWH) instead of warfarin reduces the incidence of recurrent venous thromboses from 17% to 9%. This is shown to be statistically significant. This single trial is used as the basis of recommending the use of LMWH in all cancer patients with deep vein thrombosis.

What evidence level does this trial offer?

A. Evidence level Ia
B. Evidence level Ib
C. Evidence level IIa
D. Evidence level IIb
E. Evidence level III

33   Answer on p.142.

A phlebotomist sustains a needlestick injury whilst taking blood from a HIV-positive patient.

Which one of the following has been shown to most reduce the risk of HIV transmission?

A. Thorough immediate washing of the injury site with water
B. Oral lamivudine therapy for 1 month
C. Oral zidovudine therapy for 1 month
D. Oral ritonavir therapy for 1 month
E. Oral triple therapy for 1 month

Answer on p.143.

A 75-year-old lady presents with persistent diarrhoea and weight loss. Twenty years previously she had radiotherapy for carcinoma of the ovary. Thirty years ago she lived in Hong Kong for 18 months. Her father died of cancer of the colon aged 62 years.

Hb	9.4 g/dL	(11.5–16 g/dL)
WCC	9.6×10^9/L	$(4–11 \times 10^9$/L)
Platelets	234×10^9/L	$(150–400 \times 10^9$/L)
B_{12}	153 pmol/L	(160–900 pmol/L)
Red cell folate	21 nmol/L	(130–630 nmol/L)
Ferritin	5 µg/L	(20–250 µg/L)
Erythrocyte sedimentation rate (ESR)	36 mm/hour	

Which of the following is the most likely diagnosis?

A. Radiation enteritis
B. Carcinoma of the colon
C. Crohn's disease
D. Tropical sprue
E. Acquired lactose intolerance

 Answer on p.143.

Where in the lungs is the azygous lobe?

A. Above right upper lobe
B. Above right middle lobe
C. Above lingula lobe
D. Below lingula lobe
E. Below right middle lobe

 Answer on p.144.

A 32-year-old woman presents with left loin pain and haematuria. She is known to suffer with Crohn's disease.

Which of the following is likely to be the aetiology of this presentation?

A. Hypercalciuria
B. Hyperbilirubinaemia
C. Hyperuricaemia
D. Hyperoxaluria
E. Type 1 renal tubular acidosis

37   Answer on p.145.

Which one of the following patients should not drive a motor car in the UK?

A. Coronary angioplasty performed 10 days previously
B. Implantable cardioverter defibrillator (ICD) inserted 7 months previously
C. Monocular vision for 3 years with normal acuity and visual fields in the other eye
D. Previously well-controlled epileptic, last fit was at lunchtime 9 months previously
E. Subarachnoid haemorrhage 4 months ago, with no cause found

38   Answer on p.145.

A 76-year-old gentleman is referred with an international normalized ratio (INR) of 8.4. He normally takes warfarin for a prosthetic mitral valve. He had an epistaxis lasting 15 minutes this morning. He is otherwise asymptomatic and haemodynamically stable.
   Having stopped his warfarin for tonight, which of the following is the most appropriate course of action?

A. 5 mg iv vitamin K
B. 0.5 mg orally (po) vitamin K
C. 4 units of fresh frozen plasma iv
D. 50 units/kg of prothrombin complex concentrate
E. Recheck INR in 24 hours

39   Answer on p.146.

What is the most common predisposing illness that has been related to the onset of Guillain–Barré syndrome?

A. *Campylobacter jejuni*
B. *Yersinia enterocolitica*
C. *Escherichia coli*
D. *Brucella melitensis*
E. *Chlamydia trachomatis*

40   Answer on p.147.

A 25-year-old male from Ghana has been living in the UK for 5 years. He presents with a 5-day history of painful penile ulcers. He has recently had unprotected sex with a new partner. On examination he has a cluster of 1–2 mm punched out penile ulcers. He has tender inguinal lymphadenopathy but no evidence of pus. What is the most likely diagnosis?

A. Genital herpes
B. Beçhet's disease
C. Syphylis
D. Chancroid
E. Lymphogranuloma venereum

---

41   Answer on p.147.

A 64-year-old man who suffers from haemochromatosis is seen in A&E with a 2-day history of pain and swelling in his right knee. On examination it is swollen and he has decreased range of movement. You aspirate his knee.
    What will the aspirate be most likely to show?

A. Gram-positive cocci in clusters
B. Positively bifringent crystals
C. Gram-positive cocci in chains
D. Inflammatory cells with haemosiderin deposition
E. Negatively bifringent crystals

---

42   Answer on p.148.

A 24-year-old asthmatic woman is brought into Casualty with a history of having possibly ingested as many as 50 paracetamol tablets 2 hours ago. She is on no other medicines and has no past medical history. She has a GCS of 15 and physical examination is normal.
    What should be done next?

A. Gastric lavage
B. Oral activated charcoal
C. Oral ipecacuanha
D. Await four-hour serum paracetamol levels
E. Intravenous *N*-acetyl cysteine

---

43   Answer on p.149.

A 52-year-old female is admitted following a significant paracetamol overdose. She begins treatment with *N*-acetyl cysteine but then says she wants to leave. She volunteers that she took the paracetamol to try and stop the 'dead soldiers from taunting her'. They have done this ever since she turned on the radio and realized that Mickey Mouse wanted her to assassinate Father Christmas. She wants to leave and kill herself. She refuses to stay in hospital and has pulled her venflon out.

Under which Section of the 1983 Mental Health Act should you detain her?

A. Section 2
B. Section 3
C. Section 4
D. Section 5(2)
E. Section 5(4)

44 Answer on p.150.

A 19-year-old female presents with severe tiredness. Three weeks ago she had a serious chest infection, which was treated with a full course of antibiotics.

Hb	9.3 g/dL	(12–16 g/dL)
Mean cell volume (MCV)	98 fL	(85–96 fL)
Mean cell haemoglobin (MCH)	28 g/dL	(32–35 g/dL)
White blood count (WBC)	7.8×10^9/L	(4–11×10^9/L)
Platelets	178×10^9/L	(150–400×10^9/L)
Reticulocytes	9%	(< 1%)
Monospot	Negative	
Blood film	Polychromasia, autoagglutination Microspherocytes	

Which of the following is the most likely diagnosis?

A. Infectious mononucleosis
B. Erythromycin-induced myasthenia
C. Penicillin-induced haemolysis
D. Hodgkin's disease
E. *Mycoplasma*-induced cold antibody haemolysis

45 Answer on p.150.

A 24-year-old lady is referred to outpatients. Her GP thinks she has irritable bowel syndrome.
Which of the following symptoms would most favour an alternative diagnosis?

A. Passage of mucous per rectum
B. Diarrhoea with > 6 bowel actions per day
C. Nocturnal diarrhoea with 1–2 bowel actions per night
D. Severe abdominal pain
E. A 2-year history of persisting symptoms

46
Answer on p.151.

A patient with chronic renal impairment is being assessed for either haemodialysis or peritoneal dialysis.
  Which of the following features would contraindicate peritoneal dialysis?

A. Insulin-dependant diabetes
B. Peripheral vascular disease
C. Ischaemic heart disease
D. Crohn's disease
E. On waiting list for renal transplant

47
Answer on p.153.

A 35-year-old man is due to have an elective splenectomy for immune thrombocytopenia.
  When should immunization for pneumococcus be administered?

A. 1 month prior to surgery
B. 1 week prior to surgery
C. 1 day after surgery
D. 1 week after surgery
E. 1 month after surgery

48
Answer on p.153.

Which of the following cytokines down-regulates the immunological response?

A. Interleukin-1
B. Interleukin-2
C. Interleukin-6
D. Interleukin-10
E. Interleukin-12

49
Answer on p.154.

A 60-year-old man is referred following his early retirement routine medical. He is normally very active and plays golf three times a week. His ECG shows 2:1 atrioventricular block. An exercise test is performed which shows a poor heart rate response.
  What is the most appropriate management?

A. AAI permanent pacemaker
B. VVI permanent pacemaker
C. VVIR permanent pacemaker
D. DDD permanent pacemaker
E. DDDR permanent pacemaker

50   Answer on p.156.

A 26-year-old surfer, who drifted out to sea, has been brought in by helicopter. On examination he has a GCS of 3.

Pulse   27 thready and irregular
BP   Unrecordable
Temperature   27.4°C rectal low reading thermometer

As the anaesthetist suctions his airway, the ECG changes to ventricular fibrillation. After a pulse check, he is shocked three times with no response and given 1 mg of intravenous adrenaline.
What should be done next?

A. Continue advanced life support (ALS) for 10 cycles and, if no change in rhythm, cease resuscitation
B. Continue ALS and actively rewarm to 30°C before reshocking
C. Give intravenous amiodarone and continue ALS
D. Insert pacing wire and over-ride pace until actively rewarmed
E. Continue ALS, shocking with 3×360 J every 3 minutes

51   Answer on p.156.

A 73-year-old left-handed gentleman has a non-haemorrhagic stroke. He demonstrates difficulty in finding words and is unable to write. He understands what is being said to him but has difficulty distinguishing left from right.
Where in the brain is the lesion most likely to be?

A. Right frontal lobe
B. Left frontal lobe
C. Right parietal lobe
D. Left parietal lobe
E. Right temporal lobe

52   Answer on p.157.

A 74-year-old man is referred with a 1-year history of progressive weakness. On examination he has wasting and fasciculation of his forearms. Reflexes are exaggerated in his lower limbs and plantars are upgoing. Sensation is normal throughout.
What is the most likely diagnosis?

A. Syringomyelia
B. Multiple sclerosis
C. Subacute combined degeneration of the cord
D. Amyotrophic lateral sclerosis
E. Multiple territory cerebral infarcts

53   Answer on p.158.

A group of friends meet for a dinner party. They have chicken salad and garlic bread followed by homemade profiteroles. That night they all become unwell with nausea, vomiting and abdominal cramps followed later by diarrhoea. The episode of food poisoning lasts for 24 hours.
  What is the most likely causative organism?

A. *Campylobacter jejunii*
B. *Staphylococcus aureus*
C. *Bacillus cereus*
D. *Clostridium perfringens*
E. *Vibrio cholerae*

54   Answer on p.159.

A 50-year-old female presents with tiredness. Full blood count and film are shown:

Hb	8.2 g/dL	(12–16 g/dL)
WCC	5.2×10^9/L	(4–11×10^9/L)
Platelets	342×10^9/L	(150–400×10^9/L)

Film   Macrocytes and microcytes seen
           Target cells and Howell Jolly bodies
           Irregularly contracted red cells

  What is the diagnosis?

A. Primary sideroblastic anaemia
B. Coeliac disease
C. Sickle cell disease
D. Hypothyroidism
E. Myelodysplastic syndrome

55   Answer on p.160.

A 21-year-old male attends his GP's surgery complaining of a 1-day history of gross haematuria 2 days after the onset of a sore throat and cough.
  The most likely diagnosis is which of the following?

A. Post-streptococcal glomerulonephritis
B. Urinary tract infection
C. Goodpasture's syndrome
D. IgA nephropathy
E. Minimal change nephropathy

56   Answer on p.160.

Which of the following drugs should be avoided in a patient in myaesthenia gravis?

A. Chlorpromazine
B. Gentamicin
C. Verapamil
D. Gold
E. Sulphasalazine

57   Answer on p.162.

A 72-year old man is receiving palliative chemotherapy for metastatic bowel cancer. He is taking 60 mg of MST (sustained-release morphine) twice a day.
    What dose of oramorph should be given for breakthrough pain?

A. 5 mg
B. 10 mg
C. 15 mg
D. 20 mg
E. 30 mg

58   Answer on p.162.

A 28-year-old female is admitted with abdominal pain and vomiting. She has had flu-like symptoms for 1 week. On examination she has reduced power and tone in the lower limbs together with absent ankle and knee reflexes.

Hb	10.2 g/dL	(12–16 g/dL)
WCC	6.8×10^9/L	(4–11×10^9/L)
Platelets	192×10^9/L	(150–400×10^9/L)
MCV	65 fL	(80–96 fL)
Mean cell haemoglobin concentration (MCHC)	28 g/dL	(32–35 g/dL)
Urinary δ-aminolaevulinic acid	90 mmol/day	(11–57 mmol/day)

Which of the following is the most likely diagnosis?

A. Acute intermittent porphyria
B. Alcohol abuse
C. Guillain–Barré
D. Severe bulimia, with multiple vitamin deficiencies
E. Lead poisoning

59 Answer on p.163.

What is the treatment of pityriasis versicolor?

A. Oral clotrimazole
B. Topical tioconazole
C. Topical benzyl benzoate
D. Selenium shampoo
E. Oral griseofulvin

60 Answer on p.164.

Which one of the following is associated with a finding of a shortened QTc interval on ECG?

A. Tachycardia
B. Subarachnoid haemorrhage
C. Hypercalcaemia
D. Cocaine use
E. Amitryptyline

61 Answer on p.164.

What is the treatment of choice for type 1 sphincter of Oddi dysfunction?

A. Fat-free diet
B. Sphincterotomy
C. Oral calcium channel blocker
D. Oral buscopan
E. Biliary stent

62 Answer on p.165.

A 72-year-old lady is seen in clinic with a diagnosis of thyroid cancer. Which of the following has the worst prognosis?

A. Papillary carcinoma with lymph node spread
B. Follicular carcinoma with solitary lung metastases
C. Anaplastic carcinoma as part of a goitre
D. Locally invasive medullary cell carcinoma
E. Thyroid lymphoma

63   Answer on p.166.

Patients with Sjögren's syndrome are it increased risk of which one of the following malignancies?

A. Nasopharyngeal carcinoma
B. Adenocarcinoma of the parotid gland
C. Non-Hodgkin's lymphoma
D. Oesophageal squamous cell carcinoma
E. Myeloma

64   Answer on p.167.

Which one of the following is the antigen responsible for farmer's lung?

A. *Aspergillus clavatus*
B. *Naegleria gruberi*
C. Avian proteins
D. *Micropolyspora faeni*
E. *Chlamydia psittaci*

65   Answer on p.168.

A 62-year-old female with a 20-year history of rheumatoid arthritis presents with fatigue, and swelling of the abdomen and legs. On examination she has a symmetrical, deforming polyarthropathy in the upper and lower limbs and rheumatoid nodules at both elbows. The jugular venous pressure (JVP) is raised to the earlobes and there is a four-fingerbreadth hepatomegaly, together with bilateral pitting oedema of both legs up to the knees.
   The CXR, ECG and blood gases are all normal.
   What is the most likely diagnosis?

A. Multiple pulmonary emboli
B. Tricuspid stenosis
C. Budd–Chiari syndrome
D. Constrictive pericarditis
E. Pulmonary fibrosis with cor pulmonale

66   Answer on p.169.

Which of the following treatments have been shown to improve survival in patients with adult respiratory distress syndrome (ARDS)?

A. Inhaled nitric oxide
B. Corticosteroids
C. Prostacyclin given by aerosol
D. Extracorporeal membrane oxygenation (ECMO)
E. None of the above

67   Answer on p.170.

Which one of the following is synthesized in the hypothalamus?

A. Prolactin
B. Growth hormone
C. Oxytocin
D. Follicle-stimulating hormone (FSH)
E. Melanocyte-stimulating hormone (MSH)

68   Answer on p.171.

A 65-year-old man develops a widespread symmetrical maculopapular rash following the introduction of a new medicine.
   Which of the following drugs is the most likely cause?

A. Sulphonamide
B. Penicillin
C. Barbiturate
D. Carbamazepine
E. Amiodarone

69   Answer on p.171.

A 56-year-old man has Guillain–Barré syndrome. He is managed on a general medical ward, but his condition is slowly deteriorating.
   Which of the following is the most important test to perform on a regular basis?

A. Blood pressure
B. ECG
C. Peak flow
D. Spirometry
E. Blood gases

70   Answer on p.172.

A 38-year-old lady is referred with abnormal liver function tests picked up on routine testing. Results are shown below.

Alkaline phosphatase	354 U/L	(30–150 U/L)
ALT	43 IU/L	(5–35 IU/L)
Bilirubin	15 µmol/L	(3–17 µmol/L)
IgM	3.5 g/L	(0.5–2.5 g/L)
Antimitochondrial antibodies	Positive	

Which of the following is the first-line treatment of choice:

A. Azathioprine
B. Cylcosporin
C. Prednisolone
D. No treatment as asymptomatic
E. Urosodeoxycholate

71   Answer on p.173.

A 16-year-old male presents with a 3-day history of flu-like symptoms and dyspnoea. He does not improve with penicillin and is admitted with severe right lower lobe pneumonia. On examination he has widespread blistering target lesions on his skin and signs in the right mid-zone.
Which of the following is the most likely cause of the illness?

A. Psittacosis
B. *Legionella*
C. Tuberculosis
D. *Mycoplasma*
E. *Varicella*

72   Answer on p.174.

A 32-year-old woman attends clinic with a 2-year history of recurrent urinary tract infections, with symptoms including frequency, fever and back pain.
Which one of the following investigations would be most appropriate?

A. Ultrasound
B. Retrograde urography
C. Intravenous urography
D. Micturating cystourethrogram
E. Kidneys, urethra, bladder (KUB) X-ray

73 Answer on p.175.

In which of the following conditions is an ECG most useful as an adjunct to routine follow-up?

A. Marfan syndrome
B. Polycystic kidney disease
C. Huntington's disease
D. Di George's syndrome
E. Becker muscular dystrophy

74 Answer on p.176.

In severe poisoning, haemoperfusion may be used to increase the elimination of which of the following poisons?

A. Lithium
B. Aspirin
C. Phenobarbital
D. Theophylline
E. Methanol

75 Answer on p.176.

These are the bloods of a 50-year-old man attending for a routine medical.

Na	132 mmol/L
K	4 mmol/L
Bicarbonate	20 mmol/L
Chloride (Cl)	107 mmol/L
Urea	5 mmol/L
Creatinine	118 mmol/L
Glucose	6.6 mmol/L
Albumin	38.6 mmol/L

What is the plasma osmolality?

A. 259 mOsm/L
B. 265.6 mOsm/L
C. 283.6 mOsm/L
D. 300 mOsm/L
E. 386 mOsm/L

76 Answer on p.176.

A 40-year-old male Sudanese refugee presents with recurrent *Salmonella* septicaemia.

He should be screened for which of the following concurrent infections?

A. *Trypanosoma brucei gambiense*
B. Schistosomiasis
C. Lissa virus
D. *Entamoeba histolytica*
E. *Histoplasma capsulatum*

77 Answer on p.177.

A 67-year-old man presents to A&E in urinary retention. He has known benign prostatic hypertrophy (BPH). His past medical history includes diabetes and ischaemic heart disease. He is catheterized.

Bloods taken show the following:

Na	135 mmol/L	(135–145 mmol/L)
K	4.9 mmol/L	(3.5–5 mmol/L)
Urea	34.2 mmol/L	(2.5–6.7 mmol/L)
Creatinine	426 µmol/L	(70–150 µmol/L)

Which one of the following will have to be reduced or discontinued?

A. Metformin
B. Doxazosin
C. Atorvastatin
D. Amlodipine
E. Aspirin

78 Answer on p.178.

A patient is admitted to the ward and found to have a wound infection with methicillin-resistant *Staphylococcus aureus* (MRSA).

Which of the following will be most effective in preventing spread of the infection to other patients?

A. Isolation of infected patients in a separate room
B. Hand-washing by staff in between each patient
C. Washing of walls and floor with chlorhexidine
D. Treatment of affected patient with antibiotics
E. Screening of staff colonized with MRSA and sending them home for a course of eradication treatment

79
Answer on p.178.

A 24-year-old male is admitted with central crushing chest pain during an all-night party where he has been taking cocaine.
What is the most likely mechanism of his pain?

A. Pericarditis
B. Intercostal muscle strain
C. Myocardial infarction
D. Coronary vasospasm
E. Cardiomyopathy

80
Answer on p.179.

A patient is admitted with acute renal failure. His creatinine is 1100 μmol/L. He is treated with emergency haemodialysis. After 2 hours on dialysis he has a grand mal seizure.
What is the most likely aetiology of the seizure?

A. Hypovolaemia
B. Uraemia
C. Dysequilibrium syndrome
D. Dialysis encephalopathy
E. Subdural haematoma

81
Answer on p.180.

A 19-year-old male student returned from western Uganda 4 days ago, where he spent part of his gap year doing voluntary work. He complains of a sore throat, myalgia and an intermittent fever for 3 days. On examination he has a temperature of 39.4°C, but there are no other physical signs. His FBC and three thick films for malarial parasites are normal.
Which of the following is the most appropriate course of action?

A. Intravenous quinine therapy
B. Strict isolation of the patient
C. Oral aspirin, and repeat thick films for up to 3 days
D. Serum PCR for *Ebola* virus
E. Oral praziquentel therapy

82
Answer on p.181.

Which of the following antibodies are typically found in a patient with drug-induced systemic lupus erythematosus?

A. Anti-Ro antibodies
B. Anticentromere antibodies
C. Anti-smooth muscle antibodies
D. Antihistone antibodies
E. Anti-double-stranded DNA antibodies

83   Answer on p.181.

A 28-year-old lady is seen in the antenatal clinic. She is 16 weeks pregnant. There is a strong family history of type II diabetes. Since learning of her pregnancy, she has eaten the same diet as her mother, a type II diabetic. When seen, her fasting blood glucose is 12.8 mmol/L.
   What is the most appropriate treatment?

A. Metformin
B. Insulin
C. Gliclazide
D. Acarbose
E. Continue on diet alone

84   Answer on p.182.

A 17-year-old female is referred by her GP to an asthma clinic for review of her medicines. She currently takes her salbutamol 10 times a day despite being on beclomethasone and salmeterol inhalers twice a day. Compliance has never been a problem.
   What is the next management step?

A. Oral prednisolone
B. Oral leukotriene receptor antagonist
C. Check spirometry
D. Oral theophylline
E. Check inhaler technique

85   Answer on p.182.

A middle-aged man is found collapsed in the street. You are on your own and having established it is safe to approach, you assess the man. He has a patent airway but is not breathing. There is nothing to suggest drowning or trauma.
   What is the most appropriate next step?

A. Give two rescue breaths and then check pulse
B. Check pulse and, if absent, give pre-cordial thump
C. Check pulse and, if absent, start BLS
D. Give 1 minute of BLS, then leave and call for an ambulance
E. Leave and call for an ambulance immediately

86
Answer on p.183.

A 77-year-old male is referred with gradual onset forgetfulness, deterioration in self-care and low mood. On examination, he demonstrates mild dyspraxia and executive dysfunction. There are no other localizing signs.
Which of the following is the most likely diagnosis?

A. Alzheimer's disease
B. Vascular dementia
C. Frontal lobe dementia
D. Lewy body dementia
E. Huntington's disease

87
Answer on p.184.

Which one of the following nerves exits the skull via the foramen rotundum?

A. The trochlear nerve (cranial nerve IV)
B. The ophthalmic division of the trigeminal nerve (cranial nerve V_1)
C. The maxillary division of the trigeminal nerve (cranial nerve V_2)
D. The mandibular division of the trigeminal nerve (cranial nerve V_3)
E. The abducens nerve (cranial nerve VI)

88
Answer on p.184.

Which of the following conditions can be diagnosed by routine chromosome analysis?

A. Marfan's syndrome
B. Neurofibromatosis Type I
C. Fragile X syndrome
D. Turner's syndrome
E. Williams' syndrome

89
Answer on p.186.

A 26-year-old man presents with sudden onset colicky left-sided loin pain. Urinalysis reveals microscopic haematuria +++.
What is the most likely diagnosis?

A. Acute tubular necrosis
B. Renal stone disease
C. IgA nephropathy
D. Renal artery stenosis
E. Minimal change nephropathy

90
Answer on p.187.

A 45-year-old lady transferred to the medical ward from ITU where she had been ventilated for status epilepticus. During the seizure, she is thought to have aspirated and is now being successfully treated for pneumonia. On admission to the ward, she appears jaundiced and her bloods are found to be as follows.

Total protein	69 g/L	(62–80 g/L)
Albumin	32 g	(34–48 g/L)
Bilirubin	270 μmol/L	(< 17 μmol/L)
ALP	520 IU/L	(25–115 IU/L)
Aspartate transaminase (AST)	108 IU/L	(10–40 IU/L)
Gamma-glutamyl transpeptidase (γ-GT)	242 IU/L	(11–50 IU/L)

She has a past history of epilepsy, which had been well controlled with drugs up until this admission. She does not drink alcohol. Prior to this admission she has been well.

Select the drug most likely to be causing her jaundice.

A. Halothane
B. Phenytoin
C. Paracetamol
D. Sodium valproate
E. Augmentin

91
Answer on p.188.

A 56-year-old publican feels tired all the time. He smokes 30 cigarettes a day and takes bendrofluazide for hypertension. On examination he is hypertensive (BP 180/110 mmHg) and mildly plethoric.

Hb	19.2 g/dL	(14–17.7 g/dL)
WCC	11.8×10^9/L	($4–11 \times 10^9$/L)
Platelets	407×10^9/L	($150–400 \times 10^9$/L)
Packed cell volume (PCV)	0.57 L/L	(0.42–0.53 L/L)

Which one of the following investigations should be performed next?

A. Blood gases
B. Leukocyte alkaline phosphatase
C. RBC cell mass measurement
D. Bone marrow aspiration
E. Erythropoietin levels

92   Answer on p.189.

Which one of the following side effects is most commonly associated with ribavarin therapy?

A. Pancytopenia
B. Haemolysis
C. Lupus-like syndrome
D. Myocarditis
E. Haemorrhagic cystitis

93   Answer on p.190.

A 50-year-old male presents with a deep ulcer on his shin. It initially presented as a small blister, which broke down and enlarged. On examination the ulcer has a purple coloured edge with granulation tissue in the centre. His peripheral pulses are normal.
    Which of the following is the most likely diagnosis?

A. Ischaemic ulcer
B. Venous ulcer
C. Pyoderma gangrenosum
D. Basal cell carcinoma
E. Squamous cell carcinoma

94   Answer on p.191.

A 28-year-old man attends with winging of the scapula.
    A lesion of which of the following nerves is responsible?

A. Dorsal scapular nerve
B. Suprascapular nerve
C. Long thoracic nerve
D. Thoracodorsal nerve
E. Subscapular nerve

95   Answer on p.192.

An 81-year-old male presents to his GP with a 6-month history of diarrhoea and lassitude. His only significant history is of a 'stomach operation' for an ulcer. Blood tests are as follows:

Hb	9.2 g/dL	(13–18 g/dL)
WCC	3.2×10^9/L	$(4–11 \times 10^9$/L)
Platelets	154×10^9/L	$(150–400 \times 10^9$/L)
MCV	116 fL	(76–96 fL)

Which of the following is the most likely diagnosis?

A. Absence of intrinsic factor post-gastrectomy
B. Folic acid malabsorption
C. Carcinoma of the stomach
D. Post-gastrectomy hypergastrinaemia
E. Blind loop syndrome

96   Answer on p.192.

A 45-year-old, previously fit gentleman is referred to outpatients with headaches, change of appearance and sweating. An oral glucose tolerance test showed he failed to suppress growth hormone below 1 mU/L.
Which of the following is appropriate first-line therapy of this patient?

A. Octreotide
B. Prednisolone
C. Trial of bromocriptine for 6 months
D. External radiotherapy
E. Transphenoidal hypophysectomy

97   Answer on p.193.

A 62-year-old man is referred by his GP with a history of progressive weakness of his arms and legs. On examination he has fasciculation and muscle wasting in all four limbs. He has marked upper arm weakness and is hyper-reflexic in his legs. He has evidence of bulbar involvement and his swallow time is delayed.
Which of the following is the most likely diagnosis?

A. Sporadic amyotrophic lateral sclerosis
B. Familial amyotrophic lateral sclerosis
C. Progressive muscular atrophy
D. Progressive bulbar palsy
E. Primary lateral sclerosis

98   Answer on p.194.

A 35-year-old male with a 25-year history of diabetes presents with sudden onset, painless loss of vision of the left eye. Visual acuity is markedly reduced in the affected eye and dilated fundoscopy reveals loss of red reflex with evidence of a vitreous haemorrhage. ➤

What is the most likely retinal abnormality to cause this?

A. Cotton wool spots
B. Hard exudates
C. Venous beading
D. Microaneurysm
E. Neovascularization of the optic disc

99   Answer on p.194.

Which of the following have been shown to improve survival in patients with multiple myeloma?

A. Radiotherapy
B. Autologous haematopoietic stem cell transplantation
C. Bisphosphonates
D. Thalidomide derivative CC5013
E. Alpha-interferon

100   Answer on p.195.

A 49-year-old woman presents with weakness in both legs. On examination she has brisk reflexes in the lower limbs and a sensory level at L1. Her serum calcium is 3.05 mmol/L and ALP 462 U/L.
   Which of the following is the most likely diagnosis?

A. Multiple myeloma
B. Carcinoma of the lung
C. Carcinoma of the breast
D. Primary hyperparathyroidism
E. Sarcoidosis

101   Answer on p.196.

A patient is diagnosed with osteogenesis imperfecta.
   It is caused by mutation in the genes that encode for which of the following?

A. Collagen
B. Elastin
C. Fibronectin
D. Immature osteoclasts
E. Immature osteoblasts

102   Answer on p.198.

A 28-year-old known intravenous drug user presents to casualty with shortness of breath. Examination reveals:

Pulse	100 beats/minute
BP	140/80 mmHg
Temperature	37.8°C
Respiratory rate (RR)	30/minute

There is a pan-systolic murmur at the left sternal edge. She is admitted and has a normal transthoracic echocardiogram.
Which of the following treatment options should be instigated?

A. Await results of blood cultures
B. Intravenous cefuroxime and clarithromycin
C. Intravenous flucloxacillin and fusidic acid
D. Intravenous teicoplanin and gentamycin
E. Full heparinization

103   Answer on p.198.

A 67-year-old male is seen with hypertension that is becoming resistant to treatment. His creatinine is 210 (70–150 μmol/L) and urinalysis shows protein ++. An ultrasound shows a right kidney of 9.5 cm and a left kidney of 7.7 cm diameter. There is no dilatation of the calyces.
Which of the following would be the next most appropriate investigation?

A. Intravenous urogram
B. Renal biopsy
C. Renal angiogram
D. DMSA radioisotope scan
E. Retrograde urography

104   Answer on p.199.

Which one of the following is not a pre-malignant condition?

A. Lentigo maligna
B. Bowen's disease
C. Xeroderma pigmentosa
D. Actinic keratoses
E. Keratoacanthoma

105   Answer on p.200.

In a patient with a broad complex tachycardia, a supraventricular tachycardia with bundle branch block is more likely than ventricular tachycardia when which one of the following is present? ➤

A. Axis deviation
B. QRS complexes with duration of < 0.16 seconds
C. Predominantly negative deflection in V6
D. Concordance throughout the chest leads with negative deflections throughout
E. rS complex in V1

106 Answer on p.200.

Which of the following features is associated with a better outcome in a female with anorexia nervosa?

A. Overexercising
B. Onset of symptoms before the age of 14
C. Bingeing/vomiting behaviour
D. Being in social class 1
E. Body mass index of 15

107 Answer on p.201.

A 30-year-old male presents with increasing dyspnoea and cough. He is a non-smoker and takes no medication. He has a past history of stage 2b Hodgkin's lymphoma, which was treated and at his last follow-up was in remission.
His pulmonary function tests are as follows.

Arterial blood gases (on air)		Normal range
PaO_2	8.8 kPa (66 mmHg)	11.3–12.6 kPa (85–95 mmHg)
$PaCO_2$	4.4 kPa (33 mmHg)	4.7–6.0 kPa (33–45 mmHg)
pH	7.45	
H^+	33 nmol/L	33–44 nmol/L

Pulmonary tests	Actual (litres)	Predicted (litres)	Normal range
Forced expiratory volume in 1 second (FEV_1)	2.57	3.40	2.30–4.50
Forced vital capacity (FVC)	3.02	4.60	3.20–5.70
FEV_1/FVC ratio	85%		
Vital capacity	3.02	4.60	3.20–5.70
Residual volume	1.99	2.25	1.42–3.08
Total lung capacity	5.01	6.85	5.98–8.37
CO gas transfer factor (mL/kPa per minute)	2.2	4.5	2.8–6.2

Which of the following is the most likely diagnosis?

A. Adriamycin-induced cardiomyopathy
B. *Pnuemocysis carinii* pneumonia
C. Radiation-induced pulmonary fibrosis
D. Bleomycin-induced pulmonary fibrosis
E. Relapse of Hodgkin's disease

108
Answer on p.202.

Which of the following statements regarding the reporting of adverse drug reactions to the Committee on Safety of Medicines (CSM) is true?

A. Reporting of adverse drug reactions on yellow cards is compulsory
B. Well-recognized adverse drug reactions do not need to be reported to the CSM
C. All adverse reactions to drugs marked with a black triangle in the BNF should be reported to the CSM
D. Yellow card reporting gives the CSM an accurate indication of all adverse drug reactions in the UK
E. Doctors only report 50% of adverse drug reactions that occur

109
Answer on p.203.

A 26-year-old female is brought into A&E from the local airport. She had just returned from a holiday in Thailand. At the end of the returning flight she experienced sudden-onset, left-sided, chest-wall pain. The pain was worse on inspiration and associated with dyspnoea. On examination, she has a pulse of 100/minute, but cardiovascular examination is otherwise unremarkable. Respiratory rate is 18/minute with shallow breathing to avoid pain. Auscultation of the lungs is normal. There is some local left-sided chest-wall tenderness. She has no past medical history. She has not taken malaria prophylaxis and is no regular medication.

What is the most likely diagnosis?

A. Pulmonary embolus
B. SLE pericarditis
C. Left apical pneumothorax
D. Left rib fracture
E. Malaria

110 Answer on p.204.

A 23-year-old woman presents with a right femoral deep vein thrombosis (DVT). Results of her blood tests are as follows:

Hb	13.2 g/dL	(13–18 g/dL)
WCC	5.3×10^9/L	$(4–11 \times 10^9$/L)
Platelets	125×10^9/L	$(150–400 \times 10^9$/L)
Prothrombin time	12 seconds (control 12 seconds)	
Activated partial thromboplastin time (APTT)	62 seconds (control 40 seconds)	
ANA	Negative	

Which of the following is the most likely diagnosis?

A. Protein S deficiency
B. Christmas disease
C. Antiphospholipid syndrome
D. Systemic lupus erythematosus
E. Protein C deficiency

111 Answer on p.204.

Which one of the following is not a characteristic of mitochondrial genetic disease?

A. Lactic acidosis
B. Encephalomyopathy
C. Aminoaciduria
D. Myoclonic epilepsy
E. Diabetes

112 Answer on p.205.

A 25-year-old female has a routine chest X-ray as part of a medical. It shows a bulky mediastinum, which is confirmed on computed tomography (CT) to be an anterior mediastinal mass.
    What is this most likely to be?

A. Pharyngeal pouch
B. Aortic arch aneurysm
C. Neurogenic tumour
D. Enlarged pulmonary artery
E. Thymoma

113
Answer on p.205.

A 32-year-old woman has recently returned from Mombassa in Kenya is admitted with a brief history of fever, rigors and headache, and increasing confusion. On arrival, she has a GCS of 6. A thick film reveals *Plasmodium falciparum*, with a parasitaemia of 1%.

Which one of the following is the best indicator that this patient has a poor prognosis?

A. Platelet count of 44
B. Worsening GCS
C. Serum lactate of 20 mmol/L
D. Serum bilirubin 109 μmol/L
E. Serum creatinine 245 μmol/L

114
Answer on p.206.

A 67-year-old man presents with pain in both shoulders and the pelvic girdle, and general malaise.

ALT	26 IU/L	(3–35 IU/L)
ALP	198 IU/L	(3–110 IU/L)
Bilirubin	16 μmol/L	(3–17 μmol/L)
ESR	78 mm/hour	(< 20 mm/hour)
Ca	2.6 mmol/L	(2.12–2.65 mmol/L)

Which of the following is the most likely diagnosis?

A. Carcinoma of the prostate with bony metastases
B. Paget's disease
C. Polymyositis
D. Polymyalgia rheumatica
E. Hypothyroidism

115
Answer on p.207.

What is the first-line treatment of primary focal segmental glomerulosclerosis?

A. ACE inhibitor
B. High-dose alternate day steroids
C. Cyclophosphamide
D. Cyclosporin
E. Methotrexate

116 Answer on p.207.

A 30-year-old man presents with easy bruising. Results of his blood test are as follows:

Hb	14.1 g/dL	(13.5–18 g/dL)
WCC	9.5×10^9/L	$(4–11 \times 10^9$/L)
Platelets	200×10^9/L	$(150–400 \times 10^9$/L)
Prothrombin time	13 seconds	(10–14 seconds)
APTT	60 seconds	(35–45 seconds)
Bleeding time	11 minutes	(2–7 minutes)

Which of the following is the most likely diagnosis?

A. Haemophilia A
B. Haemophilia B
C. Von Willebrand's disease
D. Alcoholism
E. Aspirin therapy

117 Answer on p.208.

Which one of the following is an example of an immune-mediated Type IV hypersensitivity reaction?

A. Rheumatoid arthritis
B. Autoimmune haemolytic anaemia
C. Grave's disease
D. Anaphylaxis
E. Sarcoidosis

118 Answer on p.210.

A 55-year-old woman presents with blisters on her skin. A skin biopsy shows patchy IgA deposition along the basement membrane.
Which of the following is the most likely diagnosis?

A. Pemphigus
B. Pemphigoid
C. Dermatitis herpetiformis
D. Linear IgA disease
E. Epidermolysis bullosa

119 Answer on p.210.

A 22-year-old man has been referred to the clinic with a recent history of haemoptysis and worsening renal function.

Which one of the following would most indicate Wegener's granulomatosis as the diagnosis?

A. Eosinophilia
B. Increased transfer factor
C. Neurological involvement
D. MPO-ANCA
E. PR3-ANCA

120 Answer on p.211.

Which of the following drugs used in the management of HIV infection is known to induce cytochrome P450?

A. Nevirapine
B. Ritonavir
C. Indinavir
D. Delavirdine
E. Amprenavir

121 Answer on p.212.

A 36-year-old man is seen in a neurology clinic with a 12-month history of headaches. He describes a severe unilateral supraorbital and temporal headache. It is intense, constant and as if someone is boring into his head. The attacks last about an hour, occurring daily for a week at the same time in the early hours of the morning. He experiences this phenomenon every 4 months. During attacks he finds his eyes water and has a blocked nose. His wife says his eyes look bloodshot.

You examine him between attacks. Examination is normal.

Which of the following is the most likely diagnosis?

A. Tension headache
B. Chronic sinusitis
C. Migraine
D. Trigeminal neuralgia
E. Cluster headache

122 Answer on p.213.

A GP referred a 54-year-old gentleman to the admissions department who had attended a well man clinic with a BP of 215/140 mmHg. He recently visited an optician as his eyesight was worsening and his wife reports he has been complaining of headaches for about 1 month.

On examination, he has bilateral retinal haemorrhages and exudates. All else is unremarkable. ➤

Which of the following would you prescribe?

A. Captopril po
B. Labetolol iv
C. Sodium nitroprusside iv
D. Nifedipine, sublingual
E. Nifedipine po

123   Answer on p.214.

A 57-year-old known alcoholic is admitted with haemetemesis. He has stigmata of chronic liver disease but no hepatomegaly. An upper GI endoscopy shows that he had bled from gastric erosions. He is also noted to have oesophageal varices.
   What is the best management to prevent variceal bleeding in this patient?

A. Oral propranolol
B. Oral omeprazole
C. Endoscopic variceal banding
D. Endoscopic variceal injection sclerotherapy
E. Insertion of a Sengstaken–Blakemore tube

124   Answer on p.215.

In which of the following patients is long-term domiciliary oxygen therapy not indicated?

A. COPD and carboxy-haemaglobin of 2%
B. Idiopathic pulmonary hypertension and PO_2 of 7.6 kPa
C. COPD with pulmonary hypertension and PO_2 of 7.9 kPa
D. Cystic fibrosis with PO_2 of 7.9 kPa and secondary polycythaemia
E. COPD with PO_2 of 7.5 kPa

   NB. COPD = chronic obstructive pulmonary disease

125   Answer on p.216.

A 32-year-old female is admitted with abdominal pain. On arrival, she has a seizure. She is wearing a medic-alert bracelet, which states that she has acute intermittent porphyria. Her airway is protected and she is being given oxygen. She is given intravenous glucose but her seizure continues.
   What is the most appropriate course of action?

A. Intravenous paraldehyde
B. Intravenous carbamazepine
C. Intravenous phenobarbitone
D. Intravenous phenytoin
E. Intravenous clonazepam

126 Answer on p.217.

Which of the following have been shown to inhibit the antiplatelet activity of aspirin?

A. Ibuprofen
B. Esomeprazole
C. Dipyridamole
D. Tranexemic acid
E. Carbimazole

127 Answer on p.218.

A 52-year-old man with non-specific chest pain is referred for an exercise ECG. In which of the following situations should the test be stopped?

A. ST segment elevation > 1 mm in a non-Q wave lead
B. Inverted U waves
C. Heart rate of 165 beats/minute at 9 minutes
D. Systolic blood pressure of 225 mmHg
E. ST segment depression of 2 mm in leads V2–6

128 Answer on p.219.

A 21-year-old male is seen in A&E suffering from shortness of breath and left-sided pleuritic chest pain. His chest X-ray confirms a small pneumothorax. During the examination it is also noted that he is very tall with disproportionately long arms, elongated fingers, pectus excavatum, flat feet and a soft systolic murmur.
On which chromosome would you expect to find an abnormality?

A. 21
B. 15
C. 7
D. 17
E. None of the above

129 Answer on p.220.

A 60-year-old lady presents to A&E with increasing shortness of breath. She has suffered from seropositive rheumatoid arthritis for 20 years. Her chest X-ray shows a moderate pleural effusion on the right. Analysis of the fluid shows the protein content to be 13 g/L. ➤

What is the most likely cause for her effusion?

A. Secondary to her rheumatoid arthritis
B. Carcinoma of the bronchus
C. Constrictive pericarditis
D. Nephrotic syndrome
E. Ovarian tumour

130 Answer on p.221.

Which of the following is not a feature of juvenile myoclonic epilepsy?

A. Precipitated by sleep deprivation
B. Precipitated by alcohol
C. Poor response to sodium valproate
D. Diurnal variation
E. Early morning twitching

131 Answer on p.221.

A 56-year-old man presents with difficulty getting out of his armchair. His symptoms have got progressively worse and he has also noticed difficulty in swallowing.

On examination he has wasting of shoulder and pelvic muscles with clear proximal muscle weakness. Affected muscles are tender. Investigations include a creatine phosphokinase of 5600 IU/L.

Which of the following is the most likely diagnosis?

A. Polymyalgia rheumatica
B. Dermatomyositis
C. Polymyositis
D. Hyperthyroidism
E. Alcoholic myopathy

132 Answer on p.222.

A 45-year-old male with known slow acetylator status is diagnosed with tuberculosis.

Which of the following changes should be made to the normal treatment regimen?

A. Reduce isoniazid dose
B. Reduce pyrazinamide dose
C. Reduce rifampicin dose
D. Increase isoniazid dose
E. Increase pyrazinamide dose

133

Answer on p.223.

A 73-year-old male presents to casualty having developed a rash. This has developed over the past week since starting zopiclone for insomnia. On examination he is red all over and hot to touch.

In addition to stopping the zopiclone, what would be the most appropriate management?

A. Oral antihistamine
B. Oral steroids
C. Topical steroids
D. Paste bandaging
E. Admit to hospital

134

Answer on p.224.

Which of the following causes a right shift in the oxygen dissociation curve?

A. A raise in pH
B. Hyperthermia
C. Carboxyhaemoglobin of 15%
D. Haemoglobin F
E. Stress polycythaemia

135

Answer on p.225.

A 17-year-old male presents with nocturnal shortness of breath. He is audibly wheezy after running a short distance, and is sometimes awoken with breathlessness and chest tightness at night. You suspect that he has asthma.

Which of the following will best confirm your clinical suspicions?

A. Trial of salbutamol
B. Trial of oral steroid
C. Spirometry alone
D. Peak flow monitoring diary
E. Arterial blood gas

136

Answer on p.226.

A 55-year-old gentleman presents to his GP with a 2-month history of tiredness and lethargy. Initial blood tests are as follows: ➤

Hb	9.2 g/dL	(13–18 g/dL)
WCC	7.1×10^9/L	(4–11×10^9/L)
Platelets	243×10^9/L	(150–400×10^9/L)
MCV	96 fL	(76–96 fL)
Total protein	78 g/L	(60–80 g/L)
Albumin	30 g/L	(35–50 g/L)
Na	133 mmol/L	(135–145 mmol/L)
K	5.5 mmol/L	(3.5–5 mmol/L)
Urea	16.4 mmol/L	(2.5–6.7 mmol/L)
Creatinine	254 µmol/L	(70–150 µmol/L)

What investigation is the most useful in gaining a diagnosis?

A. Chest X-ray
B. Short synacthen test
C. Colonoscopy
D. Plasma electrophoresis
E. 24-hour protein/creatinine ratio

137 Answer on p.226.

In sepsis-related disseminated intravascular coagulation, which of the following therapies has been shown to reduce mortality?

A. Intravenous unfractionated heparin
B. Fresh-frozen plasma
C. Recombinant activated protein C
D. Cryoprecipitate
E. Platelet infusion

138 Answer on p.228.

A 28-year-old male presents to his GP 8 weeks after returning from Peru with persistent watery diarrhoea and weight loss. A stool culture and microscopy taken 2 weeks ago was negative.
Which of the following is the most likely diagnosis?

A. Crohn's disease
B. Schistosomiasis
C. Tropical sprue
D. Ulcerative colitis
E. Giardiasis

139 Answer on p.229.

Which of the following patients with an upper gastrointestinal haemorrhage has the highest pre-endoscopy mortality risk?

A. 42-year-old on long-term haemodialysis (BP 110/76 mm/Hg, pulse 90 beats/minute)

B. 50-year-old with metastatic breast cancer (BP 105/70 mm/Hg, pulse 110 beats/minute)

C. 61-year-old with ischaemic heart disease (BP 90/70 mm/Hg, pulse 60 beats/minute)

D. 51-year-old with rheumatoid arthritis (BP 108/74 mm/Hg, pulse 92 beats/minute)

E. Previously well 79-year-old (BP 110/76 mm/Hg, pulse 95 beats/minute)

140 Answer on p.230.

A 15-year-old girl presents with a 2-day history of abdominal pain and blood-stained diarrhoea. Three days later she develops pain in her right shoulder, left ankle and knee. Examination reveals a purpuric rash on her legs and periorbital oedema. Blood pressure is 150/97 mmHg. Investigations are as follows:

Hb	10.2 g/dL	(11.5–16 g/dL)
WCC	11.9×10^9/L	(4–11×10^9/L)
Platelets	153×10^9/L	(150–400×10^9/L)
MCV	75 fL	(76–96 fL)
Na	136 mmol/L	(135–145 mmol/L)
K	5.8 mmol/L	(3.5–5 mmol/L)
Creatinine	136 µmol/L	(70–150 µmol/L)
ESR	37 mm/hour	
Clotting normal		
Urinalysis:	Blood ++, protein ++	

What is the most likely diagnosis?

A. Polyarteritis nodosa

B. Systemic lupus erythematosus

C. IgA nephritis

D. Haemolytic uraemic syndrome

E. Henoch–Schonlein purpura

141 Answer on p.231.

A patient is commenced on oral digoxin. The patient is told that the drug will not reach its full affect for a week.

Which of the following pharmacokinetic variables can explain this?

A. Plasma protein binding

B. Half-life

C. Bioavailability

D. Volume of distribution

E. Creatinine clearance

142
Answer on p.231.

A 27-year-old woman presents to her GP with a painful neck and general malaise. On examination there is local thyroid tenderness. Blood tests are as follows:

Thyroid-stimulating hormone (TSH)	0.1 mU/L	(0.3–4.0 mU/L)
Free T4	32 pmol/L	(10–22 pmol/L)

What is the most appropriate initial treatment?

A. Propranolol
B. Carbimazole
C. Propranolol and carbimazole
D. Prednisolone
E. Aspirin

143
Answer on p.232.

Which of the following clinical features makes a diagnosis of constrictive pericarditis less likely than restrictive cardiomyopathy?

A. Atrial fibrillation
B. Left ventricular hypertrophy
C. Non-pulsatile hepatomegaly
D. Normal systolic function
E. Raised JVP with prominent x and y descents

144
Answer on p.233.

A 24-year-old female complains of an 8-week history of watery diarrhoea associated with mucus production and weight loss. Three months previously she returned from Eastern Europe. Blood results are as follows:

Hb	11 g/dL	(11.5–16 g/dL)
MCV	80 fL	(76–96 fL)

Duodenal biopsies show partial villous atrophy.
Which of the following is the most appropriate treatment?

A. Oral prednisolone
B. Gluten-free diet
C. Oral metronidazole
D. Ciprofloxacin
E. Iron supplements

145
Answer on p.234.

Infective endocarditis caused by which one of the following organisms should prompt colonoscopic investigation?

A. *Pseudomonas aeruginosa*
B. *Streptococcus pyogenes*
C. *Coxiella burnetii*
D. *Streptococcus bovis*
E. *Escherichia coli*

146
Answer on p.235.

Which of the following family histories would warrant a patient referral a genetics service?

A. Patient whose father died of lung cancer at 35
B. Patient whose mother and sister both had cervical cancer under 40
C. Patient whose mother had breast cancer at 53 and uterine cancer at 60
D. Patient whose sister had breast cancer at 48
E. Patient whose sister had breast cancer at 42 and mother had ovarian cancer at 49

147
Answer on p.236.

A patient is taking 40 mg prednisolone a day but wishes to be taking fewer tablets.

What equivalent anti-inflammatory dose of dexamethasone should he have?

A. 2 mg
B. 4 mg
C. 6 mg
D. 8 mg
E. 10 mg

148
Answer on p.237.

A 64-year-old lady with end-stage renal failure, on haemodialysis was found to have the following blood results:

Hb	8.7 g/dL	(11.5–16 g/dL)
WCC	6.2×10^9/L	(4–11×10^9/L)
Platelets	168×10^9/L	(150–400×10^9/L)
MCV	79 fL	(76–96 fL)
Reticulocytes	0.6%	(0.8–2%)

➤

She started erythropoietin injections 2 weeks ago. At that time, her Hb was 10.2 g/dL.

Which of the following is the most appropriate therapy?

A. Increase erythropoietin administration
B. Transfusion of a unit of packed red cells
C. Oral iron sulphate
D. Intravenous iron sulphate
E. Referral to haematologist for bone marrow

149   Answer on p.238.

A patient presents with erythematous scarring alopecia and lesions over the face.

What is the most likely cause?

A. Discoid lupus
B. Lichen planus
C. Psoriasis
D. Trichotillomania
E. Pemphigus

150   Answer on p.239.

A 50-year-old female presents with left ear deafness and loss of balance. On examination she has loss of corneal reflex on the left and ipsilateral ataxia. Weber's test lateralizes to the right.

What is the most likely diagnosis?

A. Ramsay–Hunt syndrome
B. Otosclerosis
C. Paget's disease
D. Vertebrobasilar stroke
E. Acoustic neuroma

151   Answer on p.240.

A 58-year-old male develops sudden onset of painful swelling in the first metatarsophalangeal joint.

Which of the following is the most likely diagnosis?

A. Psoriatic arthritis
B. Gout
C. Osteoarthritis
D. Rheumatoid arthritis
E. Infective arthritis

152 Answer on p.240.

A 26-year-old woman is seen by her GP having become jaundiced and feeling generally unwell. She has a history of intravenous heroin use and has shared needles. A hepatitis screen is sent off and the results are as follows:

Anti-HAV	Negative
Anti-HBs	Positive
Anti-HbsAg	Negative
HbsAg	Negative
HbeAg	Negative
Anti-HCV	Negative
Anti-HBc	Positive

Which of the following is the most likely cause of the jaundice?

A. Acute hepatitis C
B. Chronic hepatitis B and acute hepatitis C
C. Hepatitis E
D. Chronic hepatitis E
E. Acute hepatitis B

153 Answer on p.241.

Which one of the following is true concerning cerebrospinal fluid?

A. Absorption is independent of intracerebral pressure
B. Total volume is about 300 mL
C. It is formed by the arachnoid villi
D. Daily production is 550 mL
E. It flows from the subarachnoid space into the cerebral ventricles

154 Answer on p.242.

A GP visits a 65-year-old man at home a few days after the death of his wife. She had a long illness with cancer and died peacefully at home. The GP notices the man to be low in mood and tearful. He claims to have seen his wife in the past 2 days and admits to going out at night looking for her at her favourite places.
What is your assessment of the man's mental state?

A. Abnormal grief reaction
B. Normal grief reaction
C. Depression
D. Acute neurosis
E. Acute psychosis

155

Answer on p.242.

You review a 26-year-old asthmatic male 2 weeks following his discharge from hospital. Despite frequent admissions with his asthma, he has up until now refused to give up smoking. His last admission necessitated admission to ITU overnight and a subsequent prolonged stay on the respiratory ward. At follow-up he says he has re-evaluated his life and is determined to give up smoking.

Which of the following smoking cessation techniques are most likely to help this man?

A. Nicotine replacement patches plus counselling
B. Hypnosis
C. Acupuncture
D. Buproprion plus counselling
E. Advice from the doctor

156

Answer on p.243.

A 16-year-old girl presents with a 3-month history of fatigue. She has noticed her periods have become much heavier and her mother thinks she has been intermittently jaundiced. She is taking no medication. On examination she looks anaemic and has 2 cm splenomegaly. Her blood results are as follows:

Hb	6.5 g/dL	(12–16 g/dL)
WCC	7.0×10^9/L	($4–11 \times 10^9$/L)
Platelets	342×10^9/L	($150–400 \times 10^9$/L)
Reticulocytes	10%	(<1%)
Direct Coomb's test	Negative	
Haptoglobins	Not detected	
Urinary haemosiderin	Absent	

What is the most likely diagnosis?

A. Hereditary eliptocytosis
B. Hereditary spherocytosis
C. Thalassaemia trait
D. Warm agglutinin disease
E. Paroxysmal nocturnal haemaglobinuria

157   Answer on p.244.

A 23-year-old female is brought into casualty with shortness of breath.
Blood gases on room air are as follows:

pH	7.49
PCO_2	2.3 kPa
PO_2	15.3 kPa
Bicarbonate	11 mmol/L
O_2 saturation	96%

  Which of the following is the most likely cause?

A. Acute pulmonary embolus
B. Diabetic ketoacidosis
C. Salicylate overdose
D. Chronic pulmonary emboli
E. Acute asthma

158   Answer on p.244.

The case fatality rate for meningococcal meningitis and septicaemia in the
UK is which of the following?

A. 5%
B. 10%
C. 15%
D. 20%
E. 25%

159   Answer on p.245.

A 40-year-old female presents with a 2-month history of symmetrical joint
pains and morning stiffness that lasts a few hours. She has evidence of
inflammation of the wrists and metacarpophalangeal joints. She is
rheumatoid factor negative and has no subcutaneous nodules or nail
changes.
  What is the most likely diagnosis?

A. Ankylosing spondylitis
B. Psoriatic arthritis
C. Osteoarthritis
D. Gout
E. Rheumatoid arthritis

---

160   Answer on p.245.

An 18-year-old male is admitted to the psychiatric ward with a new diagnosis of schizophrenia. He has no past medical or psychiatric history. The episode occurred rapidly after the sudden death of his mother.

Which of the following features suggest the poorest long-term prognosis?

A. Acute onset of first presentation
B. Clear precipitating factor
C. Absence of previous mental health problems
D. Agitated presenting state with bizarre delusions and hallucinations
E. Poverty of speech on admission

---

161   Answer on p.246.

A 64-year-old gentleman presents with acute renal failure and a rash. He has a monoclonal cryoglobulinaemia.

Which of the following is the most likely underlying diagnosis?

A. Hepatitis C
B. Hepatitis B
C. Mycoplasma infection
D. Multiple myeloma
E. Systemic lupus erythematosus

---

162   Answer on p.247.

A 54-year-old lady collapses on the coronary care ward with chest pain whilst visiting her husband. She has been getting chest pain on and off for the past few weeks and has self-medicated with her husband's glyceryl trinitrate (GTN) with good effect. On examination she is pale, clammy and peripherally cool. Her pulse is 40/minute and blood pressure 80/46 mmHg. She has cannon waves in her JVP.

Which of the following is the most likely diagnosis?

A. Pulmonary embolus
B. Acute inferior myocardial infarction
C. Acute anterior myocardial infarction
D. Acute aortic dissection
E. Overdose of husband's propranolol

163   Answer on p.247.

A 45-year-old woman is referred with dizzy spells. She describes seeing the room spin horizontally, especially on moving her head. On occasion they have come on a few minutes after lying down in the bed. The episodes last for a few minutes. She describes no headaches, shortness of breath or palpitations. Examination of her cranial nerves is normal.
   What is the most likely diagnosis?

A. Cerebello-pontine angle lesion
B. Vestibular neuritis
C. Menière's disease
D. Vestibular migraine
E. Benign positional vertigo

164   Answer on p.248.

A 26-year-old female is admitted with a 4-week history of bloody diarrhoea. There have been no infectious contacts and no recent travel abroad. Her bowels are open 15 times per day. On examination she looks pale, her temperature is 37.3°C, pulse 100/minute sinus rhythm and BP 110/80 mmHg. Abdominal examination is normal. Rectal examination reveals bright red blood on the glove. Abdominal radiograph is normal. Rigid sigmoidoscopy shows erythematous mucosa with some ulcers and pus. A biopsy is taken. Blood results are as follows:

Hb	9.6 g/dL	(12–16 g/dL)
WCC	12.0×10^9/L	($4.5–10 \times 10^9$/L)
Platelets	426×10^9/L	($150–400 \times 10^9$/L)
Albumin	33 g/L	(35–45 g/L)

   Which of the following is the most appropriate treatment option?

A. Empirical therapy with oral metronidazole
B. Await results of rectal biopsy and stool cultures
C. Start oral ampicillin and intravenous hydrocortisone
D. Send stool for immediate microscopy and, if negative for amoebic cysts, start intravenous hydrocortisone
E. Empirical therapy with intravenous hydrocortisone

165   Answer on p.249.

A 72-year-old long time smoker is seen by his GP with worsening dyspnoea and persistent cough. He has lost over a stone in 4 weeks. A chest X-ray shows a cavitating lesion. ➤

What is the most likely diagnosis?

A. Small cell carcinoma
B. Squamous cell carcinoma
C. Large cell carcinoma
D. Adenocarcinoma
E. Tuberculosis

166 Answer on p.250.

In a patient with hemiballismus, where in the brain is the lesion?

A. Caudate nucleus
B. Subthalamic nucleus
C. Basal ganglia
D. Red nucleus
E. Substantia nigra

167 Answer on p.250.

A 48-year-old female is referred to outpatients. She is asymptomatic, but is worried about her risk of colorectal cancer as her father has just died at the age of 68 years from metastatic carcinoma of the sigmoid colon.
  Her lifetime risk of colorectal cancer is which of the following?

A. 1 in 6
B. 1 in 10
C. 1 in 12
D. 1 in 18
E. 1 in 25

168 Answer on p.252.

A 23-year-old primigravida is seen in antenatal clinic in the 13th week of pregnancy. Her blood pressure is 148/90 mmHg and 24-hour urinary protein 1.4 g (normal < 0.2 g).
  What is the most likely cause?

A. Essential hypertension
B. Gestational hypertension
C. Pre-eclampsia
D. Normal changes of pregnancy
E. Glomerulonephritis

169

Answer on p.252.

Which of the following is characteristic of a trinucleotide repeat disorder?

A. The number of repeats is the same in affected family members
B. Clinical features appear later in subsequent generations
C. Affected individuals are infertile
D. Clinical features worsen in subsequent generations
E. Females are less severely affected than males

170

Answer on p.253.

Which of the following is the half-life of warfarin?

A. 25 hours
B. 30 hours
C. 35 hours
D. 40 hours
E. 50 hours

171

Answer on p.253.

A 13-year-old boy who lives on a farm in Wales is seen with right upper quadrant pain. An ultrasound confirms the presence of a large cyst with several 'daughter' cysts lying with it in the right lobe of the liver. A full blood count shows an eosinophilia.
   Which of the following medical treatments for this cyst should be given?

A. Praziquantel
B. Metronidazole
C. Albendazole
D. Pentamidine
E. Doxycycline

172

Answer on p.254.

Which of the following drugs is associated with the development of a positive antinuclear antibody (ANA)?

A. Penicillin
B. Isoniazid
C. Methotrexate
D. Doxazosin
E. Flecainide

---

173 Answer on p.255.

A 35-year-old man is diagnosed with Kearns–Sayre syndrome.
   Which of the following ocular abnormalities is most likely to be present?

A. Angioid streaks
B. Pigmented retinopathy
C. Optic atrophy
D. Loss of red reflex
E. Blue sclerae

---

174 Answer on p.257.

A 45-year-old female presents with a 6-month history of malaise. Results of her blood tests are:

ALT	203 U/L
ALP	267 U/L
Bilirubin	16 µmol/L
IgG	25 g/L (7.5–15 g/L)
IgM	3 g/L (0.5–2.5 g/L)
IgA	1 g/L (1–4 g/L)

   What is the most likely diagnosis?

A. Alcoholic liver disease
B. Primary biliary cirrhosis
C. Autoimmune chronic active hepatitis
D. Primary sclerosing cholangitis
E. Non-alcoholic steatohepatitis

---

175 Answer on p.258.

A 45-year-old homosexual man, known to be HIV-positive presents with fits. A CT scan shows multiple ring-enhancing lesions in the cerebral cortex.
   Which of the following would be your initial diagnosis?

A. Progressive multifocal leucoencephalopathy
B. Tuberculomas
C. Focal cryptococcal infection
D. Cerebral toxoplasmosis
E. Cerebral lymphoma

176
Answer on p.258.

A 52-year-old man presents with weakness in the right hand. On examination he has weakness in all the small muscles of the hand except the lateral two lumbricals and the muscles of the thenar eminence. There is a variable sensory loss on the medial aspect of the palmar surface of the right hand.
   Which of the following is the most likely diagnosis?

A. T1 root lesion
B. Median nerve lesion
C. Ulnar nerve lesion
D. C7 cervical disc lesion
E. Lesion of the lower trunk of the brachial plexus

177
Answer on p.259.

A 24-year-old primigravida is diagnosed with a significant pulmonary embolus at week 17 of her pregnancy.
   Which of the following is the best course of management?

A. Warfarin
B. Unfractionated heparin
C. Low-molecular-weight heparin
D. Aspirin
E. Caval filter

178
Answer on p.260.

Which of the following patients should be treated with zanamivir?

A. A 52-year-old renal transplant recipient with a 1-day history of flu-like symptoms
B. A 68-year-old with COPD and a 3-day history of flu-like symptoms
C. A 66-year-old insulin-dependent diabetic with a 4-day history of flu-like symptoms
D. A 62-year-old with hypertension and a 1-day history of flu-like symptoms
E. A 43-year-old brittle asthmatic with a 1-day history of flu-like symptoms

179
Answer on p.260.

Which of the following has a multifactorial inheritance?

A. Ankylosing spondylitis
B. Huntington's disease
C. Friedreich's ataxia
D. Acute intermittent porphyria
E. Achondroplasia

180

Answer on p.261.

In the ISIS II trial the group who received aspirin and streptokinase had a 5-week mortality rate of 8%, compared with 13.2% in the placebo group.
What is the number needed to treat for aspirin and streptokinase?

A. 19.2
B. 192
C. 5.2
D. 52
E. 25

181

Answer on p.262.

Which of the following conditions is not associated with underlying malignancy?

A. Bullous pyoderma gangrenosum
B. Migratory thrombophlebitis
C. Pathergy
D. Palmar keratoses
E. Dermatomyositis

182

Answer on p.263.

A 53-year-old gentleman who attends the haematology clinic regularly has his bloods checked. Currently he is not receiving any treatment. The results are shown below:

Hb	14.4 g/dL	(11.5–16 g/dL)
Haematocrit	0.58 L/L	(0.4–0.54 L/L)
MCV	72 fL	(76–96 fL)
WCC	12.4×10^9/L	($4–11 \times 10^9$/L)
Platelets	542×10^9/L	($150–400 \times 10^9$/L)

Which of the following procedures is the most appropriate?

A. Bone marrow
B. Cytogenetics
C. Upper GI endoscopy
D. Venesection
E. Chemotherapy

183

Answer on p.263.

A 75-year-old female presents to her GP with malaise, fatigue and polyuria. She gets progressively worse over the following week and is admitted with vomiting, abdominal pain and confusion. Her corrected calcium is 3.54 mmol/L and serum parathormone is raised.
What is the most likely cause of her hypercalcaemia?

A. Solitary parathyroid adenoma
B. Multiple parathyroid adenomas
C. Diffuse parathyroid hyperplasia
D. Metastatic bony deposits
E. Parathyroid hormone-related peptide due to malignant disease

184

Answer on p.264.

A 60-year-old man is admitted with 1-month history of haemoptysis and shortness of breath. His admission blood test results are as follows:

Na	138 mmol/L
K	4.9 mmol/L
Urea	22.3 mmol/L
Creatinine	760 μmol/L
Hb	13.4 g/dL
WBC	5.6×10^9/L
Platelets	238×10^9/L

His chest radiograph shows bilateral blotchy shadowing.
What is the most likely diagnosis?

A. Wegener's granulomatosis
B. Goodpasture's disease
C. Alveolar cell carcinoma
D. Systemic lupus erythematosus
E. Post-streptococcal glomerulonephritis

185

Answer on p.265.

What is the most common underlying cause of an infiltrating cardiomyopathy?

A. Loeffler's syndrome
B. Scleroderma
C. Sarcoidosis
D. Endomyocardial fibrosis
E. Amyloidosis

186   Answer on p.266.

Which one of the following is true concerning total parenteral nutrition?

A. Trace metal supplements should be given each week
B. Fats comprise the predominant energy source
C. Should not be given to vegans
D. Typically contains 14 g/L of D-amino acids
E. Contains heparin

187   Answer on p.267.

In gastro-oesophageal reflux disease, prior to performing a laparoscopic fundoplication, the patient must have:

A. Failed, or only partially responded to, a trial of full-dose proton pump inhibitor therapy
B. Had an upper gastrointestinal endoscopy demonstrating macroscopic evidence of reflux oesophagitis
C. Had oesophageal pH and manometry studies
D. Failed, or only partially responded to, a trial of full-dose proton pump inhibition and promotility therapy
E. Had gastric emptying studies performed

188   Answer on p.268.

An 18-year-old female with cystic fibrosis is admitted with fever and increased sputum production. She returned home a week ago from a camp for cystic fibrosis patients and their families.
    Which antibiotic should be started whilst sputum cultures are awaited?

A. Vancomycin
B. Aztreonam
C. Clarithromycin
D. Ceftazidime
E. Tobramycin

189   Answer on p.268.

A 74-year-old man is admitted for assessment of his confusion. His wife has observed a change in his personality over the past 12 months. His memory has worsened and he varies from being forgetful to drowsy and unresponsive. He seems to have visual hallucinations and she has noticed him staring at objects that are not there. His symptoms became worse when started on haloperidol. On examination he walks with a shuffling gait and has increased tone in his arms. His mini-mental state score is 19/30.

What is the likely primary brain pathology?

A. Neurofibrillary tangles
B. Multiple grey matter infarcts
C. Eosinophilic inclusion bodies
D. Pick's bodies
E. Neuritic plaques

190 Answer on p.269.

A 79-year-old man presents with a stiff jaw and spasms of the facial muscles. Four days previously, he trod on a nail whilst gardening. There is now an ulcerated lesion on the dorsum of his foot, where the nail was.

A diagnosis of tetanus in this patient should be based on which of the following?

A. History and clinical findings
B. Positive blood cultures for *Clostridium tetani*
C. ELISA for *Clostridium tetani*
D. DNA sampling for *Clostridium tetani* from the wound
E. Biopsy and cultures from ulcer

191 Answer on p.269.

Regarding migraine management, which of the following drugs is the least appropriate choice for long-term prophylaxis?

A. Propranolol 10 mg tds
B. Sodium valproate 600–2000 mg daily
C. Pizotifen 0.5–1.5 mg nocte
D. Amitriptyline 10–100 mg nocte
E. Methysergide 1–2 mg tds

192 Answer on p.270.

A 45-year-old man is referred by his GP to a gastroenterologist with anaemia. He is asymptomatic.

Hb	9.6 g/dL	(13–18 g/dL)
WCC	4.2 × 10⁹/L	(4–11 × 10⁹/L)
Platelets	158 × 10⁹/L	(150–400 × 10⁹/L)
MCV	60 fL	(76–96 fL)
Ferritin	35 µg/L	(12–200 µg/L)
Blood film	Hypochromic, microcytic	

➤

Which one of the following investigations should be performed next?

A. Upper gastrointestinal endoscopy
B. Lower gastrointestinal endoscopy
C. Antiendomysial antibodies
D. Plasma electrophoresis
E. Haemoglobin electrophoresis

193 Answer on p.271.

The enzyme defect responsible for phenylketonuria is which of the following?

A. Homogentisic acid oxidase
B. Cystathionine synthetase
C. Glucocerebrosidase
D. Phenylalanine hydroxylase
E. Phosphofructokinase

194 Answer on p.271.

A 35-year-old female with a renal transplant is seen in outpatients. She has noticed a change in her mouth, which concerns her. On examination she has marked gingival hypertrophy.
    What is the most likely cause of these changes?

A. Tacrolimus
B. Nifedipine
C. Cyclosporin
D. Methotrexate
E. Acute myeloid leukaemia induced by immunosuppression

195 Answer on p.272.

A 48-year-old patient with longstanding rheumatoid arthritis develops worsening dyspnoea.
    What is the most likely cause?

A. *Pneumocystis carinii* pneumonia
B. Pulmonary embolus
C. Pulmonary fibrosis
D. Pulmonary nodules
E. Pulmonary oedema

196
Answer on p.273.

A 45-year-old male with known depression is admitted having taken an overdose. Which of the following suggests the greatest likelihood that he will try to kill himself again?

A. He wrote a suicide note
B. He washed the tablets down with alcohol
C. He has a history of diabetes
D. He lives alone
E. He had his dog put down the day before the attempt

197
Answer on p.274.

A randomized controlled trial is being set up to compare two different treatments. Which of the following statements is incorrect?

A. To increase the power of a study, a larger sample size is required
B. A larger sample size is required, if there is a small difference in results to be measured
C. A larger sample size will be required, if there is a precise outcome measure
D. A Type 1 error is the chance of detecting a statistically significant difference when there is no real difference between treatments
E. A Type 2 error is the chance of not detecting a significant difference when there really is a difference

198
Answer on p.275.

A 62-year-old woman is investigated as an outpatient for palpitations. Her blood tests show no endocrine or electrolyte abnormality and her ECG is normal. A 24-hour ECG shows three distinct episodes of atrial fibrillation, which revert spontaneously to sinus rhythm.
    Which is the most appropriate drug to prevent recurrent atrial fibrillation?

A. Digoxin
B. Sotalol
C. Flecainide
D. Disopyramide
E. Amiodarone

199
Answer on p.275.

A 58-year-old gentleman is brought in to A&E after being found slumped in a doorway. He is unable to give a history, although he is rousable. When transferring to a trolley, it is noted that he is unsteady on his feet and stands with his feet widely apart. He is not cooperative with an examination; however, it is noted that nystagmus is present. ➤

Which of the following is the most appropriate initial course of action?

A. Aspirin
B. CT head
C. 50 mL of 50% dextrose iv
D. Thiamine iv
E. Hydroxycobalamin iv

---

200 Answer on p.276.

A skin biopsy is examined by direct immunofluorescence. Which of the following findings suggest a diagnosis of bullous pemphigoid?

A. Fibrinogen along the dermoepidermal junction
B. IgG and C3 along the dermoepidermal junction
C. IgM and C3 along the dermoepidermal junction
D. IgA and C3 in the dermal papillae
E. Intercellular IgG and C3

---

201 Answer on p.276.

Which of the following tests is the best indicator of severity of disease in Goodpasture's syndrome?

A. Anti-GBM antibody titres
B. ESR
C. Decreased transfer factor
D. Eosinophil levels
E. Increased transfer factor

---

202 Answer on p.277.

In which of the following conditions is the nitroblue tetrazolium test used for screening?

A. Chronic granulomatous disease
B. Wiskott–Aldrich syndrome
C. Di George's syndrome
D. X-linked agammaglobulinaemia
E. Hyperimmunoglobulinaemia E-recurrent infection syndrome

---

203 Answer on p.278.

A 35-year-old man is admitted with a stiff jaw and inability to open his mouth. Three days previously he was immunized with tetanus toxin following a laceration to his arm in the garage.

On examination he was unable to open his mouth and showed 'risus sardonicus'. His arm laceration was swollen, erythematous and exuding pus.

Which of the following is the best immediate management?

A. Oral penicillin V
B. Intramuscular human anti-tetanus immunoglobulin
C. Intravenous pancuronium
D. Debridement and cleaning of wound
E. Injection of tetanus antitoxin into wound

---

204 Answer on p.279.

A 21-year-old male is admitted with an extensive vesciculopapular rash all over his body. He is febrile and has many shallow painful ulcers on his buccal mucosa.

What is the most likely diagnosis?

A. Kaposi's varicelliform eruption
B. Stevens Johnson syndrome
C. Bullous pemphigus
D. Primary *Varicella zoster* infection
E. Staphylococcal toxic shock syndrome

---

205 Answer on p.280.

A 15-year-old female is admitted to hospital with a fever. On examination she has swelling and erythema of her right knee and left elbow. She has a pink rash on her right arm. The PR interval on ECG measures 0.28.

Which of the following is the most likely diagnosis?

A. Still's disease
B. Lyme disease
C. Acute rheumatic fever
D. Henoch Schonlein purpura
E. Systemic lupus erythematosis

---

206 Answer on p.281.

A 40-year-old man with ankylosing spondylitis develops a deep vein thrombosis following a long-haul flight. In view of starting warfarin, his diclofenac is stopped, but his back pain returns and he feels unable to cope without NSAIDs. ➤

Which of the following is the safest to prescribe him?

A. Indomethacin
B. Diclofenac
C. Naproxen
D. Ibuprofen
E. Rofecoxib

207

Answer on p.281.

A 25-year-old male presents with a tremor in his right hand. It is normal at rest, but worse when he uses his hand for writing or holding a cup. He has a history of asthma and takes regular inhalers. He has noticed the tremor improves on drinking alcohol. He is on no other medication. His father has a similar problem.

Neurological examination reveals the following:

- there is no tremor at rest but he develops a tremor in the right hand on out-stretching his arms
- coordination, power and sensation are normal
- his gait is normal and he demonstrates no signs of ataxia.
- he also has a mild rhythmical nodding of his head.

What is the likely diagnosis?

A. Benign essential tremor
B. Parkinson's disease
C. Huntington's chorea
D. Salbutamol-induced tremor
E. Delirium tremens

208

Answer on p.282.

A 50-year-old man is referred, by the rheumatologists, for investigation of dyspnoea. Chest radiograph reveal upper lobe lung fibrosis.

What is the most likely primary diagnosis?

A. Rheumatoid arthritis
B. Ankylosing spondylitis
C. Scleroderma
D. Systemic lupus erythematosus
E. Asbestosis

209

Answer on p.282.

A 35-year-old woman is seen by her GP with symptoms of frequency and dysuria. She recently attended with severe right-sided back pain, radiating to her groin. This lasted 12 hours and then passed.

Urinalysis shows: blood ++, protein +, pH 9.
Which of the following is the most likely organism causing her symptoms?

A. *Escherichia coli*
B. *Proteus mirabilis*
C. *Pasturella multocida*
D. *Candida albicans*
E. *Enterococcus faecalis*

---

210   Answer on p.283.

Which of the following patients does not have diabetes mellitus?

A. A 74-year-old man complaining of blurred vision with a random venous blood glucose of 14.6 mmol/L
B. A 54-year-old woman with a fasting glucose of 6 mmol/L and glucose of 13.2 mmol/L 2 hours after an oral load of 75 g glucose
C. A 38-year-old man with glycosuria, plasma glucose of 6.8 mmol/L fasting and 10.8 mmol/L 2 hours after an oral load of 75 g glucose
D. A 84-year-old woman with an initial fasting blood glucose of 8.8 mmol/L and subsequent fasting blood glucose of 8.1 mmol/L
E. A 69-year-old male with tingling in his feet and a random venous blood glucose 11.8 mmol/L

---

211   Answer on p.284.

Which of the following has been shown to improve the mortality from acute variceal haemorrhage?

A. Intravenous terlipressin
B. Intravenous broad-spectrum antibiotics
C. Injection sclerotherapy
D. Oesophageal banding
E. Transjugular intrahepatic portosystemic shunt (TIPS)

---

212   Answer on p.285.

A 26-year-old male is diagnosed with Hodgkin's lymphoma.
Which of the following features indicates the worst prognosis?

A. Pruritus
B. Fever
C. Superior vena caval obstruction
D. Enlarged mediastinal lymph nodes
E. Mixed cellularity histological subtype

213
Answer on p.286.

A 62-year-old female is treated for hypercalcaemia with intravenous fluids and zoledronate.

Which of the following best describe the mode of action of zoledronate?

A. Decreases gastrointestinal absorption of calcium
B. Stimulates calcitonin secretion
C. Increases absorption of calcium into bone
D. Inhibits osteoclast activity
E. Increases osteoblast activity

214
Answer on p.287.

A 56-year-old lady with metastatic breast cancer has bone pain from known spinal and rib secondaries. She is currently receiving modified-release morphine 120 mg twice a day with oromorph 40 mg for breakthrough pain. Her pain is controlled but she is drowsy. Previous attempts to decrease the dose of morphine resulted in a return of pain but increased her drowsiness.

What is the most appropriate management?

A. Convert morphine to 75 µg/hour fentanyl patch
B. Convert morphine to 50 µg/hour fentanyl patch
C. Add naproxen 500 mg bd
D. Add naproxen 500 mg bd and decrease morphine to 100 mg bd
E. Stop modified-release morphine and retitrate dose with prn oromorph

215
Answer on p.287.

A 24-year-old female is admitted with palpitations. Her ECG shows a narrow complex tachycardia, which spontaneously settles. The resting ECG shows a PR interval of 0.08 but no delta wave.

What is the most likely cause of her tachycardia?

A. Wolf–Parkinson–White Type A
B. Wolf–Parkinson–White Type B
C. Lown–Ganong–Levine
D. Romano–Ward
E. Jervell–Lange–Nielson

216

Answer on p.288.

Which of the following is true of mitochondrial diseases?

A. They show anticipation
B. They are inherited from the mother
C. They are inherited from the father
D. They are caused by mutations in imprinted genes
E. They only affect women

217

Answer on p.289.

A 52-year-old man is investigated for recurrent chest infections and a 1-year history of intermittent diarrhoea. Clinical examination is normal. His bloods are as below:

Full blood count	Normal	
Electrolytes	Normal	
Total protein	57 g/L	(60–80 g/L)
Albumin	49 g/L	(35–50 g/L)
IgG	3.8 g/L	(7.5–15 g/L)
IgA	0.2 g/L	(1.2–4.0 g/L)
IgM	0.3 g/L	(0.5–1.5 g/L)

What is the most likely diagnosis?

A. Kartagener's syndrome
B. Yellow nail syndrome
C. Hodgkin's lymphoma
D. Acquired hypogammaglobulinaemia
E. Non-Hodgkin's lymphoma

218

Answer on p.291.

A 50-year-old male presents with progressive weakness.
Which of the following most favours a diagnosis of Lambert–Eaton syndrome rather than myasthenia gravis?

A. Response to steroids
B. Presence of a thymic tumour
C. Autoantibodies against acetylcholine receptors
D. HLA B8 tissue type
E. Autoantibodies against voltage-gated calcium channels

219 Answer on p.291.

A 28-year-old attends dermatology in outpatients with a 2-week history of painful bruising of both shins. A chest X-ray shows bilateral hilar lymphadenopathy.

How should this patient be managed?

A. Prednisolone 30 mg for 3 weeks and reassess
B. No treatment
C. Immediate referral to haematologist
D. 2-week course of erythromycin
E. Rifampicin 600 mg and isoniazid 300 mg for 6 months

220 Answer on p.292.

A 76-year-old man attends cardiology outpatients and reports that he has had dyspnoea, dizziness, fatigue and confusion following the insertion of a single-chamber right ventricular pacemaker for symptomatic bradyarrhythmia 2 months ago. On examination his pulse is 70 beats per minute and he has cannon a waves in the JVP. His ECG shows a paced ventricular rhythm with retrograde P waves.

Which of the following is the most likely diagnosis?

A. Pulmonary embolism
B. Previously unrecognized tricuspid stenosis
C. Infective endocarditis
D. Pacemaker syndrome
E. Failure to capture, with an underlying complete heart block

221 Answer on p.292.

A 54-year-old female is seen in casualty after returning from South Africa where 6 weeks previously she had a splenectomy following a road traffic accident. She feels generally unwell and has had rigors.

On examination:

Pulse 116/minute
BP 90/50 mm Hg
Temperature 38.2°C

Which of the following is the most likely diagnosis?

A. Malaria
B. Subphrenic abscess
C. Post-transfusion HIV seroconversion
D. Streptococcal sepsis
E. Yellow fever

222   Answer on p.292.

You are the SHO in the endocrinology clinic. You see a 51-year-old patient who has recently been diagnosed with acromegaly. A screening colonoscopy, performed last week was normal.

What would you recommend to this patient in terms of colonoscopy follow-up?

A. No follow-up needed unless symptoms occur
B. Colonoscopy every 2 years
C. Flexible sigmoidoscopy every 2 years
D. Measurement of IGF-1 every 3 years and, if raised, proceed to colonoscopy
E. Colonoscopy every 5 years

223   Answer on p.293.

A 33-year-old woman presents with a 2-month history of lower back pain. Her blood test results are as below:

Na	138 mmol/L	(135–145 mmol/L)
K	3.3 mmolL	(3.5–5 mmol/L)
Cl	118 mmol/L	(95–105 mmol/L)
Bicarbonate	13 mmol/L	(24–30 mmol/L)
Urea	6.8 mmol/L	(2.5–6.7 mmol/L)
Creatinine	108 µmol/L	(70–150 µmol/L)
Corrected Ca	2.1 mmol/L	(2.12–2.65 mmol/L)
PO_4	0.69 mmol/L	(0.8–1.45 mmol/L)
Urine dipstick:	Blood++, pH 5.9	

Which of the following is the most likely diagnosis?

A. Idiopathic hypercalciuria
B. Bartter's syndrome
C. Glomerulonephritis
D. Distal (type 1) renal tubular acidosis
E. Osteoporosis

224   Answer on p.294.

Regarding hepatitis D, which of the following statements is correct?

A. The hepatitis D virion contains a DNA genome and the hepatitis D antigen
B. It is commonly transmitted by blood transfusion
C. Vertical transmission is rare
D. Coinfection with hepatitis B causes chronic progressive liver disease in over 50%
E. A patient who is hepatitis B surface antigen negative cannot have hepatitis D infection

225

Answer on p.295.

A 22-year-old patient with anorexia nervosa is started on nasogastric feeding. After 4 days she has a grand mal seizure. The day previously her blood tests were as follows.

Na	136 mmol/L	(135–145 mmol/L)
K	3.2 mmol/L	(3.5–5.0 mmol/L)
Urea	1.2 mmol/L	(2.5–6.6 mmol/L)
Creatinine	56 µmol/L	(60–120 µmol/L)
Albumin	28 g/L	(35–50 g/L)
Calcium	2.0 mmol/L	(2.12–2.65 mmol/L)
Magnesium	0.7 mmol/L	(0.75–1.05 mmol/L)

What is the most likely cause of this patient's seizure?

A. Cerebral oedema
B. Hypokalaemia
C. Hypocalcaemia
D. Hypophosphataemia
E. Previously unrecognized craniopharyngioma

226

Answer on p.295.

A 75-year-old woman presents to A&E with melaena. She is known to have atrial fibrillation for which she takes warfarin. Her blood results are as follows:

Hb	10.6 dg/L	(13.5–18.0 dg/L)
INR	6.2	

One week previously the patient saw her GP for upper abdominal/lower chest discomfort.

Which of the following drugs did the GP most likely prescribe?

A. Lanzoprazole
B. Rofecoxib
C. Celecoxib
D. Cocodamol
E. Omeprazole

227

Answer on p.296.

A 6-year-old child is investigated for easy bruising, and has the following blood results:

Prothrombin time	13 seconds	(12–15.5 seconds)
APTT	86 seconds	(30–46 seconds)
Thrombin time	12 seconds	(15–19 seconds)
Bleeding time	6 minutes	(2–8 minutes)

What is the most likely diagnosis?

A. Haemophilia A
B. Haemophilia B
C. Von Willebrand's disease
D. Chronic liver disease
E. Bernard–Soulier syndrome

228   Answer on p.297.

A 35-year-old male postal worker is admitted with fever, shortness of breath and non-productive cough. He is a non-smoker. On examination he has a respiratory rate of 28, BP 130/75 mmHg, pulse 92/minute. Auscultation reveals bronchial breathing in the right base.

Hb	13 g/dL
WCC	14.2×10^9/L (90% neutrophils)
Platelets	234×10^9/L

Which of the following is the most appropriate antibiotic treatment?

A. Intravenous benzyl penicillin
B. Oral amoxycillin and erythromycin
C. Intravenous amoxycillin and erythromycin
D. Oral quinolone
E. Intravenous cefuroxime and erythromycin

229   Answer on p.298.

A 17-year-old girl presents to her GP with arthralgia and a rash on her face. Four weeks earlier she had given birth to her first child.
Which of the following is the most likely diagnosis?

A. Polyarteritis nodosa
B. Rubella
C. Systemic lupus erythematosus
D. Parvovirus B19
E. Rheumatoid arthritis

230   Answer on p.299.

A 56-year-old female is admitted having been found collapsed at home by her husband. She had felt generally unwell and took to her bed 3 days ago with a headache. She had just completed a course of antibiotics for a UTI. She is conscious but has reduced power in her limbs. A lumbar puncture was performed and the CSF was noted to congeal quickly. Results are as follows: ➤

Pressure	19 cmH$_2$O	(6–15 cmH$_2$O)
Protein	4.6 g/L	(0.15–0.45 g/L)
Colour	Obvious xanthochromia	
	Non-turbid	

What is the most likely diagnosis?

A. Tuberculous meningitis
B. Tumour obstructing CSF flow
C. Hydrocephalus complicating recent subarachnoid haemorrhage
D. Acute subarachnoid haemorrhage
E. Partially treated bacterial meningitis

---

231   Answer on p.299.

A new drug for the treatment of ulcerative colitis is tested on 60 patients. Each patient was allocated to receive drug A (standard treatment) or drug B (new treatment) for 4 weeks. There was then a 2-week washout period and then the patients were allocated to receive the other treatment for 4 weeks. Response to treatment was assessed by documenting the number of times patients opened their bowels in 24 hours after 4 weeks therapy. The results showed a Gaussian distribution.

Which of the following statistical tests is best for comparing the effects of the two treatments?

A. Paired t-test
B. Unpaired t-test
C. Mann–Whitney U-test
D. Wilcoxon test
E. McNemar's test

---

232   Answer on p.300.

A 55-year-old male with type 2 diabetes is seen in clinic for annual review. Fundoscopy reveals scattered exudates 1.5 disc spaces away from the fovea. His blood pressure is 150/95 mmHg.

What is the correct management?

A. Review in 12 months
B. Review in 3 months
C. Routine referral to ophthalmologist
D. Urgent referral to ophthalmologist
E. Immediate referral to ophthalmologist

233 Answer on p.301.

A medical student counts the number of café au lait spots on successive patients with neurofibromatosis. Results are as follows:

6, 7, 7, 7, 8, 8, 9, 9, 11
Mean = 8.0
Standard deviation = 1.8

What is the standard error of the mean?

A. 0.4
B. 0.6
C. 0.8
D. 1.0
E. 1.2

234 Answer on p.301.

Which of the following have been shown to reduce the mortality from Barrett's oesophagus?

A. Long-term proton pump inhibitor therapy
B. Antireflux surgery
C. Yearly screening endoscopy
D. 3-yearly screening endoscopy
E. None of the above

235 Answer on p.302.

A 38-year-old man presents with right renal colic and loin pain. Plain radiography demonstrates a stone in the right pelviureteric junction.
What is the most likely cause of the stone?

A. Chronic infection
B. Hyperparathyroidism
C. Idiopathic hypercalciuria
D. Xanthinuria
E. Hyperuricuria

236 Answer on p.302.

A 26-year-old female presents to her GP 4 days after the birth of her first child. She reports low mood and feelings of inability to cope. The midwife reports mood swings, tearfulness and irritability. ➤

Which of the following is the most likely diagnosis?

A. Maternity blues
B. Acute mania
C. Post-natal depression
D. Puerperal psychosis
E. Pseudocyesis

237   Answer on p.304.

A 73-year-old woman is admitted with a history of progressive confusion
and diarrhoea. She is unable to give a history, but her GP surgery
confirms that she is being treated for bipolar affective disorder and
hypothyroidism. On examination she appears confused and unkempt.
She is apyrexial, clinically dry but haemodynamically stable. She is noted
to have a coarse tremor and dysarthric speech.
   Which of the following will be the most useful initial investigation?

A. Urgent psychiatric assessment
B. Serum electrolytes
C. Serum lithium levels
D. Thyroid function tests
E. CT scan of brain

238   Answer on p.305.

Which of the following antiretroviral agents is classed as a non-nucleoside
reverse transcriptase inhibitor?

A. Zidovudine
B. Nevirapine
C. Didanosine
D. Ritonavir
E. Lamivudine

239   Answer on p.305.

A 42-year-old nurse is admitted for investigation of dizzy spells and
nocturnal fits. Three separate early morning glucose samples (analysed in
the laboratory) were as follows:

Day 1   1.3 mmol/L
Day 2   2.2 mmol/L
Day 3   2.8 mmol/L

C-peptide after 24-hour fast taken at day 2   1.9 nmol/L (0.2–0.6 nmol/L)
Proinsulin percentage   16% (10–20%)

What is the most likely diagnosis?

A. Insulinoma
B. Surreptitious sulphonylurea self-administration
C. Phaeochromocytoma
D. Maturity-onset diabetes in the young
E. Surreptitious insulin self-administration

240   Answer on p.306.

Which of the following pharmacokinetic parameters remains normal in chronic renal failure?

A. Renal metabolism of drug
B. Hepatic metabolism of drug
C. Gastrointestinal absorption of drug
D. Bioavailability of drug following intravenous administration
E. Volume of distribution

241   Answer on p.306.

Hereditary tylosis is associated with a 95% lifetime risk of developing which one of the following internal malignancies?

A. Nasopharyngeal carcinoma
B. Oesophageal carcinoma
C. Duodenal carcinoma
D. Pancreatic carcinoma
E. Anal carcinoma

242   Answer on p.307.

A patient is thought to have Creutzfeldt–Jacob disease (CJD).
   Which of the following features suggests a diagnosis of variant CJD rather than sporadic CJD?

A. Dementia
B. Upgaze paresis
C. Myoclonus
D. Presentation at 60 years of age.
E. Periodic spike and wave complexes on EEG

243 Answer on p.308.

Concerning hereditary angioedema, which one of the following is correct?

A. Attacks are often precipitated by danazole
B. It is an autosomal recessive condition
C. Serum C2 levels are reduced
D. Urticaria is a common clinical finding
E. Responds well to adrenaline and hydrocortisone

244 Answer on p.309.

A 74-year-old woman was admitted to the coronary care unit with cardiac chest pain. The ECGs showed anterior T-wave inversion and the troponin I was positive. She asks you about her prognosis.

Which of the following is not true compared to a patient with a Q-wave infarction?

A. Higher incidence of early re-infarction
B. Higher mortality at 1 year
C. Lower in-hospital mortality
D. Lower incidence of heart failure
E. Lower incidence of post-infarction angina

245 Answer on p.309.

A 76-year-old male with a history of Type 2 diabetes is admitted with pneumonia. He gives a history of rapidly progressing shortness of breath and purulent bloodstained sputum. Chest radiograph demonstrates left upper lobe consolidation with a bulging fissure.

Which of the following is the most likely diagnosis?

A. Streptococcal pneumonia
B. Psittacosis
C. *Klebsiella* pneumonia
D. *Mycoplasma* pneumonia
E. Influenza pneumonia

246 Answer on p.310.

An 80-year-old man presents with a 6-month history of increasing dysarthria, recurrent falls and emotional lability. On examination he has impaired tongue movement, normal gag reflex, increased jaw jerk and upper motor neuron signs in both legs.

Which is the most likely diagnosis?

A. Syringomyelia
B. Motor neurone disease
C. Multiple sclerosis
D. Pontine glioma
E. Multiple bilateral cerebrovascular events

247   Answer on p.310.

A 15-year-old patient with a history of severe asthma, hay fever, recurrent sinus and gastrointestinal infections is admitted following a road traffic accident. He develops a severe anaphylactic reaction to a cross-matched transfusion.

What is the most likely immunological explanation for the transfusion reaction?

A. ABO incompatibility
B. Rhesus incompatibility
C. Presence of anti-IgA antibodies in recipient
D. Presence of anti-IgA antibodies in donor blood
E. Presence of Lewis antibodies in recipient

248   Answer on p.311.

A 53-year-old lady who has suffered from rheumatoid arthritis for 25 years, presents to A&E with an acutely painful left hip. She is currently being treated for a flare of her disease with prednisolone and methotrexate. On examination there is decreased range of movement. X-rays are unremarkable (anterior/posterior views). A joint aspirate from the hip is negative on microscopy.

Which of the following is the most likely diagnosis?

A. Avascular necrosis of the femoral head
B. Septic arthritis
C. Posterior subluxation
D. Osteomyelitis
E. Flare of arthritis

249   ◦   Answer on p.312.

A 64-year-old man is admitted having taken an overdose of propranolol. On examination he appears unwell. His pulse is 34/minute and blood pressure 70/40. ➤

What is the most appropriate initial management?

A. External pacing
B. Intravenous atropine
C. Intravenous isoprenaline
D. Intravenous adrenaline (epinephrine)
E. Intravenous glucagon

250 Answer on p.312.

The presence of which one of the following autoantibodies would most support the diagnosis of systemic sclerosis?

A. Centromere
B. Jo-1
C. Sm
D. Histones
E. SCL-70

251 Answer on p.313.

What is the initial treatment for a MALT lymphoma of the stomach?

A. Course of antibiotics
B. Chemotherapy
C. Total gastrectomy
D. Radiotherapy
E. Course of steroids

252 Answer on p.313.

A 27-year-old diabetic woman is admitted to intensive care unwell with diabetic ketoacidosis (DKA). She was found unconscious on the couch in the same clothes from the previous nights clubbing with her friends. Her ECG shows J waves.
   What is the most likely cause?

A. Hypokalaemia
B. Hypothyroidism
C. Hypothermia
D. Hypomagnesaemia
E. Hypocalcaemia

253 Answer on p.314.

A 34-year-old man presents with unilateral visual disturbance. He was diagnosed with HIV disease 5 years ago, since which time he has been taking zidovudine therapy.

Which of the following is the most helpful in the diagnosis of this patient's eye symptoms?

A. Formal assessment of visual acuity and visual fields
B. MRI scan of the brain and orbits
C. Fundoscopy
D. IgG anti-*Toxoplasma gondii* serology
E. IgG anti-cytomegalovirus serology

254   Answer on p.315.

Which of the following drugs exhibits zero-order kinetics?

A. Phenytoin
B. Amitriptyline
C. Paracetamol
D. Salbutamol
E. Frusemide

255   Answer on p.315.

A 47-year-old gentleman is seen at his GP's surgery complaining of tiredness and facial tingling. Blood tests were sent and the results are shown below:

Calcium	1.42 mmol/L	
Corrected calcium	1.46 mmol/L	(2.2–2.6 mmol/L)
Phosphate	1.1 mmol/L	(0.7–1.4 mmol/L)
Albumin	38 g/L	(35–50 g/L)
ALP	134 U/L	(30–150 U/L)
Parathormone	0.02 pmol/L	(0.8–8.5 pmol/L)

Which one of the following would be compatible with the above results?

A. Magnesium deficiency
B. Vitamin D deficiency
C. Pseudohypoparathyroidism
D. Renal disease
E. Di George's syndrome

256 Answer on p.316.

Which of the following HLA antigens is associated with the development of narcolepsy?

A. B27
B. DR2
C. DR3
D. DR4
E. Dw3

257 Answer on p.317.

A healthy 24-year-old female is seen for her first appointment in the antenatal clinic. She is 13 weeks pregnant. She mentions that her brother has cystic fibrosis (CF) and she is concerned about the chances of her child inheriting the condition. The carrier frequency of CF is 1/25.

What is the chance that the child will have the condition?

A. 1/150
B. 1/50
C. 1/200
D. 2/75
E. 1/100

258 Answer on p.319.

A 53-year-old man has a hemicolectomy for a Dukes B colorectal carcinoma.

Which of the following tumour markers is most appropriate to check at his follow-up appointments?

A. CA-125
B. CA 19-9
C. CEA
D. β-HCG
E. PSA

259 Answer on p.320.

A known asthmatic attends A&E with progressive breathlessness and wheeze over the last 2 days. He normally takes a regular steroid inhaler and salbutamol when he feels short of breath. His normal peak flow is 550 L/minute. Examination reveals the following:

Oxygen saturation	90%
Respiratory rate	32/minute
Pulse	120 beats/minute
Peak flow	180 L/minute

He is on 60% oxygen and has been given two salbutamol nebulizers, one containing ipratropium, and 40 mg of prednisolone. There is still no improvement.

The next step in his management is:

A. iv salbutamol infusion
B. Further salbutamol nebulizer
C. iv magnesium sulphate
D. iv aminophylline
E. Chest X-ray

260   Answer on p.320.

Which of the following pathological changes are characteristic of Wernicke–Korsakoff's syndrome?

A. Central pontine myelinolysis
B. Cerebral atrophy
C. Cerebellar atrophy
D. Mamillary body atrophy
E. Third ventricle dilatation

261   Answer on p.321.

A 32-year-old male is admitted with shortness of breath and swollen ankles. He has a large left pleural effusion. Past medical history includes asthma and a new diagnosis of Hodgkin's disease 1 week previously. Urinalysis shows protein +++ and a 24-hour urinary protein concentration of 5 g (<0.2).

Which one of the following is most likely to be found on renal biopsy?

A. Membranous nephropathy
B. Minimal change nephropathy
C. AA amyloid
D. IgA nephropathy
E. Kimmelsteil–Wilson nodules

262   Answer on p.322.

A 74-year-old man is seen in the Medical Admission Unit. He complains of not being able to see properly. On examination his visual fields were as follows: ➤

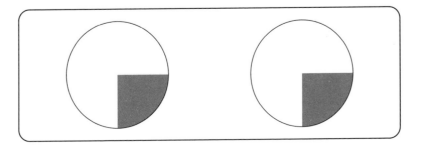

Where is the lesion?

A. Left occipital lobe
B. Right parietal lobe
C. Left parietal lobe
D. Right temporal lobe
E. Left temporal lobe

263 Answer on p.323.

A 29-year-old known iv drug user is admitted febrile, with headache, photophobia and neck stiffness. He describes a 24-hour history of progressive generalized headache and photophobia. The GP who sent him in diagnosed bacterial meningitis and gave him 2 g cefotaxime iv. On examination, he has a temperature of 39°C and appears unwell. He has no rash but shows signs of meningeal irritation. A lumbar puncture is performed and the results are as follows:

Appearance	Clear	
Cell count	368/mm^3	(5/mm^3)
Lymphocyte	Predominant	
Protein	4.2 g/L	(0.2–0.4 g/L)
CSF blood glucose ratio	40%	(2/3–1/2 of blood glucose)

Which of the following is the most appropriate treatment?

A. Cefotaxime
B. Acyclovir
C. Cefotaxime 4 g tds, ampicillin 400 mg/kg daily and vancomycin 60 mg/kg in 4 divided doses
D. Amphotericin and flucytosine
E. Isoniazid, rifampicin, pyrazinamide, streptomycin plus pyridoxine

264 Answer on p.324.

These are the routine blood tests of a 65-year-old male with a long history of dyspnoea:

Na	128 mmol/L	(135–145 mmol/L)
K	5.3 mmol/L	(3.5–5 mmol/L)
Cl	89 mmol/L	(95–106 mmol/L)
Bicarbonate	32 mmol/L	(22–30 mmol/L)
Urea	11.2 mmol/L	(2.5–6.7 mmol/L)
Creatinine	112 µmol/L	(70–150 µmol/L)
Glucose	5.2 mmol/L	(3.5–5.5 mmol/L)

What is the most likely explanation for these results?

A. Addison's disease following previous steroid use
B. Chronic pulmonary emboli
C. Compensated respiratory acidosis
D. Long-term diuretic therapy
E. ACE inhibitor therapy

265   Answer on p.325.

A 40-year-old male is referred with pain and numbness in his left arm. He has experienced pain in his neck and left axilla for several years, which is worse on movement. His symptoms are worse at night and on occasion wake him. He smokes 20 cigarettes a day. On examination he has weakness of abductor pollicis brevis.
   What is the most likely diagnosis?

A. Pancoast's tumour
B. Cervical rib
C. Carpal tunnel syndrome
D. Radial nerve compression
E. C6 radiculopathy

266   Answer on p.326.

A patient with polymyalgia rheumatica has been on oral prednisolone 5 mg/day for 12 years. The disease has burnt itself out and a decision has been made to withdraw steroid therapy.
   Which of the following is the most appropriate course of action?

A. Reduce prednisolone dose by 1 mg/month until she is off them
B. Short synthacten test
C. Long synthacten test
D. Early morning serum ACTH levels
E. Random serum cortisol levels

267   Answer on p.326.

A 42-year-old gentleman presents with an unsteady gait and bilateral gynaecomastia. Which one of the following could be the cause?

A. Kleinfelter's syndrome
B. Therapy with phenytoin
C. Bronchial carcinoma
D. Corticosteroid therapy
E. Kallmann's syndrome

268 Answer on p.327.

Which of the following illnesses/pathogens and vectors are correctly paired?

A. *Loa loa* and *Chrysops silicea*
B. Malaria and *Aedes* mosquitoes
C. Onchocerciasis and *Glossina morsitas*
D. Relapsing fever (*Borrelia duttoni*) and Ixodid ticks
E. *Leptospira interrogans* and rats

269 Answer on p.327.

Which of the following is most likely to be found in a patient presenting with a unilateral T1 spinal cord lesion?

A. Ipsilateral loss of temperature sensation below T1
B. Normal superficial abdominal reflexes
C. Ipsilateral loss of proprioception and vibration sense below T1
D. Contralateral brisk knee reflex and upgoing plantar
E. Contralateral lower motor neuron paralysis at level of lesion

270 Answer on p.328.

A patient is suspected of having acute osteomyelitis.
  Which of the following is the most important organism to cover with antibiotics?

A. *Streptococcus*
B. *Staphylococcus*
C. *Salmonella*
D. *Haemophilus*
E. Tuberculosis

271 Answer on p.328

A new blood test to screen for deep vein thrombosis is performed on 100 people. Of 15 people eventually diagnosed with DVT, 12 of them tested positive with the blood test. Five people without DVT tested positive with the blood test.
  What is the sensitivity and specificity of the test?

A. Sensitivity 94%, specificity 80%
B. Sensitivity 80%, specificity 80%
C. Sensitivity 98% specificity 94%
D. Sensitivity 80%, specificity 94%
E. Sensitivity 83%, specificity 85%

272

Answer on p.329

A 76-year-old gentleman presents to his GP with weight loss and anorexia. Examination reveals splenomegaly. Blood tests are as follows:

Hb	10.8 g/dL	(13–18 g/dL)
WCC	95.9×10^9/L	($4–11 \times 10^9$/L)
Platelets	125×10^9/L	($150–400 \times 10^9$/L)
Blood film	Myelocytes, metamyelocytes and myeloblasts	

Which of the following abnormalities is he most likely to have on cytogenetic studies?

A. Translocation (9, 22)
B. Translocation (15, 17)
C. Translocation (8, 14)
D. Deletion of chromosome 7
E. Duplication of chromosome 17

273

Answer on p.329

Which of the following best describes the mechanism of action of unfractionated heparin?

A. Stimulates antithrombin III
B. Activates plasminogen
C. Increased production of faulty Factor VIIIc
D. Increased production of protein C
E. Increased production of faulty Factors II, VII, IX and X

274

Answer on p.330

A 27-year-old female develops erythematous lesions on her legs. A skin biopsy shows a panniculitis.
Which of the following is the most likely diagnosis?

A. Lichen planus
B. Erythema nodosum
C. Pyoderma gangrenosum
D. Cutaneous vasculitis
E. Dermatitis herpetiformis

A 38-year-old nurse is referred with symptoms of tiredness, nausea and a change in weight. Her thyroid function tests are as follows:

T3	3.4 nmol/L	(0.9–2.8 nmol/L)
T4	177 nmol/L	(55–144 nmol/L)
TSH	1.2 mU/L	(0.35–5.0 mU/L)
TBG	37 mg/L	(12–30 mg/L)

These results are consistent with which of the following?

A. Autoimmune hyperthyroidism
B. Sick euthyroid syndrome
C. Papillary carcinoma of the thyroid
D. Pregnancy
E. Surreptitious thyroxin ingestion

An obese 60-year-old male is admitted with a myocardial infarction. He has a family history of non-insulin diabetes and cholesterol of 6.2 mmol/L. He has decided to stop smoking.

Which of the following interventions is most likely to prolong survival?

A. Aspirin
B. Propranolol
C. Pravastatin
D. Ramipril
E. Decrease body mass index from 30 to 20

A 34-year-old 16/40 pregnant lady is found to have asymptomatic bacteriuria of *E. coli* on screening.

Which of the following is the most appropriate action?

A. None, no treatment required
B. Trimethoprim
C. Doxycycline
D. Nitrofurantoin
E. Ciprofloxacin

278   Answer on p.334

In which of the following cardiomyopathies is digoxin contraindicated?

A. Dilated cardiomyopathy
B. Hypertrophic obstructive cardiomyopathy
C. Restrictive cardiomyopathy
D. Alcoholic cardiomyopathy
E. Amyloid cardiomyopathy

279   Answer on p.334

A 32-year-old is diagnosed with epilepsy. She is commenced on epilepsy medication but develops alopecia and weight gain.
   Which drug is most likely to have caused this?

A. Valproate
B. Phenytoin
C. Gabapentin
D. Vigabatrin
E. Carbamazepine

280   Answer on p.335

Which of the following is not a notifiable disease in the UK?

A. Rabies
B. Measles
C. Human immunodeficiency virus
D. Anthrax
E. Marburg's disease

281   Answer on p.335

An 82-year-old lady is admitted with central, crushing chest pain, similar to her angina pain. It started 1 hour previously and was not relieved by GTN but was with diamorphine. Two years previously she suffered a myocardial infarction, 1 year ago she had a 'ministroke' and is currently on amiodarone for 'a heart rhythm problem'. Her ECG shows ST elevation in leads V3–V6 and nothing else.
   Which of the following is the least appropriate course of action?

A. Request patient's old notes urgently
B. Thrombolysis
C. Computer tomography of thorax
D. Therapeutic low-molecular-weight heparin therapy
E. Transthoracic echocardiogram

282
Answer on p.336

A 48-year-old female is admitted with painless jaundice. On examination she has xanthelasma but no other stigmata. An abdominal ultrasound demonstrates a dilated common bile duct and so an endoscopic retrograde cholangiopancreatogram (ERCP) is arranged. It shows a dilated common bile duct and pancreatic duct.
   Which of the following is the most likely diagnosis?

A. Carcinoma of the head of the pancreas
B. Gallstones
C. Primary biliary cirrhosis
D. Cholangiocarcinoma
E. Portal lymphadenopathy

283
Answer on p.337

A new pregnancy test is trialled in 100 people suspected of being pregnant. Of these, 70 are actually pregnant. A total of 66 of these have a positive result with the new test. Of the 30 who are not pregnant, two test positive.
   What is the positive predictive value of the new test?

A. 66%
B. 70%
C. 87.5%
D. 94%
E. 97%

284
Answer on p.337

A 56-year-old lady with a family history of osteoporosis has a bone mineral density test. She has a Z score of 0 and a T score of −0.9.
   Which of the following statements is correct?

A. She has osteoporosis
B. She has osteopenia
C. She is at risk of fractures
D. She has a normal bone mineral density for her age
E. She has a low bone mineral density for her age

285
Answer on p.338

A patient is diagnosed with carcinoma of the lung, following a routine chest X-ray. The tumour appears respectable on CT.

Which of the following presenting features would be a contraindication to surgery?

A. Hypercalcaemia
B. Pleural effusion
C. $FEV_1 < 1.2$ L
D. Bone pain
E. Hyponatraemia

---

286   Answer on p.339

A 75-year-old man presents with nasal regurgitation, dysphagia and a hoarse voice. On examination he has a right ptosis. The pupils are unequal, the right pupil being smaller than the left. On protrusion his tongue deviates to the right and he has wasting of his right trapezius muscle.
  Where is the lesion?

A. Right lower brainstem
B. Right-sided sympathetic chain in the high cervical region
C. Right jugular foramen, inside the skull
D. Right jugular foramen, outside the skull
E. Foramen magnum

---

287   Answer on p.340

Malaria is currently a risk to travellers returning from which one of the following areas?

A. Israel
B. Singapore
C. Maldives
D. Sri Lanka
E. Cook Islands

---

288   Answer on p.341

A 32-year-old woman is seen in clinic with a BP of 200/110 mmHg. Her blood results are as follows:

Na	143 mmol/L	(135–145 mmol/L)
K	3.1 mmol/L	(3.5–5.0 mmol/L)
Urea	7.2 mmol/L	(2.5–6.7 mmol/L)
Creatinine	108 µmol/L	(60–120 µmol/L)

  Which of the following would be the most appropriate test?

A. ACTH stimulation test
B. Pituitary magnetic resonance imaging (MRI)
C. Adrenal scintillation scan
D. Plasma aldosterone and renin levels
E. Abdominal CT

289

Answer on p.342

Burr cells are found in which one of the following conditions?

A. Alcohol dependence syndrome
B. End-stage chronic liver disease
C. Acute myeloid leukaemia
D. Chronic renal failure
E. Myelofibrosis

290

Answer on p.342

Which of the following diseases has a reduced incidence in smokers?

A. Autoimmune thyroiditis
B. Addison's disease
C. Ulcerative colitis
D. Psoriasis
E. Insulin-dependent diabetes mellitus

291

Answer on p.343

A 45-year-old male is referred with hypertension. On examination he has multiple cutaneous nodules and nine café au lait spots. What is the most likely mechanism of his hypertension?

A. Vasculitis
B. Nephritis
C. Renal artery stenosis
D. Phaeochromocytoma
E. Acromegaly

292

Answer on p.344

A 35-year-old Nigerian lady had been treated in a field hospital for *falciparum* malaria with a parasitaemia of 24%. Her initial treatment involved 3 days of intravenous quinine and a course of Fansidar. She remains well over the course of the next week and represents on Day 5 in London. No parasites are detectable in a peripheral blood film and her haemoglobin has fallen from 13.5 to 7.
Which of the following tests should be performed to aid diagnosis?

A. Upper GI endoscopy
B. Parasite F test for histidine rich protein
C. G6PD levels
D. Faecal occult bloods
E. *Schistosoma* serology

A young woman is brought into A&E. On initial inspection she is lying on the bed. She does not respond when asked questions, but swears when her BP is being taken. When you apply pressure at her nail bed she opens her eyes, flexes her elbow and adducts her shoulder.

Her Glasgow Coma Scale is which of the following?

A. 8
B. 9
C. 10
D. 11
E. 12

A 48-year-old female has received radiotherapy for an inoperable spinal cord meningioma of the lumbar region. She is wheelchair bound and will not walk again. She has never worked and was widowed last year. Her 22-year old daughter has agreed to care for her at home.

Which of the following benefits does the patient qualify for?

A. Disability living allowance
B. Carers allowance
C. Attendance allowance
D. DS-1500
E. Incapacity benefit

An 18-year-old female took to her bed 2 days ago following an all night party. Her boyfriend reports that she has complained of myalgia and headache, and that she has become increasingly confused with headache and musical hallucinations. On examination she is febrile and demonstrates an expressive dysphasia with bouts of aggression, making detailed neurological examination impossible.

Which of the following is the most likely diagnosis?

A. Drug-induced psychosis
B. Malignant hyperpyrexia
C. *Herpes simplex* encephalitis
D. Cocaine-induced cerebrovascular event
E. Variant Creutzfelt–Jakob disease

---

296 Answer on p.347.

Which of the following does not have an established place in the management of Crohn's disease?

A. Elemental diet
B. Methotrexate
C. 6-Mercaptopurine
D. Cyclophosphamide
E. Anti-TNF receptor antibodies

---

297 Answer on p.347.

A 29-year-old journalist quits smoking. She has smoked 40 cigarettes per day since she was 18 and started at the age of 14 years.
   Provided she continues to abstain from tobacco products, which of the following is true?

A. She has a nearly normal life expectancy
B. She has an increased risk of fatal coronary artery disease at age 50 of 25% more than a lifelong non-smoker
C. Her lifetime risk of developing lung cancer is 25% more than a lifelong non-smoker
D. Her risk of developing oesophageal cancer is no greater than a lifelong non-smoker
E. Her risk of developing COPD by the age of 80 years is no greater than a lifelong non-smoker

---

298 Answer on p.348.

A 36-year-old man is seen in clinic for investigation of suspected obstructive sleep apnoea. He has the characteristic clinical features of acromegaly.
   What is the most appropriate test to confirm the diagnosis?

A. Growth hormone level with oral glucose tolerance test
B. Insulin tolerance test
C. 9 am serum growth hormone level
D. MRI of the pituitary
E. IGF-1 level

---

299 Answer on p.349.

A 70-year-old man presents with a 2-week history of bilateral temporal headache. He has noticed worsening of his longstanding neck pain, which now radiates to the occiput. He has also noticed bilateral masseter pain when eating. A recent X-ray of his neck shows degenerative changes and his ESR is 90 mm in the first hour.

What is the most likely diagnosis?

A. Polymyalgia rheumatica
B. Polyarteritis nodosa
C. Cervical spondylitis
D. Rheumatoid arthritis
E. Giant cell arteritis

---

300   Answer on p.350.

In a 12-lead ECG, the isoelectric limb lead is lead AVF. The limb lead with the greatest positive deflection is lead I and that with the greatest negative deflection is lead AVR.
What is the cardiac axis?

A. −90 degrees
B. −30 degrees
C. Zero
D. +90 degrees
E. +150 degrees

---

301   Answer on p.351.

A 32-year-old female develops a right deep vein thrombosis.
Which of the following drugs is most likely to have increased her risk of venous thromboembolism?

A. Amitriptyline
B. Levonorgestrel/ethinylestradiol combination pill
C. Norethisterone/ethinylestradiol combination pill
D. Gestodene/ethinylestradiol combination pill
E. Phenytoin

---

302   Answer on p.352.

Which of the following is the most common cardiac abnormality associated with Down's syndrome?

A. Ventricular septal defect
B. Ostium primum atrial septal defect
C. Tetralogy of Fallot
D. Ostium secundum atrial septal defect
E. Atrioventricular septal defect

303
Answer on p.352.

A 38-year-old female is referred with hypertension. Renal biochemistry is normal. Urinalysis shows blood ++. She has no past medical history but her mother died aged 40 from a cerebral haemorrhage.
  Which of the following is the most likely diagnosis?

A. Renovascular disease
B. Takayasu's arteritis
C. Adult polycystic kidney disease
D. Phaeochromocytoma
E. Von Hippel–Lindau disease

304
Answer on p.353.

A 74-year-old male presents to an orthopaedic pre-clerking clinic awaiting his total hip replacement. He is otherwise fit and well. Examination is unremarkable. His blood results are as follows:

Hb	17.2 g/dL	(13–18 g/dL)
WCC	29×10^9/L	(4–11×10^9/L)
Platelets	180×10^9/L	(150–400×10^9/L)
MCV	90 fL	(76–96 fL)

Differential:

Lymphocytes	16.4×10^9/L	(1.3–3.5×10^9/L)
Neutrophils	6.5×10^9/L	(2–7.5×10^9/L)

What therapy should this patient receive?

A. Chlorambucil
B. No therapy
C. Cyclophosphamide
D. Allopurinol
E. Polyvalent human immunoglobulin

305
Answer on p.354.

A 28-year-old woman with a history of treatment for depression is brought into Casualty with a Glasgow Coma Score of 3. On examination she smells of alcohol, pulse 160, BP 90/60, pupils not constricted. The ECG shows sinus tachycardia with QRS complexes of 170 milliseconds.
  Her airway is secured.
  Which of the following interventions is most appropriate next?

A. Intravenous naloxone
B. Intravenous sodium bicarbonate
C. Intravenous calcium gluconate
D. Intravenous flumazenil
E. Intravenous fluids

306 Answer on p.355.

A 44-year old female is referred with iron-deficiency anaemia. She has a past history of mouth ulcers and irritable bowel syndrome. She had a hysterectomy 6 months ago for menorrhagia due to fibroids. She has two adult children and was anaemic during both pregnancies. Her irritable bowel syndrome has been bad recently but responded to merbeverene, prescribed by her GP. She eats a normal diet.

Blood results are as follows:

Hb	9.9 g/dL	(11.5–16 g/dL)
MCV	68 fL	(76–96 fL)
Platelets	240×10^9/L	($150–400 \times 10^9$/L)
ESR	12 mm/hour	

Which of the following is the most likely cause of the anaemia?

A. Carcinoma of the colon
B. Crohn's disease
C. Coeliac disease
D. Previous blood loss from menorrhagia
E. Small bowel bacterial overgrowth

307 Answer on p.355.

A patient is diagnosed with dermatitis herpetiformis.

What is the most appropriate initial treatment to achieve a prompt clinical response?

A. Oral prednisolone
B. Oral acyclovir
C. Oral gancyclovir
D. Oral dapsone
E. Intravenous acyclovir

308 Answer on p.356.

In which of the following is venesection of no therapeutic benefit?

A. Polycythaemia secondary to chronic obstructive pulmonary disease
B. Polycythaemia rubra vera
C. Iron overload in β thalassaemia major
D. Iron overload in porphyria cutanea tarda
E. Genetic haemochromatosis, with a ferritin of 250

309

Answer on p.357.

A 56-year-old man presents with new-onset flaccid paraplegia, retention of urine and loss of pain and temperature sensation. He has a sensory level at T6. Light touch and joint position sense are unaffected.
  Which of the following is the most likely diagnosis?

A. Spinal cord compression secondary to malignant infiltration
B. Prolapsed intervertebral disc
C. Anterior spinal artery thrombosis
D. Spinal meningioma at T6
E. Syringomyelia

310

Answer on p.358.

These are the lung function tests of someone under investigation for dyspnoea:

FEV$_1$	1.5 L
FVC	1.8 L
TLCO	55% predicted
KCO	60% predicted

  Which of the following is the most likely diagnosis?

A. Cryptogenic fibrosing alveolitis
B. Motor neurone disease
C. Goodpasture's disease
D. Guillain–Barré syndrome
E. Previous thoracoplasty for tuberculosis

311

Answer on p.359.

A 70-year-old male is referred to clinic for assessment of a systolic heart murmur, picked up during a routine medical. He is asymptomatic but ECG shows LVH with strain. Echocardiogram shows peak aortic valve gradient of 90 mmHg.
  What is the correct management?

A. Urgent aortic valve replacement
B. Routine aortic valve replacement
C. Aortic valvuloplasty
D. Regular outpatient review
E. Anticoagulation

312　Answer on p.359.

A 62-year-old gentleman presents to his GP complaining of spinal pain, not relieved with NSAIDs. Routine biochemistry is shown below.

Albumin	40 g/L	(35–50 g/L)
Total protein	65 g/L	(62–80 g/L)
Ca	2.32 mmol/L	(2.12–2.65 mmol/L)
PO_4	0.85 mmol/L	(0.8–1.45 mmol/L)
ALP	641 U/L	(30–150 U/L)
ALT	32 U/L	(5–35 U/L)
Bilirubin	16 µmol/L	(3–17 µmol/L)

Which of the following is the most likely cause of his pain?

A. Polymyalgia rheumatica
B. Paget's disease
C. Osteomalacia
D. Metastatic prostatic carcinoma
E. Myeloma

313　Answer on p.360.

Which of the following tests should be used to give a prompt diagnosis in a patient with suspected *Legionella pneumophilia* infection?

A. Sputum culture
B. Bronchial washings direct immunofluorescence
C. Bronchial washings PCR
D. Pleural aspirate microscopy after H and E staining
E. *Legionella* urinary antigen

314　Answer on p.361.

A 56-year-old man with metastatic colorectal cancer is admitted with symptomatic hypercalcaemia (corrected calcium 3.6 mmol/L). He is a nauseated and unable to keep oral medication down. He is on modified-release morphine sulphate 60 mg bd for bone pain. He is started on intravenous fluids to be followed by intravenous bisphosphonate.
What is the best way to manage his bone pain?

A. Change morphine to fentanyl patch 25 µ/hour
B. Change morphine to fentanyl patch 50 µ/hour
C. Change morphine to diamorphine syringe driver 60 mg in 24 hours
D. Change morphine to diamorphine syringe driver 40 mg in 24 hours
E. Change morphine to diamorphine syringe driver 10 mg in 24 hours

315

Answer on p.361.

Which of the following antibiotics is bactericidal?

A. Trimethoprim
B. Erythromycin
C. Isoniazid
D. Tetracycline
E. Chloramphenicol

316

Answer on p.362.

In which of the following conditions is permanent pacemaker insertion a recognized indication?

A. Asymptomatic 2:1 block MobitzType I (Wenckebach phenomenon)
B. Complete heart block complicating an inferior myocardial infarction
C. Asymptomatic bifascicular block
D. Hypertrophic obstructive cardiomyopathy
E. Wolf–Parkinson–White

317

Answer on p.362.

A 67-year-old male has started amiodarone for paroxysmal atrial fibrillation.
   Which of the following complications is he most likely to get?

A. Hyperthyroidism
B. Hypothyroidism
C. Corneal microdeposits
D. Peripheral neuropathy
E. Pulmonary fibrosis

318

Answer on p.363.

Which of the following poisons and toxins is not dialysable?

A. Lithium
B. Aspirin
C. Theophylline
D. Lead
E. Methanol

Answer on p.363.

A 63-year-old lady is seen with a 2-week history of feeling generally unwell, arthralgia and temperature. Three weeks previously she had received a course of amoxicillin for a urinary tract infection.
Routine blood tests are shown below.

Hb	12.4 g/dL	(11.5–16 g/dL)
WCC	12.8×10^9/L	($4–11 \times 10^9$/L)
Neutrophils	10.5×10^9/L	($2–7.5 \times 10^9$/L)
Lymphocytes	1.7×10^9/L	($1.3–3.5 \times 10^9$/L)
Eosinophils	1.3×10^9/L	($0.04–0.44 \times 10^9$/L)
Na	136 mmol/L	(135–145 mmol/L)
K	5.4 mmol/L	(3.5–5 mmol/L)
Urea	26.7 mmol/L	(2.5–6.7 mmol/L)
Creatinine	492 μmol/L	(70–150 μmol/L)

What is the most likely diagnosis?

A. Acute tubulointerstitial nephritis
B. Acute pyelonephritis
C. Churg–Strauss
D. Post-streptococcal glomerulonephritis
E. Renal abscess

Answer on p.364.

A patient under investigation for hypertension is found to have markedly raised 24-hour urinary catecholamines, supporting a diagnosis of phaeochromocytoma.
Which of the following investigations would best localize the tumour?

A. Metaiodo-benzylguanidine (MIBG) scintiscan and selective angiography of renal vasculature
B. Magnetic resonance imaging and selective angiography of renal vasculature
C. Magnetic resonance imaging and metaiodo-benzylguanidine scintiscan
D. Computerized tomography scan abdomen and selective angiography of renal vasculature
E. Computerized tomography scan abdomen and metaiodo-benzylguanidine scintiscan

321   Answer on p.365.

What is the first clinically detectable sign in a patient with a left acoustic neuroma?

A. Loss of hearing on the left
B. Loss of the corneal reflex on the left
C. Left LMN VII palsy
D. Ataxia on the left side, worse in the upper limb
E. Diplopia on left lateral gaze

322   Answer on p.366.

A 72-year-old female is receiving palliative chemotherapy for metastatic breast cancer.
  Which of the following clinical features most suggests the development of hypercalcaemia?

A. Confusion
B. Nausea
C. Lethargy
D. Prolonged QT interval
E. Trousseau's sign

323   Answer on p.367.

Which of the following best describes a palpable circumscribed skin lesion measuring 0.4 cm?

A. Macule
B. Papule
C. Vesicle
D. Nodule
E. Pustule

324   Answer on p.367.

A 76-year-old man with idiopathic Parkinson's disease, well controlled on Sinemet, becomes jaundiced and is found to have inoperable carcinoma of the pancreas. He has a biliary stent inserted at ERCP and his jaundice improves but he experiences persistent nausea, which is only relieved by intermittent large-volume vomits.
  What is the most appropriate antiemetic for his symptoms?

A. Cyclizine
B. Metoclopramide
C. Levomepromazine
D. Prochlorperazine
E. Domperidone

In which of the following is a reversed splitting of the second heart sound found?

A. Right bundle branch block
B. Left bundle branch block
C. Ventricular septal defect
D. Atrial septal defect
E. Some normal adolescents

A 26-year-old lady is referred by her GP. She presented with general malaise and was found to have an early diastolic murmur at the lower left sternal edge. Urine dipstick shows haematuria + and proteinuria +. Blood results are as follows.

Na	138 mmol/L
K	5.3 mmol/L
Urea	14.2 mmol/L
Creatinine	230 µmol/L
ESR	98 mm in the first hour
CRP	4 mg/L

She has no previous medical history and had a medical examination for insurance purposes 3 months ago. At this time she had no documented murmur and her creatinine was 84 µmol/L.
What is the unifying diagnosis?

A. Atrial myxoma
B. Bacterial endocarditis
C. Rheumatic fever
D. Marantic endocarditis
E. Libman–Sacks endocarditis

A 24-year-old man, diagnosed with HIV 6 years previously presents with right-sided weakness and visual disturbances. On further questioning, his partner describes a gradual deterioration in mental capacity over the last few months. Examination reveals right-sided weakness and a homonymous hemianopia.
Investigations are as follows.

CD4 count	52/mm^3 (350–2200/mm^3)
CT	Multiple lesions in the white matter, no mass effect
CSF	No cells
	Protein = 0.45 g/L (0.15–0.45 g/L) ➤

What virus is most likely to be responsible for this patient's symptoms?

A. JC virus
B. HIV
C. CMV
D. *Herpes simplex* type 2
E. BK virus

328

Answer on p.370.

A 64-year-old male presents with sudden weakness of his left arm, which resolves completely after 7 hours. He has had two previous similar episodes over the past 3 months. On examination he is normotensive but is in atrial fibrillation (rate 78/minute). CT of the brain given with intravenous contrast is normal.

What is the most appropriate management?

A. Dipyridamole
B. Disopyramide
C. Aspirin
D. Warfarin
E. Digoxin

329

Answer on p.371.

A 76-year-old gentleman who is receiving renal replacement therapy by dialysis is seen in admissions with a right ileofemoral DVT. Bloods at this time are unremarkable. He is initially started on intravenous unfractionated heparin. On day 6 of admission he complains of a painful, cold, left foot. You are unable to feel any pulses.

Investigations now show the following results:

Hb	9.2 g/dL	(13.5–18 g/dL)
WCC	6.8×10^9/L	(4–11×10^9/L)
Platelets	16×10^9/L	(150–400×10^9/L)

What intervention should be carried out immediately?

A. Embolectomy
B. Stop unfractionated heparin and give low-molecular-weight heparin
C. Platelet transfusion
D. Stop unfractionated heparin
E. Stop unfractionated heparin and give intravenous protamine sulphate

330 Answer on p.371.

A 52-year-old man with known epilepsy and previous history of alcoholism is admitted confused having been found by his social worker. On examination he is not oriented in time or person. However, his GCS is 14/15. He has nystagmus on right lateral gaze.
What is the most appropriate investigation?

A. Serum thiamine levels
B. Serum phenytoin levels
C. CT brain
D. Skull X-ray
E. Lumbar puncture

331 Answer on p.372.

There is a recognized association between bronchogenic carcinoma and exposure to which one of the following?

A. Beryllium
B. Coal dust
C. Silica dust
D. Cotton dust
E. Uranium

332 Answer on p.373.

A young man is brought into casualty, unable to give a history. On examination he is drowsy.

Pulse	110 beats/minute
BP	105/65 mmHg
Temperature	36.2°C

Arterial blood gas on 100% oxygen:

pH	7.1
PCO_2	2.4 kPa
PO_2	25.2 kPa
Bicarbonate	12 mmol/L
Na	144 mmol/L
K	5.4 mmol/L
Cl	106 mmol/L
Urea	7.2 mmol/L
Creatinine	117 μmol/L
BM	5.6 mmol/L

➤

Which of the following is the most likely cause of his condition?

A. Diabetic ketoacidosis
B. Salicylate poisoning
C. Paracetamol overdose
D. Severe alcohol poisoning
E. Renal tubular acidosis

333 Answer on p.375.

Which one of the following conditions is associated with coeliac disease?

A. Sjögren's syndrome
B. Kleinfelter's syndrome
C. Primary sclerosing cholangitis
D. Type 1 renal tubular acidosis
E. Cancer of the right hemicolon

334 Answer on p.376.

A 50-year-old female is admitted following an adverse reaction to her medicine. She has been started on a new tablet for her rheumatoid arthritis and has noticed a loss of taste and developed a rash. Investigations reveal thrombocytopenia and proteinuria.
   Which drug has she been started on?

A. Gold
B. Penicillamine
C. Sulphasalazine
D. Methotrexate
E. Hydroxychloroquine

335 Answer on p.376.

A 38-year-old male is investigated for hypertension and palpitations. He is found to have a phaeochromocytoma. As part of his pre-operative work-up you are asked to ensure his blood pressure is controlled prior to surgery. Which of the following is the most appropriate drug as initial therapy?

A. Atenolol
B. Labetalol
C. Nifedipine
D. Phenoxybenzamine
E. Hydralazine

336

Answer on p.377.

A 73-year-old female is assessed for worsening falls. Her daughter says that she has become incontinent of urine and has become progressively muddled and forgetful. On examination she walks with a broad-based gait. Tone is normal and plantars are downgoing.

What is the likely diagnosis?

A. Multi-infarct dementia
B. Parkinson's disease
C. Alzheimer's disease
D. Normal pressure hydrocephalus
E. Frontal lobe tumour

337

Answer on p.378.

Which of the following cells is responsible for the secretion of somatostatin in the pancreas?

A. Acinar cells
B. α cells
C. β cells
D. δ cells
E. PP cells

338

Answer on p.378.

Which of the following drugs is most likely to result in the blood results below?

Na	141 mmol/L	(135–145 mmol/L)
K	3.3 mmol/L	(3.5–5.0 mmol/L)
Cl	118 mmol/L	(95–106 mmol/L)
Bicarbonate	13 mmol/L	(22–30 mmol/L)
Urea	6.8 mmol/L	(2.5–6.7 mmol/L)
Creatinine	108 µmol/L	(70–150 µmol/L)

A. Bendrofluazide
B. Acetazolamide
C. Aspirin
D. Voltarol
E. Gentamicin

Answer on p.379.

A 19-year-old insulin-dependent diabetic student returns to the UK from rural eastern Thailand where he spent his gap year working on a farm. He has a 4-day history of fever, cough and right upper quadrant pain. He has a temperature of 38.7°C and 12 cm tender hepatomegaly.

Hb	9.4 g/dL
WCC	8.5×10^9/L
Platelets	134×10^9/L
Malaria film	Negative

An abdominal ultrasound scan shows multiple small liver and splenic abscesses.

Which of the following is the most likely diagnosis?

A. Amoebiasis
B. Meilioidosis
C. Typhoid fever
D. Metastatic *Streptococcus milleri* infection
E. Malaria

340 Answer on p.380.

Which of the following side effects is most frequently seen in patients receiving long-term cyclosporin therapy?

A. Alopecia
B. Hirsuitism
C. Hypertrichosis
D. Myopathy
E. Neuropathy

341 Answer on p.381.

Which of the following oral hypoglycaemic agents have been shown to reduce cardiovascular mortality in Type 2 diabetes mellitus?

A. Metformin
B. Glibenclamide
C. Gliclazide
D. Rosiglitazone
E. Chlorpropramide

342 Answer on p.382.

A 67-year-old man is admitted with a myocardial infarction. He is currently taking frusemide and ramipril. On examination he has a pulse of 80 beats/minute and BP 100/65 mmHg.

Which of the following drugs is most likely to improve future morbidity?

A. Aspirin
B. Isosorbide mononitrate
C. Propranolol
D. Bendrofluazide
E. Nifedipine

343   Answer on p.383.

A 62-year-old female is referred to the Parkinson's clinic for assessment. She has a slow monotonous voice, bradykinesia, rigidity, tremor and loss of upward gaze. She is normotensive with no postural drop. She has a shuffling gait and has diminished armswing on walking.
What is the most likely diagnosis?

A. Idiopathic Parkinson's
B. Progressive supranuclear palsy
C. Multiple system atrophy
D. Cerebrovascular disease
E. Drug-induced

344   Answer on p.383.

A 21-year-old woman is seen in clinic complaining of dysuria and vaginal discharge. An mid-stream urine test is negative. An endocervical swab was taken which showed intracellular diplococci.
What is the best treatment for this patient?

A. Metronidazole
B. Doxycycline
C. Amoxicillin and probenecid
D. Benzylpenicillin intramuscularly
E. Cefuroxime intramuscularly

345   Answer on p.384.

A 75-year-old gentleman is admitted with gradually worsening dyspnoea. He has severe chronic obstructive pulmonary disease, and has been housebound for 6 months. He takes nebulized salbutamol and atrovent via a home nebulizer. In addition, he takes oral aminophylline, prednisolone and has domiciliary oxygen that he uses 16 hours per day. His wife says that he has been producing small amounts of white sputum.

PO_2	7.1 kPa (10–13.3 kPa) on 2 L of oxygen via nasal prongs
PCO_2	7.4 kPa (4.8–6.1 kPa)
CXR	Overexpanded, but no focal signs

➤

Which of the following is the most appropriate management for this patient?

A. Oral slow-release morphine sulphate
B. BIPAP
C. Intravenous aminophylline, omitting the loading dose
D. Referral to a specialist centre for consideration of lung reduction surgery
E. Intravenous corticosteroids

---

346 Answer on p.385.

A 55-year-old man is concerned about his risk of venous thromboembolism. Each year he travels by air from the UK to Australia to visit relatives.

His air travel will increase his annual risk of venous thromboembolism by which of the following?

A. 0.1%
B. 2%
C. 6%
D. 12%
E. 21%

---

347 Answer on p.385.

A 30-year-old gentleman presents with oral and genital mucocutaneous ulcerations. He has a past history of DVT.

Which of the following HLA associations is most strongly linked with his condition?

A. HLA A3
B. HLA B51
C. HLA B27
D. HLA DR3
E. HLA DR4

---

348 Answer on p.386.

A 78-year-old male is referred for consideration of chemotherapy for small-cell lung cancer. He has a past history of COPD and has home help once a day. He washes, dresses and cooks his own meals independently. He potters around the house but rarely goes out due to dyspnoea.

What is his WHO performance status?

A. Performance status 0
B. Performance status 1
C. Performance status 2
D. Performance status 3
E. Performance status 4

349

Answer on p.386.

A patient presents with a complete homonymous hemianopia.
Which of the following is the most likely diagnosis?

A. Retinal artery occlusion
B. Pituitary macroadenoma
C. Temporal lobe infarction
D. Parietal lobe infarction
E. Occipital cortex infarction

350

Answer on p.387.

A 54-year-old man is admitted with haematemesis. He awoke the morning
after an all-day drinking binge feeling nauseated. He vomited twice with
limited relief of his symptoms. On vomiting for a third time, he brought up
what he thought was a cupful of fresh blood.
What is the most likely source of his bleeding?

A. Oesophageal varices
B. Gastric erosions
C. Gastric ulcer
D. Oesophageal erosions
E. Mallory–Weiss tear

ANSWERS

A

Answer B
Systemic lupus erythematosus

This lady has nephrotic syndrome. Nephrotic syndrome is characterized by heavy proteinuria (> 3 g/day), hypoalbuminaemia and oedema. She has a low serum C_3, which indicates that the disease is probably immune mediated.

Causes of renal failure and low C_3
- Systemic lupus erythematosis
- Mesangiocapillary glomerulonephritis
- Post-streptococcal glomerulonephritis
- Bacterial endocarditis

Cause of renal failure and low C_4
- Cryoglobulinaemia

Although **diabetes** can cause nephrotic syndrome, it is an unlikely cause in this case, as it is not immune mediated. Furthermore, nephrotic syndrome is usually a late complication of diabetes typically occurring 15 years onwards after initial diagnosis.

Minimal change glomerulonephritis is the commonest cause of nephrotic syndrome in children. In adults it accounts for about a quarter of all causes of nephrotic syndrome. As the name suggests, there are no changes to be seen on light microscopy and the only changes present on electron microscopy are fusion of the podocytes. It is associated with Hodgkin's disease and asthma, and can run in families; however, on the whole, no cause is found. It does not seem to be immune mediated and does not cause a drop in C_3 levels.

Rheumatoid arthritis is a chronic multisystem disease. It can affect the kidneys in a variety of ways:

- amyloidosis
- glomerulonephritis
- drug-induced disease, e.g. penicillamine.

Rheumatoid arthritis could cause nephrotic syndrome with a low C_3. However, it is uncommon as an initial presentation and with no symptoms of arthritis.

Systemic lupus erythematosus (SLE) is an immune-mediated multisystem inflammatory disease. It affects the kidneys in a multitude of ways. Most types of glomerulonephritis can occur in this disease, including membranous, proliferative and mesangiocapillary. SLE predominantly affects women between the ages of 20 and 40. There is ➤

a decrease in C_3 levels as this is an immune-mediated process. SLE would also explain the moderately low haemoglobin, which is due to anaemia of chronic disease. Thus, this is the correct answer.

Answer C
Legionella pneumonia

A previously fit and well man presents with confusion, abdominal pain, respiratory symptoms, hyponatraemia and renal impairment. The most likely diagnosis is **_Legionella_ pneumonia**. It is a fastidious organism present in water, particularly institutional and hotel water supplies. Infection is by breathing in contaminated water droplets.

Symptoms include a prodromal illness of headaches, myalgia and pyrexia. Abdominal pain is a common feature. Neurological symptoms, including confusion, hallucinations, myelitis, cerebellar syndrome and peripheral neuropathy, may occur. Renal impairment is due to either pre-renal dehydration or acute interstitial nephritis or a combination of both. Hyponatraemia is secondary to syndrome of inappropriate antidiuretic hormone secretion (SIADH), salt-losing nephropathy or gastrointestinal losses. The blood film shows a relatively normal WCC with a lymphopenia.

Diagnosis is by urinary antigen, IgM for *Legionella* (acute and convalescent sera) and direct immunofluorescent antibody test. The treatment of choice is erythromycin and if there is little initial response add in rifampicin.

Churg–Strauss is a small-vessel granulomatous vasculitis that presents with rash, symptoms of asthma, neuropathy and eosinophilia. Males are more affected than females and in particular those in their thirties. It tends to be a milder disease than some of the other vascilitides, renal involvement being uncommon. This gentleman has renal involvement, is pyrexial and has no wheeze.

Sarcoidosis often presents with respiratory symptoms, erythema nodosum, arthralgia, anterior uveitis and CXR changes. Hyponatraemia and renal involvement do not tend to be features. It affects females more than males and in particular Afro-Caribbeans.

Mycoplasma is another atypical pneumonia that would not respond to an initial course of amoxicillin, as it has no cell wall. Symptoms include dry cough, dyspnoea, pleuritic chest pain and erythema multiforme. Complications include SIADH, myositis, cold autoimmune haemolytic anaemia, thrombocytopenia, myocarditis, pericarditis, encephalitis, transverse myelitis, Guillain–Barré and peripheral neuropathy. Pneumonia is normally seen in a lobar pattern on the chest film and it less commonly causes SIADH.

Pneumocystis carinii is unlikely, given there is no history of immunosuppression. It presents with a dry cough and increasing shortness of breath. Often there are no changes on the CXR. Diagnosis is by silver staining induced sputum or a bronchoalveolar lavage specimen.

Answer E
Oral bendrofluazide

Trials published in the early 1990s examined the outcome of treatment of hypertension in people over the age of 65. All trials reported a reduction in mortality from cardiovascular events for patients aged 65–80.

The evidence for treatment above the age of 80 is equivocal. However, if treatment has already been started before this age, it is continued.

Isolated systolic hypertension, as this gentleman has, is present in 50% of the population above 60. In this group there is a marked increase in the number of cardiovascular complications, e.g. CCF and dementia.

A low-dose **thiazide diuretic** has been shown to reduce cardiovascular mortality significantly (SHEP trial) as have dihydropyridine calcium-channel antagonists (second-line choice in those unable to tolerate thiazides). In contrast, β-**blockers** seem only to reduce the number of stroke events. They also tend to be poorly tolerated in the elderly.

ACE inhibitors for the treatment of hypertension have not been studied in the elderly.

Answer C
Excision of remaining mole with a clear margin of skin

Malignant melanoma is a serious killer of young adults, particularly in those in the Southern Hemisphere where advertisement campaigns have targeted awareness of this condition. The incidence of melanoma is rapidly increasing in the UK.

In anyone suspected of having a melanoma, an initial excision biopsy is performed by either a surgeon or a dermatologist. There should be a 2 mm margin of clearance laterally. The histology of this specimen determines further management and prognosis.

Staging, treatment and prognosis of melanoma

TNM stage	Breslow thickness (mm)	Treatment	5-year survival (%)
I	Up to 0.75	Re-excision of mole	95
	0.76–1.5	Re-excision with 1 cm margin	85
II	1.51–4.0	Re-excision of wound with 3 cm margin	65
III	> 4.0	Re-excision	45
		Chemotherapy/interferon	
	Nodal disease	Re-excision and lymph node clearance	40
		Chemotherapy/interferon	
IV	Metastases	Re-excision	< 10
		Radiotherapy/chemotherapy	
		Interferon	

Answer B
Give 1 L of normal saline over 30 minutes

This patient has features of diabetic ketoacidosis and should be treated as an emergency.

The pathogenesis of ketoacidosis in the diabetic is caused by a deficiency of insulin. This means there is reduced uptake of glucose by the tissues and cells have to use another form of energy substrate, i.e. lipids. This results in ketosis, metabolic acidosis and hyperkalaemia together with hyperglycaemia, glycosuria and an osmotic diuresis.

Aims of treatment are:

- normoglycaemia
- rehydration
- correction of acidosis.

The principles of management are fluids and insulin therapy.

Immediate fluid therapy will address the problems of dehydration, hyperglycaemia, and hyperkalaemia, whereas an **insulin sliding scale** will only address the problems of hyperglycaemia and hyperkalaemia. She will need both fluid and insulin; however, as is often the case, they cannot be set up together practically as there is only one nurse present and so it is a case of prioritization.

Treatment with **calcium gluconate** is unnecessary unless there are electrocardiographic signs of hyperkalaemia or arrhythmias. The potassium will fall with both the fluid and insulin therapy, and patients can often become hypokalaemic and require potassium replacement. Thus regular blood samples will need to be taken over the course of her treatment, particularly in the first 24 hours.

ECG features of hyperkalaemia
- Tall tented T waves
- Widened QRS complexes
- Flattened P waves

Blood gases are an important tool in the assessment and management of diabetic ketoacidosis. However, initiation of treatment should not be delayed by waiting for blood gas results.

For exam purposes, **intravenous bicarbonate** should not be given for correction of diabetic ketoacidosis as it can lead to a paradoxical increase in intracerebral acidosis. Do not forget that acidosis can result in significant gastroparesis, and a drowsy patient may need a nasogastric tube to decompress the stomach and drain gastric contents, lessening the risk of aspiration.

Answer A
Cardioversion

This patient has ischaemic colitis. This is a condition caused by relative ischaemia to the watershed area of the middle and inferior mesenteric arteries. It is commonly seen in elderly patients who are hypotensive from another cause and is more common in patients with vascular disease. Typically, the patient complains of mild to moderate lower abdominal pain with plum-coloured stools. The diagnosis is based on a high index of clinical suspicion in a patient who is sick from another cause, e.g. prolonged cardiac arrhythmia, sepsis or hypovolaemia. The plain abdominal X-ray can sometimes be helpful as occasionally mucosal oedema can be seen in the left side of the colon particularly around the splenic flexure (thumb printing).

Treatment is generally supportive and is aimed at restoring appropriate blood flow and, in this case, the best way of doing that is by **cardioversion**. **Digoxin** is a less reliable and slower method of optimizing cardiovascular stability.

Ninety-five per cent of patients with ischaemic colitis settle spontaneously once the circulating volume has been restored. Up to 10% of patients develop a subsequent stricture in the watershed area at the splenic flexure. Perforation of the colon is rare and is the only indication for **surgery** in a patient with ischaemic colitis.

Ischaemic colitis needs to be clearly distinguished from acute small bowel ischaemia or infarction. In small bowel ischaemia/infarction the patient typically complains of very severe central abdominal pain and usually there are very few signs in the abdomen. It is caused by either emboli or vascular disease (or a combination of both) in the territory of the superior mesenteric artery. The treatment of choice is a laparotomy, as delay will lead to a gangrenous bowel, perforation and peritonitis.

In this case, the history is typical of ischaemic colitis particularly in view of the timing of the symptoms and the fact that the atrial fibrillation is of new onset. **Anticoagulation** is of no proven benefit in either condition.

	Acute small bowel ischaemia	Ischaemic colitis
Aetiology	Embolic	Hypotension
Site of pain	Generalized/mid-abdomen	Lower abdomen
Severity of pain	Severe	Mild, may be absent
Blood and diarrhoea	Usually absent	Plum coloured
Age range	Variable	Elderly
Plain abdominal X-ray	Unhelpful	Occasional oedema at splenic flexure
Treatment	Laparotomy	Stabilize blood pressure

Answer D
Systemic lupus erythematosus

There are two main tests used in syphilis serology, namely:

- venereal disease reference laboratory (VDRL)
- *Treponema pallidum* haemagglutination assay (TPHA).

VDRL is non-specific as it tests for antiphospholipid antibodies. The titre will relate to disease activity.

TPHA is a treponemal-specific IgG antibody test and will remain positive lifelong after syphilis or a related treponemal infection, such as **yaws**, pinta or bechel, even after effective therapy has been given.

In **primary syphilis**, the TPHA becomes positive first, followed by the VDRL.

In **secondary syphilis**, the TPHA remains positive, and the VDRL titres will peak and then fall.

In **tertiary** or late-stage syphilis, the TPHA remains positive with a low VDRL titre.

As already mentioned, VDRL is non-specific to syphilis infection and a positive result may occur in several other conditions as listed below.

Causes of a positive VDRL
- Syphilis (*Treponema pallidum* subsp. *pallidum*)
- Yaws (*Treponema pallidum* subsp. *pertenue*)
- Bejel (*Treponema pallidum* subsp. *endemicum*)
- Pinta (*Treponema pallidum* subsp. *carateum*)
- Leptospirosis
- Epstein–Barr virus
- Mycoplasma
- Bacterial endocarditis
- Systemic lupus erythematosus
- Sjögren syndrome
- Hashimoto's disease
- Human immunodeficiency virus (HIV)

Answer E
Posterior communicating artery aneurysm

Examination of this man reveals a IIIrd cranial nerve palsy. Common causes of a IIIrd cranial nerve palsy include:

- aneurysm of the posterior communicating artery
- infarction of the third nerve commonly caused by either diabetes or atheroma
- midbrain infarction
- midbrain tumour.

Some of these causes can be explained by understanding the anatomy and course of the nerve within the skull. It starts from between the cerebral peduncles, running anteriorly between the posterior cerebellar and the superior cerebellar artery. From here it runs parallel to the posterior communicating artery until it enters the cavernous sinus. The nerve then enters the orbit through the superior orbital fissure. It supplies the superior, medial and inferior recti, inferior oblique, levator palpebrae superioris and sphincter pupillae.

Signs of a IIIrd cranial nerve lesion include:

- complete ptosis
- fixed and dilated pupil
- 'down and out' eye.

Compression from the posterior communicating artery is the most common cause of a painful IIIrd cranial nerve palsy. This man needs urgent referral to a neurosurgical unit for angiography and surgery.

The presentation of a **subarachnoid haemorrhage** is classically described as thunderclap headache, mostly occipital that can be associated with vomiting and loss of consciousness. This man does have a headache of sudden onset; however, with subarachnoid haemorrhage, if the cranial nerves are affected, it tends to be the VIth.

Multiple sclerosis can be a difficult diagnosis to make, as there is an unlimited number of ways it can present; nevertheless, there are patterns in its presentation. It commonly affects the eyes by way of optic neuritis, an internuclear ophthalmoplegia or a VIth cranial nerve palsy. Pain is not a feature.

Cavernous sinus thrombosis is rare but most frequently occurs after local sepsis of the face or paranasal sinus. It presents with a painful, congested eye, proptosis and exophthalmus. Usually there is a VIth cranial nerve palsy, as this nerve runs through the middle of the sinus and is the most vulnerable in this situation.

Optic nerve gliomas tend to produce a visual field defect, characteristically a 'hole', which can occur anywhere in the fields; however, at the time of diagnosis, there is usually established optic atrophy. This tends not to be acutely painful.

9 Question on p.6.

Answer A
Isosorbide mononitrate

Sildenafil is a phosphodiesterase type-5 inhibitor licensed for the treatment of erectile dysfunction. ➤

The mechanism of penile erection involves the release of nitric oxide by nerve endings in the corpus cavernosum, in response to sexual stimulation. This, in turn leads to the formation of cyclic GMP, which produces smooth muscle relaxation in the corpora cavernosa. Sildenafil selectively inhibits the metabolism of cyclic GMP by phosphodiesterase type-5. It reaches its peak effect 1 hour after oral ingestion and has a half-life of 3–5 hours.

Because phosphodiesterase is also involved in the vasodilator response to nitrates, sildenafil can potentiate, to a dangerous degree, the vasodilating and hypotensive effects of these drugs. Sildenafil is absolutely contraindicated in patients taking nitrates.

10

Question on p.6.

Answer B
Raised intracranial pressure

Electroconvulsive therapy is a therapy in which the patient receives an electrical current across the brain in order to induce a seizure. This is done under a general anaesthetic and with muscle relaxants.

It is used for the following situations:

* severe depression
* grave suicide risk
* refusal to eat or drink
* failure of other treatment methods.

It is usually administered twice a week for 4 weeks. Recognized side-effects include short-term amnesia, headaches, seizures between treatments, delirium in the elderly and arrhythmias.

The only absolute contraindication to ECT is **raised intracranial pressure**.

The other relative contraindications are based upon anaesthetic risk, and this needs to be weighed-up against continuing anguish and potential mortality from not treating. Relative contraindications include:

* recent myocardial infarction
* recent cerebrovascular event
* recent ventricular arrhythmia
* brain tumour
* Severe pulmonary disease.

11

Question on p.6.

Answer C
DR4

This patient has rheumatoid arthritis, splenomegaly and leucopenia, a combination that is highly suggestive of Felty's syndrome. Up to 3% of patients with rheumatoid arthritis have Felty's syndrome. As they are neutropenic they are at increased risk of bacterial infections, which can be severe and fatal. The risk of sepsis correlates with the degree of neutropenia. Patients with Felty's also usually have evidence of a mild anaemia and thrombocytopenia.

Rheumatoid arthritis is associated with HLA haplotypes **DR1** and **DR4**. Ninety per cent of patients with Felty's syndrome are HLA DR4. This compares to 70% of patients with rheumatoid and 30% of the general population. Patients with Felty's are particularly likely to be DW4 and DW14 positive.

Patients with **DR3** are less likely to have rheumatoid arthritis than the general population.

B27 is associated with seronegative spondylarthritides and not with rheumatoid or Felty's syndrome.

DQ2 is associated with coeliac disease.

---

12 Question on p.7.

Answer A
Methotrexate

All of the drugs mentioned are used in the treatment of rheumatoid arthritis. The question is really asking whether you know which drugs are associated with pulmonary fibrosis. They are listed below. As you can see, they are mainly chemotherapy agents or drugs that may be used in the treatment of rheumatoid.

Drugs causing pulmonary fibrosis
- Busulphan
- Bleomycin
- Cyclophosphamide
- Melphelan
- Methotrexate
- Sulphasalazine
- Gold
- Nitrofurantoin
- Amiodarone

It is also important to be familiar with other respiratory problems seen in rheumatoid arthritis, such as pleural disease, cricoarytenoid arthritis, rheumatoid nodules, Caplan's syndrome, pulmonary fibrosis and obliterative bronchiolitis.

Pleural thickening and **effusions** are the most common lung complications seen. They are covered in more detail in the question about pleural effusions (Question 129, p. 43). ➤

Disease involvement of the cricoarytenoid joints (**cricoarytenoid arthritis**) may cause dyspnoea, stridor and hoarseness. Occasionally, it leads to severe airways obstruction necessitating a tracheostomy.

Rheumatoid nodules may be seen as single or multiple lesions on the chest X-ray. Their size varies from a few millimetres to centimetres. They usually cause no symptoms but can cavitate. They may give rise to a pneumothorax or pleural effusion.

Obliterative bronchiolitis is rare. It presents as progressive dyspnoea with evidence of irreversible airflow limitation. Corticosteroids may slow down progression.

Caplan's syndrome used to be a favourite of the MRCP examiners. It is the presence of pulmonary nodules (usually 0.5–5 cm in diameter) in individuals with pneumoconiosis from dust inhalation. It is usually seen in coal workers' pneumoconiosis, but is also associated with silica and asbestos inhalation. It may occur without prior evidence of pneumoconiosis before nodules become apparent.

Pulmonary fibrosis is recognized in rheumatoid arthritis and is considered a variant of the cryptogenic form of the disease.

13 Question on p.7.

Answer C
Intravenous calcium gluconate

This patient is in renal failure with dangerously high potassium. The presence of ECG changes indicates a need for immediate treatment because the myocardium will be unstable. The patient could die from a cardiac arrhythmia at any time and so the most important treatment is to first give intravenous calcium gluconate.

Calcium gluconate stabilizes the myocardium from the toxicity of hyperkalaemia and works immediately. Its effects last for about an hour, so further intervention may be required. It does not decrease the potassium levels and another method will be needed to achieve this.

Insulin and dextrose is commonly used in clinical practice for mild hyperkalaemia. Insulin induces cellular uptake of potassium by activating Na/K-ATPase and the dextrose prevents hypoglycaemia. This is unlikely to reduce the potassium to a safe level in this case and the patient could succumb to myocardial toxicity before it works.

Nebulized salbutamol also induces cellular uptake of potassium by activating Na/K-ATPase. It is not the best choice for the same reasons given for insulin/dextrose. Also the β_2-agonist effects of salbutamol may worsen myocardial instability.

Calcium resonium removes potassium from the body by binding in the gastrointestinal tract. It works too slowly in an emergency situation and is unpalatable to many. It can constipate and on occasion lead to perforation. Therefore, regular concomitant laxative therapy is imperative.

Haemodialysis is the quickest and most effective way of treating hyperkalaemia. It removes potassium from the body by diffusion across a semi-permeable membrane. It is likely that this patient will need dialysis once he is stable. If he were dialysed prior to receiving calcium gluconate, he would probably have a cardiac arrest.

14Question on p.7.

Answer C
They are a useful indicator of severity of ischaemic heart disease

Troponins are regulatory elements of the contractile apparatus in muscle. Specific cardiac isoforms exist that are highly sensitive and can be readily checked at the bedside. Cardiac troponins are normally very low or undetectable in the blood. They can be detected 4–6 hours after myocardial damage, rising to peak levels at 24 hours. They may remain detectable in the blood for up to 14 days.

Troponins are not solely indicators of myocardial infarction. Up to 30% of patients with unstable angina may have raised troponins and a positive test is associated with a higher risk of myocardial infarction or death. Higher levels are associated with a worse prognosis.

They are useful in the assessment of patients with unstable angina because they will help the clinician select patients who would benefit most from more aggressive treatment. Likewise, negative troponins associated with clinical and ECG criteria may help identify patients suitable for earlier discharge.

15Question on p.8.

Answer D
Failure to wash bedding

Scabies is a condition caused by infestation of the mite *Sarcoptes scabiei*. Transmission is by skin-to-skin contact. It can occur at any age but most commonly young adults (from intimate contact), institutionalized patients and healthcare workers. Clinical presentation may take several weeks from infection because sensitization to the mite takes time. Many of the clinical features are likely to be present and include the following:

- Pruritus – most noticeable at night
- Scabetic burrows
  - Flexor surfaces of wrists
  - Between webs of fingers
  - Axillae
  - Penile shaft
  - Lateral borders of hands and feet
- Scabetic nodules around the groin, waist and thighs
- Urticaria.

Treatment involves topical application of either **malathion, permethrin** or **benzoyl benzoate** from the neck down. Treatment of the head is not necessary in adults unless the patient is elderly, immunocompromised or following treatment failure.

Since transmission is from skin-to-skin contact, **all members of the household or ward should be treated simultaneously**. Any intimate contacts should also be treated even if asymptomatic.

With regards to malathion, the risk of systemic effects associated with 1–2 applications is low. Application for more than three consecutive weeks or at intervals of less than a week should be avoided and has no improved benefit of eradication.

Treatment failure or re-infection is common and several of the possible answers to the question are correct.

Malathion is the first-line treatment for scabies and resistance is unlikely. Hence A is incorrect.

Since this man is neither elderly nor immunocompromised, B is unlikely to be correct. E is not only incorrect but also potentially dangerous.

So that leaves C or D. **Clothes and bedding** should be washed as the mite can survive up to 72 hours off the host. The 'underpants option' is less likely because the patient will have to keep the malathion on his body for 24 hours and, even if he can cope with wearing a pair of pants during this time, the scabies will not.

D is the most likely correct answer.

---

16 Question on p.8.

Answer B
Metformin

Polycystic ovary syndrome is characterized by anovulation, infertility and hyperandrogenism. It is a common cause of anovulatory infertility. Other clinical features include irregular periods, hirsutism and acne. Insulin resistance is common and up to 40% of patients have type II diabetes, which is worsened by obesity.

The initial treatment of choice for patients with polycystic ovary syndrome who have anovulatory infertility is diet, exercise and weight loss. This approach is, however, frequently unsuccessful as patients find weight loss very difficult.

In patients who fail to become pregnant after such lifestyle modification, the next treatment of choice is **metformin**. A recent meta-analysis has shown that metformin induces ovulation in 46% of patients, compared to 24% who took placebo. Metformin also has beneficial effects on the metabolic problems by reducing blood pressure, insulin resistance and low-density lipoproteins. Metformin has no effect on weight loss. Treatment should be continued for 6–12 months. If the patient becomes pregnant, the drug should be stopped immediately, as its safety in the first trimester of pregnancy has not been established.

If the patient fails to become pregnant on metformin alone, **clomiphene** should be added. On this combination, up to 75% of patients will ovulate.

Third-line therapies for patients who fail to conceive using the above strategies include ovarian drilling, **gonadotrophins** and **assisted conception techniques**.

Orlistat is used in the treatment of morbid obesity. It is licensed (NICE guidelines 2001) for short-term use in patients with a body mass index of > 30 kg/m^2 and in patients with a body mass index of > 28 kg/m^2 who have significant comorbidities (e.g. diabetes, hypertension and hypercholesterolaemia), which persist despite standard treatment. Its place in the treatment of anovulation in patients with polycystic ovary syndrome is unknown.

17
Question on p.8.

Answer C
Cystic fibrosis

The polymerase chain reaction (PCR) is a rapid and versatile method for amplifying specific DNA sequences in the laboratory. The reaction involves sequential cycles composed of three steps:

1. denaturation at high temperature, typically ~95°C
2. reannealing at temperatures around 50–70°C
3. DNA synthesis, typically at about 70–75°C.

Since the technique is designed to allow selective amplification of specific target DNA sequences, it is necessary to know some DNA sequence information in advance so appropriate primers for the reaction can be designed. In addition to the primers and the DNA being tested, the reaction requires a suitably heat-stable DNA polymerase and DNA precursors (dATP, dCTP, dGTP, dTTP).

PCR is the basis of many of the tests carried out in a molecular genetics laboratory, including screening for uncharacterized mutations in disease genes when a particular diagnosis is suspected and testing relatives for known familial mutations. Common examples include testing for mutations that cause **cystic fibrosis, Huntington disease** and **Duchenne muscular dystrophy**.

Cytogenetic techniques are used in the investigation of chromosomal disorders (see Question 272, p. 89). Down's syndrome is due to trisomy 21, the presence of an extra copy of chromosome 21 and there is a well-recognized relationship with maternal age.

Turner's syndrome is caused by the presence of only one sex chromosome resulting in a 45,X karyotype. Clinical features include short stature, characteristic facies, lymphoedema, webbed neck, low posterior hairline, broad chest with widely spaced nipples, gonadal dysgenesis (streak ovaries) and an increased incidence of renal and cardiovascular defects such as coarctation of the aorta. ➤

Di George's syndrome was originally described as a combination of congenital heart disease with thymic and parathyroid hypoplasia. It was previously thought to be distinct from the velocardiofacial (Shprintzen's) syndrome (a combination of congenital heart disease, characteristic facies, cleft palate and velopharyngeal insufficiency). Since the development of fluorescent *in situ* hybridization (FISH), both conditions have been found to be due to a microdeletion of chromosomal material from the long arm of chromosome 22 and are more commonly called the 22q11 deletion syndrome.

Phenylketonuria (PKU) is an autosomal recessive inborn error of metabolism with a frequency of around 1 in 10 000 births in the UK and a carrier frequency of 1 in 50. It is due to deficiency of the enzyme phenylalanine hydroxylase, which converts phenylalanine to tyrosine. If left untreated, it can lead to severe mental retardation as a result of accumulation of phenylalanine but, with appropriate dietary modification, most of those affected can achieve normal development and lead active healthy lives. The majority of cases of PKU are now detected by newborn screening programmes, which involve the collection of a spot of blood on to a piece of filter paper during the first week of life. Blood phenylalanine levels can then be analysed and appropriate treatment can be initiated promptly for affected individuals.

18

Question on p.8.

Answer D
Leishmania braziliensis

Dermatobium hominis is a common cause of human myiasis also known colloquially as bot fly lava. Though capable of causing a superficial ulcer with visible maggots it is unlikely to disseminate to the nasopharynx.

Trypanosoma cruzi or Chagas disease is commonly transmitted by the reduviid or assassin bug (*Triatoma infestans* being the most important vector in South America). It has rarely been reported in Belize and is not an important public health issue in this country. The answer is false, as the pathogen does not localize to the nasopharynx.

Leishmaniasis is endemic to Belize and considered an occupational hazard of operational importance to the British Army. The disease is transmitted by the bite of an infected female *Phlebotomus* sandfly (particularly lutzomyia species). *Leishmania mexicana* commonly causes an isolated skin lesion (Bay sore) and Chiclero's ulcer – a destructive lesion of the pinna. *Leishmania braziliensis* on the other hand disseminates and localizes to the nasopharynx, and causes widespread destruction or espundia; hence, it is the correct answer.

Dracunculiasis is caused by *Dracunculus medinensis* – also known as guinea worm. The parasite is an important cause of morbidity in much of Africa and India. Recently, there has been a World Health Organization (WHO) Programme that aims to eradicate the disease completely and currently few infections are reported outside of Sudan. The Programme has been particularly successful in Asia, where it is thought the disease has been eradicated.

19
Question on p.9.

Answer C
Elbow pronation

The radial nerve is formed from the terminal branch of the posterior cord of the brachial plexus. The posterior cord is made up of upper, medial and lower trunks. It contains roots from C5–8.

Damage to the nerve in the axilla often comes from the incorrect use of crutches whereby the weight of the patient is taken in the axilla and not the heel of the hand. Damage here causes weakness of all of the muscles supplied by the radial nerve. Damage further down may be caused by sleeping with the arm hanging over a chair, the so-called 'Saturday night palsy'. This is so named as it occurs in those who have had a deep alcohol-induced sleep. Damage may also occur from fractures of the midshaft of the humerus. The injury here is lower down the radial nerve and tends to spare the innervation of the triceps.

Pronation is performed by the pronator teres, innervated by the median nerve.

A table of the major upper limb nerves and their innervation is given below.

	Radial	Median	Ulnar
Root supply	C5–8	C6–T1	C8–T1
Sensory	Dorsal forearm and hand	Lateral palm, thumb and 2½ fingers	Medial palm and 1½ fingers
Motor supply	Triceps C6,7,8	Pronator teres C6,7	Wrist flexor C7,8,T1
	Wrist extensors C7,8	Wrist flexors C6,7	All other small muscles of hand C7,8,T1
	Finger extensors C7,8	Long finger flexors C8,T1	
	Brachioradialis C5,6	Abduct thumb C8,T1	
	Supinator C6,7	Oppose thumb C8,T1	
Damage from	Crutch palsy	Carpal tunnel	Supracondylar #
	Saturday night palsy	syndrome	Olecranon #
	# Humerus		

#, fracture.

20
Question on p.9.

Answer B
Domperidone

Lactation is stimulated by the anterior pituitary hormone, prolactin. Prolactin secretion is controlled by the hypothalamus through the release ➤

of dopamine, which inhibits the process. There is no known hypothalamic prolactin-releasing hormone. Although both thyrotrophin-releasing hormone (TRH) and vasoactive intestinal polypeptide (VIP) stimulate prolactin secretion, it is not thought that this is physiologically important.

Griseofulvin and **spironolactone** may cause gynaecomastia but do not affect prolactin concentrations leading to galactorrhoea.

Bromocriptine is a dopamine agonist and will therefore decrease prolactin levels.

Cimetidine causes gynaecomastia and may cause rises in prolactin concentrations, but only when given intravenously. The question states oral medicine, so cimetidine is not the correct answer.

Domperidone is a dopamine antagonist and leads to large rises in prolactin concentrations and hence is the correct answer.

Causes of gynaecomastia
Drugs:
- Cimetidine
- Digoxin
- Spironolactone
- Griseofulvin
- Methyldopa
- Chlorpromazine

Other causes:
- Kleinfelter's syndrome
- Chronic liver disease
- Dialysis
- Acromegaly
- Lymphoma
- Bronchial carcinoma
- Oestrogen-secreting tumour

Causes of galactorrhoea
- Pregnancy
- Prolactinoma
- Oestrogen
- Chronic renal failure
- Hypothyroidism
- Ectopic prolactin secretion from renal or lung tumours
- Pituitary mass lesion – causing inhibition of blood flow from the hypothalamus
- Dopamine-antagonizing drugs

21

Question on p.9.

Answer D
14 mmol/L

$$\text{Anion gap} = \{(Na) + (K)\} - \{(bicarbonate) + (Cl)\}$$
$$= \{(138) + (4)\} - \{(20) + (108)\}$$
$$= 14 \text{ mmol/L}$$

The anion gap is caused by negatively anions in the serum, which are not normally measured with the urea and electrolytes. They consist of negatively charged particles carried by albumin, lactate and phosphate. The reference range for a normal anion gap can easily be remembered as the teenage years 13–19.

There are a number of causes of an increased anion gap including the following.

Type	Accumulating anions
Lactic acidosis	Lactate
Type A (caused by sepsis/organ failure)	
Type B (iatrogenic, e.g. metformin)	
Diabetic ketoacidosis	Organic acids
Renal failure	Sulphate
	Phosphate

Most patients with an increased anion gap have an associated metabolic acidosis.

22

Question on p.10.

Answer B
Angle of needle bevel inserted horizontally

Post-lumbar puncture headache occurs after 10% of lumbar punctures. The headache is a low-pressure headache, which is worse on standing and improved by lying down. Symptoms tend to resolve in a few days. Treatment involves bed rest, adequate fluid intake and simple analgesia.

Incidence of headache is not related to the amount of cerebrospinal fluid (CSF) taken but rather a continuous leak of CSF from the hole made in the dura. Therefore, incidence is related to the size of the hole. ➤

> **Predictors of post-lumbar puncture headache**
> - Gauge of needle
> - Number of attempts
> - Angle of bevel insertion:
>   - Horizontal insertion will part dural fibres
>   - Vertical insertion will slice through dural fibres
> - Replacing the introducer stylet will decrease the incidence of headache
>
> **Contraindications to lumbar puncture**
> - Signs or symptoms of raised intracranial pressure without imaging
> - Focal neurological signs without imaging
> - Local infection, e.g. skin, bone, pustular acne
> - Thrombocytopenia
> - Clotting abnormality

23

Question on p.10.

Answer C
Continue aspirin and start dipyridamole

Long-term antiplatelet therapy has been shown to reduce the risk of vascular events following stroke or TIA by a quarter: about 36 serious vascular events will be avoided over 36 months among 1000 patients.

Aspirin appears safe in the acute phase of stroke, and is the initial treatment for secondary prevention of a stroke or TIA. No significant difference has been found between the protective effects of high-dose aspirin (500–1500 mg per day) and of medium aspirin dosage (75–325 mg per day). Medium-dose aspirin therapy is the most widely tested antiplatelet regimen and no other regimen appears to have a greater protective effect. Higher doses are associated with increased adverse events, and so answer A would not help and may have adverse effects.

Other **antiplatelet drugs** (apart from ticlopidine, which is very expensive) alone have not been shown to be more effective than aspirin alone. Data from one randomized controlled trial shows that **dipyridamole** has an independent effect equal to low-dose aspirin and some additive effect when used in combination.

Warfarin reduces the relative risk of further ischaemic strokes in patients with atrial fibrillation to the same relative extent as its primary preventative action in atrial fibrillation. There is no evidence to suggest that warfarin reduces the risk of further TIAs in patients in sinus rhythm. There is an increase risk of bleeding if warfarin is started in a patient already taking aspirin with no proven benefit.

Answer D
Aldosterone

The adrenal glands consist of the outer cortex and an inner medulla. The cortex consists of three anatomically distinct zones. Starting from the outermost, they are as follows.

- The **zona glomerulosa** which is the site of mineralocorticoid production, e.g. aldosterone. It is mainly regulated by angiotensin II, potassium and adrenocorticotrophic hormone (ACTH). In addition, dopamine, atrial natriuretic peptide (ANP) and other neuropeptides modulate adrenal zona glomerulosa function.
- The central **zona fasciculata** is mainly responsible for glucocorticoid synthesis, which is regulated by ACTH. In addition, several cytokines [interleukin-1 (IL-1), IL-6, tumour necrosis factor (TNF) and neuropeptides] influence the biosynthesis of glucocorticoids.
- The inner **zona reticularis** is the site of adrenal androgen secretion [predominantly dihydroepiandrostenedione (DHEA), DHEA sulphate and androstenedione], as well as some glucocorticoid production (cortisol and corticosterone).

The medulla produces adrenaline and noradrenaline. It should be noted that only a small proportion of circulating noradrenaline is derived from the adrenal gland, most coming from sympathetic nerve endings.

Answer B
Variegate porphyria

It is sometimes difficult to know where to start with porphyrias as there are so many areas candidates can be examined on. If you learn anything from this answer, learn the essential facts below.

- All porphyrias have **autosomal dominant** inheritance except congenital porphyria.
- Only the **acute porphyrias** develop **neurological** consequences.
- All porphyrias are **photosensitive**, except acute intermittent porphyria.
- If the name sounds **'inherited'**, e.g. congenital porphyria or hereditary coproporphyria, then it is **extremely rare**.

The porphyrias are a group of inherited diseases resulting from deficiencies in the haem biosynthetic pathway. They are classified as the following. ➤

Acute porphyrias
- Acute intermittent porphyria
- Variegate porphyria
- Hereditary coproporphyria.

Non-acute porphyrias
- Cutaneous hepatic porphyria
- Congenital porphyria
- Erythropoietic protoporphyria.

The haem biosynthetic pathway is complicated and, if you have a spare evening and want to learn it, go for it. If you want to learn and understand the basics, then here are the absolute essentials.

- All porphyrias have an increased aminolaevulinic acid synthase, leading to an overproduction of porphyrins and their precursors.
- In acute porphyrias, the level of porphobilinogen deaminase is reduced or normal and so the main compound that accumulates is δ-aminolaevulinic acid (δ-ALA).
- δ-Aminolaevulinic acid is thought to be neurotoxic, which explains why the acute porphyrias have neurological features.
- The non-acute porphyrias also have raised porphobilinogen (PBG) deaminase activity. This leads to excess PBG and δ-ALA being converted to porphyrins further down the pathway.

The following table shows which porphyrins are raised in different porphyrias. Brackets signify the results during an acute attack.

	Urine δ-ALA/PBG	Urine porphyrins	Faeces porphyrins
Acute intermittent	+ (++)	+ (++)	—
Variegate	— (+)	— (+)	+ (+)
Cutaneous hepatic	—	+	—
Congenital erythropoietic	—	+	+
Erythropoietic protoporphyria	—	—	+

This particular question could be solved by applying the four essential facts alone. The wrist drop, i.e. neurological involvement, indicates an acute porphyria. The presence of a blistering rash rules out acute intermittent. This leaves variegate or hereditary. Hereditary is extremely rare and so statistically it is more likely to be variegate.

Alternatively, you could learn the table and arrive at the same answer, remembering that these results were obtained during an acute attack.

Answer D
Non-alcoholic steatohepatitis

Non-alcoholic steatohepatitis (NASH) is the commonest cause of a persistently raised ALT in a patient with no risk factors for chronic liver disease. It is commoner in patients with obesity, diabetes and hypercholesterolaemia, but is often found in people with none of these.

It used to be thought that the natural history of NASH was benign, but evidence is beginning to emerge that a small proportion of these patients can progress to cirrhosis. Diagnosis is by liver biopsy, which shows increased fat deposition and a necro-inflammatory response in the hepatocytes.

The next most likely diagnosis is **chronic hepatitis C**, which can present as an isolated rise in transaminases with no other symptoms. Most patients with chronic hepatitis C give no history of a prodromal/hepatitic illness and approximately 40% have no discernible risk factors, which predispose to hepatitis C infection.

Answer D
To assess safety of the drug in the patient population

Post-marketing surveillance of a newly marketed drug is essential to assess ongoing patient safety. Although the drug in question will have gone through several pre-marketing clinical trials, there are limitations to the certainty that they will pick up on all potential adverse drug events.

Limitations of pre-marketing clinical trials include the following.

- **Short duration** – effects that develop with chronic use or those that have a long latency period are impossible to detect.
- **Narrow population** – generally do not include special groups (e.g. children or the elderly) and to a large degree are not always representative of the population that may be exposed to the drug after approval.
- **Narrow set of indications** – those for which efficacy is being studied and do not cover actual evolving size.
- **Small size** – generally include 4000 subjects and effects that occur rarely are unlikely to be detected.

Type A adverse drug events are predictable events that are an extension of an individual drug's known pharmacological properties. These are responsible for the bulk of adverse drug events recorded and are likely to be picked up in Phase 1, 2 and 3 drug trials. ➤

Type B adverse drug events are the bizarre and unpredictable events that may occur. These include idiosyncratic reactions, allergic reactions and carcinogenic/teratogenic events.

Drug effectiveness will have already been assessed. A drug company is not going to release a drug on to the market without knowing whether it works. Part of the marketing will involve results of trials, convincing doctors how affective the new drug is.

The acceptability of a treatment or **patient satisfaction** will have been assessed during the pre-marketing trials. It is important that, before releasing a new drug, the pharmaceutical company knows that patients will comply with it.

28   Question on p.12.

Answer A
Anti-Ro

Systemic lupus erythematosus is a multisystem inflammatory disease. It is characterized by a widespread vasculitis with an underlying autoimmune pathological basis. Autoantibodies that are present are as follows:

Antinuclear antibody (ANA)	Positive in 95%
dsDNA	Antibodies present in 50%, highly specific
Anti-Ro	Positive in 25%
Anti-La	
Rheumatoid factor	Positive 40%
Complement	Low C3 levels
Immunoglobulins	Both IgG and IgM normally raised

Patients with SLE who become pregnant are at risk of multiple problems. Some patients have difficulties conceiving or recurrent abortions, particularly in relation to **antiphospholipid syndrome**. Secondly, they frequently suffer from the complications of pregnancy such as spontaneous abortions, intrauterine death and congenital abnormalities. Finally, medications that are used to treat the condition are highly toxic, e.g. immunosuppressives and steroids.

Anti-Ro antibodies are particularly associated with fetal complete heart block and other bradyarrythmias.

29   Question on p.12.

Answer E
Karposi's sarcoma

The Epstein–Barr virus (EBV) is a human DNA virus in the herpesvirus family. It is widespread in humans and primary infection usually occurs in childhood, where it remains clinically silent. Age of transmission is greater in areas with better hygiene. It persists as a latent infection in a few circulating B-lymphocytes and as a productive lytic infection in intraepithelial B cells of the mouth and pharynx, and possibly the urogenital tract and salivary glands. It is shed into the saliva and transmission is by droplet spread.

The most common disease associated with EBV is infectious mononucleosis, which may occur in the 50% of people not infected with the virus during childhood. It is transmitted by close salivary contact and has earned the name 'the kissing disease'. Other diseases are associated with EBV infection are listed below.

- **Burkitt's lymphoma.** This is a B-cell tumour found most commonly in parts of Africa and Papua New Guinea. EBV is considered an essential factor to the development of the tumour. Another cofactor identified is malaria, which is endemic in many of these areas, spread by the *Anopheles* mosquito. It is predominantly a disease of childhood and extremely rare over the age of 14 years. In the endemic areas, it is more common than all other childhood tumours added together.

  The tumour is usually multifocal and the symptoms depend entirely on the anatomical location. Jaw tumours are present in 70 per cent of patients but are almost always accompanied by tumours elsewhere. They give a rapidly growing mass with loosening of teeth and exophthalmos from orbital spread. It characteristically does not involve the spleen or peripheral lymph nodes.

  It is also seen early on in the course of HIV disease.
- **Nasopharyngeal carcinoma.** This rare tumour occurs in the post-nasal space, where it arises from squamous epithelial cells. It has a high incidence in southern China, Malaysia, Vietnam, North Africa and the Philippines. The tumour usually occurs in middle or old age, but in North Africa it has bimodal age peaks, one involving young people up to 20 years of age and a second much later in life. Irrespective of geographical region, nasopharyngeal carcinoma cells always carry the EBV genome.
- **Hodgkin's lymphoma.** Within 5 years of infectious mononucleosis, there is a 4–6-fold increase in the likelihood of developing Hodgkin disease. There is now evidence that, in Hodgkin's lymphomas, EBV DNA is carried and expressed in both the Reed–Sternberg and the mononuclear Hodgkin's cells.
- **Hairy leukoplakia.** This is usually seen in people with HIV or other immunosuppressed individuals, usually presenting as painless white patches on the tongue or on the lateral buccal mucosa. The lesions are slightly raised, poorly demarcated, and have a 'hairy' or corrugated surface. The patches are usually multiple and measure up to 3 cm in diameter. The squamous epithelial cells of this condition contain large amounts of actively replicating EBV. Treatment is with acyclovir.
- **Large cell lymphoma.** These are also seen in patients with AIDS or the immunosuppressed. Their distribution is extranodal, involving many unusual sites, most commonly the central nervous system. There is a strong association with EBV (100% in cerebral tumours).

Kaposi's sarcoma is associated with human herpesvirus type 8 and not EBV.

Question on p.12.

Answer D
Transient global amnesia

The history is classic for **transient global amnesia** (TGA). Transient global amnesia has been a well-described phenomenon for more than 40 years. Clinically, it manifests with a paroxysmal, transient loss of memory function. Immediate recall ability is preserved, as is remote memory; however, patients experience striking loss of memory for recent events and an impaired ability to retain new information. In some cases, the degree of retrograde memory loss is mild. In this patient's case, the bewilderment and amnesia with preservation of sense of self and intellectual functioning without clouding of consciousness is characteristic.

Many patients are anxious or agitated, and may repeatedly ask questions concerning transpiring events. On mental status examination, language function is preserved, which indicates a preservation of semantic and syntax memory. Attention is spared, visual-spatial skills are intact and social skills are retained. Symptoms typically last less than 24 hours. As the syndrome resolves, the amnesia improves, but the patient may be left with a distinct lapse of recollection for events during the attack.

The precise pathophysiology of TGA is not clear. On positron emission tomography (PET), and diffusion-weighted magnetic resonance imaging (DWI), blood flow to specific brain areas that involve memory appears to be disrupted transiently during TGA. This includes the thalamus and/or medial temporal structures (in particular, the amygdala and hippocampus). However, patients do not seem at higher risk of stroke or epilepsy, and recurrence is low (approximately 5% per annum).

It does not require investigation and the mainstay of treatment is reassurance.

                                                      Question on p.12.

Answer D
Malignant infiltration of bone marrow

The results suggest leucoerythroblastic anaemia, characterized by immature granulocytes and red cells (normoblasts) in the peripheral blood. This occurs when the bone marrow is replaced by another substance, e.g.

- malignant cells
- cells containing metabolic products of storage disorders
- fibrous tissue
- bone.

All the answers could give the blood picture and so the key to finding the best answer lies with choosing one, which fits the clinical picture and is most common.

Gaucher disease is a lysosomal storage disease most commonly seen in Ashkenazi Jews (1:2500 births). Patients typically have hepatosplenomegaly and large glucocerebroside containing reticuloendothelial histiocytes (Gaucher cells) in the bone marrow. It usually presents with hepatosplenomegaly in childhood with splenic complications (infarction, torsion and thrombocytopenia) and the clinical picture described makes this rare condition unlikely to be the correct answer.

Myelosclerosis, also known as **myelofibrosis**, is a myeloproliferative disorder characterized by anaemia and abnormal proliferation of haemopoietic precursors associated with a variable degree of fibrosis of the bone marrow, and myeloid metaplasia of the spleen, liver and other organs. Its presentation is variable but the first symptoms are often associated with splenomegaly, which is often the only clinical finding.

Osteopetrosis or **marble bone disease** is characterized by a widespread increase in bone density. The defect lies with osteoclast in ability to resorb mineralized bone. Two forms exist: the recessively inherited severe form, which causes death in childhood; and the dominantly inherited mild form, which is diagnosed on radiological grounds. Bony replacement of bone marrow results in a leukoerythroblastic anaemia.

Severe infection can give a leukaemoid reaction but the clinical picture does not describe a severe infection. It does not explain the anaemia either as there is nothing in the blood results to suggest haemolysis or a history of bleeding.

The most likely answer is **malignant infiltration of bone marrow**. Leukaemias, lymphoma, adenocarcinoma, myeloma and myeloproliferative disease are all capable of malignant infiltration. In this case, the patient has a large irregular liver suggesting liver metastases most probably from an unknown primary.

Causes of a leukoerythroblastic anaemia
- Malignant infiltration
- Storage disorders, e.g. Gaucher's disease
- Myelosclerosis
- Osteopetrosis
- Leukaemoid reaction secondary to severe infection

---

32 Question on p.13.

Answer B
Evidence level Ib

The key to evidence statements and grades of recommendations are outlined below. ➤

Statements of evidence
Ia. Evidence obtained from meta-analysis of randomized controlled trials.
Ib. Evidence obtained from at least one randomized controlled trial.
IIa. Evidence obtained from at least one other type of well-designed controlled study without randomization.
IIb. Evidence obtained from at least one other type of well-designed quasi-experimental study.
III. Evidence obtained from well-designed non-experimental descriptive studies, such as comparative studies, correlation studies and case studies.
IV. Evidence obtained from expert committee reports or opinions and/or clinical experiences of respected authorities.

The evidence in this trial comes from one randomized controlled trial and so the answer must be Ib.

Grades of recommendations
A. Requires at least one randomized controlled trial as part of a body of literature of overall good quality and consistency addressing the specific recommendation.
(Evidence levels Ia, Ib)
B. Requires evidence from well conducted clinical studies but no randomized clinical trials on the topic of recommendation.
(Evidence levels IIa, IIb, III)
C. Requires evidence obtained from expert committee reports or opinions and/or clinical experiences of respected authorities. Indicates an absence of directly applicable clinical studies of good quality.
(Evidence level IV)

33 Question on p.13.

Answer E
Oral triple therapy for 1 month

The risk of transmission of HIV via a needlestick injury is 0.3%. Following a needlestick injury from a HIV-positive patient, the wound should be thoroughly washed with water and the healthcare worker referred to the occupational health department. Oral zidovudine therapy for 1 month following the needlestick injury has been shown to reduce the risk of transmission by 80%. Oral triple therapy taken for the same duration is even more effective.

It is vital to read this question carefully. In this question you are asked what has been shown to decrease the risk of transmission. If you are asked 'what should the recipient of the needlestick injury do first', the answer is wash the hands thoroughly.

Question on p.14.

Answer A
Radiation enteritis

This patient's blood test results indicate small bowel disease with anaemia, a low vitamin B_{12}, red cell folate and ferritin. **Radiation enteritis** can occur at any time following radiotherapy and it is not unusual for it to present 20 years later. The radiation damage to the small bowel is due to a progressive endarteritis obliterans, which results in scarring and fibrosis of the bowel wall. Small bowel strictures are common, as is abnormal motility of the small bowel. Bacterial overgrowth is a common associated finding.

Treatment of these patients can be difficult. Major strictures can be resected, but may recur as the disease progresses. Associated motility and bacterial overgrowth can be treated with appropriate antibiotics and promotility agents. Associated vitamin and nutritional deficiencies should be treated with appropriate replacement therapy.

This patient is unlikely to have **carcinoma of the colon**, as she has a B_{12} and red cell folate deficiency, which indicate small bowel pathology.

Crohn's disease can present in the elderly for the first time, in fact there is a second peak in incidence in the sixth and seventh decades which mirrors that in early adulthood, but is less pronounced. Crohn's disease is unlikely in this patient, given the profound abnormalities of B_{12}, folate and ferritin, this could only be seen in extensive small bowel Crohn's disease. If this were the case, one would expect the ESR to be markedly elevated.

Tropical sprue can present in an identical manner to this patient, and sometimes decades after spending time in an endemic area, such as equatorial Africa. Hong Kong is not an endemic area and, therefore, this diagnosis is incorrect.

Acquired lactose intolerance is due to a (sometimes temporary) acquired deficiency of lactase in the small bowel brush border. It characteristically follows a severe gastrointestinal infection. Severe B_{12} and red cell folate deficiency is usually not seen.

 Question on p.14.

Answer A
Above right upper lobe

The azygous lobe is an anatomical variation seen in 0.5% of people. It is positioned superiomedially to the right upper lobe. It is not a true lobe as it does not have a separate bronchial tree. The radiographic appearance of the azygous lobe is that of a teardrop at about the level of T5, there is a soft convex line protruding from the midline, this represents the parietal and visceral pleura. The azygous lobe is of no clinical consequence.

36 Question on p.14.

Answer D
Hyperoxaluria

Crohn's disease is not just a disease of the gastrointestinal system. Primarily, it is a transmural, focal, subacute or chronic inflammatory disease affecting any part of the intestinal system from mouth to anus. It has a predilection for the terminal ileum. The histopathology shows characteristic non-caseating epithelioid cell granulomata.

The extraintestinal manifestations of Crohn's disease include the following.

- Skin:
  - pyoderma gangrenosum
  - erythema nodosum
  - enterocutaneous fistula.
- Musculoskeletal:
  - sacroileitis
  - ankylosing spondylitis
  - large joint oligoarthritis
  - symmetrical small joint polyarthritis.
- Ocular:
  - iritis
  - uveitis
  - episcleritis.
- Renal:
  - oxalate stones.
- Biliary:
  - gallstones
  - primary sclerosing cholangitis.
- Miscellaneous:
  - amyloidosis – rare.

Hyperbilirubinaemia is seen in haemolytic anaemia where it predisposes to pigmented gallstones.

Hypercalciuria predisposes to calcium calculi. Nearly 10% of the male population have been shown to excrete more than 7.5 mmol of calcium in 24 hours; however, not all of these develop stones. Causes of hypercalciuria include hypercalcaemia, excess dietary intake and idiopathic.

Hyperuricaemia accounts for about 5% of all renal calculi. This is predisposed to by increased cell turnover, e.g. myeloproliferative disease, gout and dehydration.

Oxalate stones are found in those who have increased intake (e.g. rhubarb and spinach, restriction of dietary calcium), and those with gastrointestinal disease (e.g. Crohn's). This is associated with increased oxalate absorption.

Answer D
Previously well-controlled epileptic, last fit was at lunchtime 9 months previously

The rules for fitness to drive are complex, and there are major differences between the rules for group 1 and group 2 drivers.

Group 1 drivers: motor cars and motor cycles
Group 2 drivers: lorries and buses

Patients with epilepsy should not drive a motor car for 1 year after a daytime fit. They must also not drive for a year after a nocturnal fit, unless they have had an attack whilst asleep more than 3 years ago and have not had any awake attacks since that sleep attack.

Patients with epilepsy may not drive a lorry or a bus for 10 years after any epileptic attack. For such patients to regain their licence, they must have not required any medication to treat their epilepsy for 10 years and be deemed to 'not be a source of danger whilst driving'.

	Group 1	Group 2
Coronary angioplasty	No driving for 1 week	No driving for 6 weeks
ICD	No driving for 6 months post-implantation Implant not fired for 6 months Miscellaneous[a]	Permanent loss of licence
Monocular vision	May continue driving if: • Normal visual acuity • Normal visual fields • Driver has adapted	Permanent loss of licence
Subarachnoid haemorrhage (no cause found)	May continue driving if cerebral angiography is normal	No driving for 6 months

[a]The reader is advised to consult the document *At a glance guide to the current standards of fitness to drive* (DVLA, Swansea, 2001). This document gives full details of the fitness to drive rules. These rules are lengthy and complex, and beyond the scope of this text.

Answer E
Recheck INR in 24 hours

Recommendations from the British Society of Haematologists are in the British National Formulary (BNF), and are based on the INR and the presence or absence of major bleeding, minor bleeding or risk factors. They are as follows: ➤

Major bleeding	Stop warfarin
	Give 5 mg iv vitamin K
	50 units/kg prothrombin complex concentrate **or** fresh frozen plasma (FFP) 15 mL/kg
INR > 8	No bleeding or minor bleeding: stop warfarin and restart when INR < 5
	If other risk factors for bleeding: 0.5 mg iv vitamin K **or** 5 mg po vitamin K
	Repeat if INR still too high after 24 hours
INR 6–8	No bleeding or minor bleeding: stop warfarin and restart when INR < 5
INR < 6 or > 0.5 above target INR	Reduce dose **or** stop warfarin and restart when INR < 5

If bleeding occurs within the therapeutic range, the possibility of an occult malignancy needs to be investigated.

As this gentleman has an INR > 8 with a minor bleed and no other risk factors, treatment would be to withhold warfarin, monitor the INR and restart when INR comes below 5.

39
Question on p.15.

Answer A
Campylobacter jejuni

Guillain–Barré is a common cause of acute polyneuropathy. It presents on the whole 2–3 weeks after an initial infection, the most common being *Campylobacter*. Up to 30% give a history of *Campylobacter* infection in the preceding 6 weeks.

Yersinia has been associated with acute watery diarrhoea and abdominal pain; however, it has also been seen to be a herald infection in seronegative spondylarthritides and possibly Graves' disease.

E. coli causes a variety of infections acutely but may also precipitate the haemolytic uraemic syndrome (HUS), possibly by causing endothelial damage. HUS is characterized by microangiopathic haemolysis, thrombocytopenia and renal failure.

Brucella causes both a septic and a reactive arthritis. It tends to present as part of a chronic infection.

Seronegative spondylarthritis is a reactive arthritis that occurs in susceptible individuals (i.e. those who are B27-positive) after an initial infection with bacillary dysentery or non-specific urethritis. Bacteria that are capable of doing this include *Salmonella, Shigella, Yersinia* and *Chlamydia*. Molecules from these bacteria have been found in the inflamed synovium, indicating a possible antigenic link between infection and inflammation.

Question on p.15.

Answer A
Genital herpes

Primary genital herpes is normally caused by infection from *Herpes simplex* virus 2 (HSV-2), although infection HSV-1 also occurs. It follows recent exposure to a sexual partner with active lesions. Exposure is common, with 25–60% of people showing serological evidence of infection. Initial infection (unlike a cold sore) is often severe, with 50% presenting with excruciatingly painful shallow ulcers. Tender inguinal lymphadenopathy is common. Ulcers develop between 3 and 14 days post-exposure. Crusting of lesions normally occurs at day 10 after ulcer formation, and the course lasts 18–22 days. The virus then lays dormant in the sacral ganglia and reoccurs at intervals.

The differential diagnosis includes:

Syphilis	Painless ulcers
Chancroid	Incubation 4–7 days, deeper ulcers than HSV
	Common in the Tropics
Lymphogranuloma venereum	Painless ulcers, common in Africa and India
Granuloma inguinale	Painless 'beefy red' heaped up ulcers
	Common in the Tropics
Behçet's	Very rare
	Other features of disease would be present, if this was the diagnosis

                                          Question on p.16.

Answer B
Positively bifringent crystals

Haemochromatosis is an inherited (autosomal recessive) disorder of iron metabolism. There is an increase in the iron that is absorbed from the gut. This leads to an increase in the deposition of iron in many organs. Particularly affected are the liver, pancreas, heart and skin. It tends to present earlier in men because of the protective effect of menstrual loss in women.

There is an association between haemochromatosis and chondrocalcinosis, a deposition of calcium pyrophosphate crystals. These are rhomboidal, **positively bifringent** crystals when viewed under polarized light. Currently, there is no explanation for the correlation between these two conditions.

Urate crystals causing gout are **needle-shaped negatively bifringent crystals.**

Haemochromatosis does not predispose to **septic arthritis.**

Haemosiderin is an insoluble complex formed by the breakdown of haemoglobin. It may indicate a recent haemarthrosis.

Question on p.16.

42

Answer D
Await serum paracetamol levels

As little as 10–15 g (20–30 tablets) of paracetamol taken within 24 hours may cause severe hepatocellular necrosis.

Gastric lavage is not indicated here as 2 hours have elapsed since the drug was taken. In addition to being an extremely unpleasant procedure, with risk of oesophageal trauma, research has suggested that the lavage process may actually push some remaining drugs from the stomach into the duodenum.

Oral ipecacuanha is also inappropriate here. This highly emetogenic drug induces vomiting with the intention of expelling remaining tablets. Since 2 hours have elapsed, a significant amount of paracetamol will already be in the bloodstream.

Oral activated charcoal binds poisons in the gastrointestinal system preventing their absorption. It needs to be given as soon as possible, as it becomes less effective if the drugs have been ingested more than an hour ago. It will be of little use in this patient and giving activated charcoal may prevent other oral medications working if they need to be given, e.g. oral methionine.

Paracetamol is metabolized in the liver to N-acetyl-p-benzoquinamine, which is a toxic to liver. It is then conjugated with glutathione to a non-toxic metabolite. There is a finite store of glutathione that is rapidly used up when a paracetamol overdose occurs. Once glutathione stores are exhausted, N-acetyl-p-benzoquinamine accumulates and binds irreversibly to hepatic cell membranes, ultimately causing hepatic necrosis.

N-**Acetyl cysteine** supplies glutathione intravenously, preventing the accumulation of toxic metabolites. Some patients experience an anaphylactoid reaction, with wheezing, hypotension and rash. It can also cause significant bronchospasm in asthmatics and should not be given unnecessarily. In the patient in the question you should wait for her **4-hour paracetamol** levels before deciding to use it. If she is above the treatment line she will not be at additional risk by waiting for the levels.

Patients are considered at high risk of developing liver damage if they are known to be in any of the following categories:

• taking medicines that induce hepatic enzymes
• has been taking alcohol or has a history of alcohol abuse
• malnourished.

Their paracetamol levels should be compared with the high-risk treatment line.

Often there is doubt about the timing of the overdose and what other substances have been ingested. In such cases, always err on the side of caution and, if the patient is anywhere near the lower treatment line, give N-**acetyl cysteine.**

Answer D
Section 5(2)

The patient in question was admitted voluntarily. She is clearly psychotic and demonstrating some First Rank symptoms. She has expressed an intention to kill herself and needs medical treatment to prevent her death. As a doctor, you can impose a Section 5(2) pending a psychiatric opinion.

The Mental Health Act is complex and the account below is by no means a comprehensive overview. Its intention is to provide you with the basics on each of the main sections that medical practitioners may encounter.

Section 2
Admission for assessment
Duration up to 28 days
Two medical recommendations required
Patient must have a mental disorder
Ought to be detained in interest of patient's own health or safety of others.

Section 3
Admission for treatment
Up to 6 months
Two medical recommendations required
Patient must have a mental illness, which is appropriate to be treated in hospital
Often follows a Section 2
Cannot be imposed if the nearest relative objects.

Section 4
Section 4 is intended for emergency admissions, where if it were not for the extreme urgency, a Section 2 would be appropriate.
72 hours duration
Only one medical recommendation required
Patient must have a mental disorder
Ought to be detained in interest of patient's own health or safety of others.

Section 5(2)
This Section contains powers for a doctor to prevent someone who is otherwise a voluntary patient from leaving hospital
72 hours duration
The registered medical practitioner who exercises the doctor's holding power must be the doctor who is in charge of the person's care
It would usually be followed up by a Section 2 or 3

Section 5(4)
A person who is a voluntary patient in hospital can be legally detained there if it appears to a suitably qualified nurse that the conditions below are met. ➤

Up to 6 hours duration by which time a doctor will have arrived to impose a Section 5(2)

Patient must be suffering from a mental disorder and a risk of harm to himself or others.

---

44 Question on p.17.

Answer E
Mycoplasma-induced cold antibody haemolysis

This patient has haemolytic anaemia. The clue lies in the blood film that shows autoagglutination. This is characteristic of 'cold agglutinin' disease. This is haemolytic anaemia caused by IgM antibodies that cause haemolysis at temperatures lower than 37°C. When the blood film is analysed in the laboratory at room temperature autoagglutination is seen. Warming the slide to body temperature reverses this effect.

> **Causes of cold agglutinin haemolytic anaemia**
> - Infectious mononucleosis
> - *Mycoplasma pneumoniae*
> - Lymphoma
> - Paroxysmal cold haemoglobinuria

Infectious mononucleosis is not the correct answer. The Monospot is negative, and she would have been very unlikely to have received antibiotics for her initial illness.

Penicillin-induced haemolysis does occur but usually at the time or very shortly after the course of treatment. Cold agglutination is not seen.

Hodgkin's disease is a possibility but is much less likely than *Mycoplasma*-induced cold antibody haemolysis, given the history of a severe chest infection.

---

45 Question on p.17.

Answer C
Nocturnal diarrhoea with 1–2 stools per night

Irritable bowel syndrome (IBS) is a functional bowel problem that can start at any age, but often starts in the late teens or early adulthood. It is a very common clinical problem and affects approximately 5% of men and 13% of women in the UK. IBS is either constipation predominant or diarrhoea predominant, but often there is a combination of both these symptoms which alternate. Abdominal pain is almost universally present, although the spectrum of severity is vast: from trivial minor discomfort to pain that is severe and profoundly affects the quality of life. The patient's pain is frequently relieved by defaecation. The severity of pain is, therefore, not a particularly helpful diagnostic discriminator.

Patients with IBS may have a wide constellation of symptoms, and frequently the patient may have had intermittent or persistent symptoms for many months or years before seeking medical advice or onward referral to a gastroenterologist. Common symptoms include abdominal bloating and the passage of mucous per rectum. Rectal mucous discharge therefore does not help distinguish IBS from other organic pathology.

Distinguishing organic pathology from IBS

Distinguishing organic pathology from IBS is a common clinical dilemma. There are a number of ground rules that are helpful in doing this. Applying the following rules will avoid unnecessarily overinvestigating patients with IBS on the one hand, and missing organic pathology on the other.

1. **Nocturnal diarrhoea** is almost always an indication that the patient has significant organic disease and should prompt appropriate investigation.
2. In patients who present for the first time at **> 40 years of age**, always image the colon at an early stage. If you do not, you will miss cancer of the colon.
3. Never ignore **weight loss**, for obvious reasons.
4. Never ignore **rectal bleeding**. However, in younger patients remember that its positive predictive value of underlying pathology is surprisingly low.
5. Systemic symptoms such as **arthralgia, and iritis** should raise the possibility of inflammatory bowel disease
6. **Mouth ulceration and anaemia** should raise the possibility of coeliac disease. Remember that the commonest mode of presentation of adult coeliac disease is iron-deficiency anaemia. Furthermore, coeliacs are often misdiagnosed as having IBS before definitive diagnosis

Always check full blood count (FBC), ESR, C-reactive protein (CRP), thyroid function test (TFT) and anti-endomysial antibodies. In patients with IBS, the ESR and CRP are frequently elevated. Occasionally, hyperthyroidism presents as diarrhoea-predominant irritable bowel.

---

46 Question on p.18.

Answer D
Crohn's disease

For patients to be suitable for peritoneal dialysis (PD), they must be capable of carrying out the dialysis or have someone who can do it for them. PD is often favoured by patients since it allows more independence. It does not require attendance at hospital 3–4 times a week and allows the patients more freedom in manipulating their fluid balance. ➤

Patients often drop their blood pressure on haemodialysis, and it is a less favoured option for patients with **ischaemic heart disease** and **peripheral vascular disease**. PD is preferred for these patients. **Insulin-dependent diabetics** often prefer PD as well. They can give the insulin intraperitoneally, allowing better glycaemic control.

Many patients on renal replacement therapy will be on a **waiting list for transplant**. Being on PD does not preclude this. However, it is important to note that patients on PD tend to have a poorer nutritional status (owing to protein loss from the peritoneal dialysate) and the quality of dialysis is poorer than with haemodialysis. Often, when a patient is being 'worked up' for a transplant, the renal team will convert the patient to haemodialysis prior to an operation to optimize their outcome.

A history of inflammatory bowel disease, such as **Crohn's disease** or ulcerative colitis, would contraindicate peritoneal dialysis for several reasons:

- inflammation within the peritoneum will impede effective dialysis
- previous abdominal surgery will affect the logistics of peritonal access and effective dialysis
- acute exacerbations of inflammatory bowel disease may be masked and mistaken for continuous ambulatory peritoneal dialysis (CAPD) peritonitis.

Contraindications to peritoneal dialysis are either relative or absolute:

Absolute contraindications for peritoneal dialysis include:
- Documented loss of peritoneal function or extensive abdominal adhesions that limit dialysate flow
- In the absence of a suitable assistant, a patient who is physically or mentally incapable of performing peritoneal dialysis
- Uncorrectable mechanical defects that prevent effective peritoneal dialysis or increase the risk of infection (e.g. surgically irreparable hernia, omphalocele, gastroschisis, diaphragmatic hernia and bladder extrophy)

Relative contraindications for peritoneal dialysis include:
- Fresh intra-abdominal foreign bodies (e.g. 4-month wait after abdominal vascular prostheses, recent ventricular–peritoneal shunt)
- Peritoneal leaks
- Body size limitations
- Intolerance to peritoneal dialysis volumes necessary to achieve adequate peritoneal dialysis dose
- Inflammatory or ischemic bowel disease
- Abdominal wall or skin infection
- Morbid obesity (in short individuals)
- Severe malnutrition
- Frequent episodes of diverticulitis

Answer A
1 month prior to surgery

The current recommendations are that patients undergoing elective splenectomy should receive the following immunizations at least 2 weeks prior to surgery:

- pneumococcal vaccine
- *Haemophilus influenza* B (HIB) vaccine
- *Meningococcus* C conjugate vaccine.

The reason that the vaccines are given at least 2 weeks before surgery is that it has been shown that doing this produces the optimal immunological response. If it is not possible to give the immunizations at least 2 weeks prior to surgery (e.g. in patients requiring emergency splenectomy), the above vaccinations should still be given at the time of surgery. The pneumococcal vaccination should be repeated on a 5-yearly basis.

Patients who have had a splenectomy should also receive prophylactic antibiotics for 2 years or until the age of 16, whichever is longer. At this time the need for continuing antibiotics should be reviewed and continued indefinitely in certain patient groups such as those at increased risk of infection (e.g. patients who are immunosuppressed or who have lymphoproliferative disease). The antibiotics most commonly used are penicillin V, amoxycillin or erythromycin in patients sensitive to penicillin. The dose is 250 mg bd, but this should be increased to the normal treatment dose at times of intercurrent infection.

Patients who have had a splenectomy are at increased risk of developing malaria when travelling to an endemic country. They should be advised to take appropriate antimalarial chemoprophylaxis. Furthermore, splenectomized patients who do contract malaria often develop fulminating disease. They should therefore be advised about this prior to travel and to weigh the risks of travel carefully before embarkation. In addition, patients without a spleen are more prone to tick-borne diseases and should take appropriate precautions when travelling, and seek early medical advice should they be bitten.

Answer D
Interleukin-10

Interleukins are cytokines produced by immunologically competent cells. They have an important role in mediating the inflammatory response. Most interleukins are pro-inflammatory and up-regulate the inflammatory response. ➤

IL-10 is produced by T cells and down-regulates the production of gamma-interferon, TNF-alpha and B cell growth and differentiation. It has an important role in regulating the gut mucosal response to normal gut flora. In IL-10 knockout mice, where no IL-10 is produced, the gut 'falls to pieces'. The action of IL-10 may prove to be of benefit in patients with inflammatory bowel disease. Research in this area is still ongoing.

IL-1 stimulates prostaglandin release and cytokine production by macrophages and T cells.

IL-2 activates cytotoxic T cells and induces proliferation of B cells and antibody production.

IL-6 induces antibody production and differentiation of cytotoxic T cells.

IL-12 activates B and T cells and induces gamma-interferon production.

49
Question on p.18.

Answer E
DDDR permanent pacemaker

The nomenclature of permanent pacemakers is becoming increasingly complicated and codes have been used since the 1970s to describe the system in place. Initially, the coding system contained three letters but recently, as newer programmable units are developed, the code may involve up to five. A basic understanding of the nomenclature is expected but it is highly unlikely that the examiners would expect you to know the more complex codes.

Regarding the three letter system:

• first letter indicates the chamber paced
• second letter indicates chamber sensed
• third letter indicates the pacemaker response to the sensed impulse.

The pacemaker code table is summarized on facing page. For completeness, the fourth and fifth letters are included.

Most pacemakers are designed to pace and sense the ventricles. They are called VVI units because they pace the ventricle (V), sense the ventricle and are inhibited (I) by a spontaneous ventricular signal.

Sometimes an atrial pacemaker will be implanted (AAI), e.g. in symptomatic sinus bradycardia.

Another system involves sensing and pacing both (dual) chambers (DDD). It paces both chambers (D), senses both chambers (D) and reacts in two ways. Spontaneous atrial and ventricular signals inhibits pacing in the same chamber. However, spontaneous atrial events will trigger ventricular ventricular pacing.

The patient in question has 2:1 block with poor heart rate response to exercise. He is relatively young and enjoys an active energetic lifestyle. It would be appropriate to provide him with a dual-chamber system to maintain AV synchrony and a rate responsive pacemaker to optimize exercise capacity because he will need to increase his heart rate appropriately on exertion.

Code letter position	1st	2nd	3rd	4th	5th
Category	Chamber(s) paced	Chamber(s) sensed	Mode of pacemaker response	Programmable functions	Tachyarrhythmia functions
Letters used	V = ventricle A = atrium D = dual	V = ventricle A = atrium D = dual	T = triggered I = inhibited D = dual T/I = atrially triggered and ventricularly inhibited	P = programmable (rate and/or output only) M = multiprogrammable 0 = none R = rate responsive	B = burst N = normal rate competition S = scanning E = controlled external

➤

A summary of optimum pacing modes is given below.

Condition	Ideal choice	Second choice
Sinoatrial disease	AAIR	AAI
Sinoatrial disease plus AV block	DDDR	DDD
Atrioventricular block	DDD	VVI
Chronic AF plus AV block	VVIR	VVI
Carotid sinus syndrome	DDD	VVI
Malignant vasovagal syndrome	DDD	VVI

50
Question on p.19.

Answer B
Continue ALS and actively rewarm to 30°C before reshocking

Standard ALS protocols should be followed initially. However, ventricular fibrillation (VF) in a hypothermic patient may not respond to defibrillation if the core temperature is below 30°C. If there is no response to 3 initial shocks, cardiopulmonary resuscitation (CPR) should be continued until the core temperature rises above 30°C. The patient should be intubated and actively rewarmed with warm bladder irrigation, nasogastric warming, active rewarming blanket and warm fluids. If the department has the expertise, intraperitoneal or extracorporal rewarming may be carried out. Once the core temperature reaches 30°C, the patient should be reassessed for a pulse.

VF is easily precipitated in hypothermic patients. Actions such as moving the patient from the ambulance to a hospital bed or airway suction commonly precipitate this.

At this temperature, the heart may be unresponsive to **cardioactive drugs**, **defibrillation** and **pacemaker** stimulation. Bradycardia tends to be physiological and pacemakers are not required unless the bradycardia persists after rewarming. Any metabolism in this situation is reduced, as is the efficacy at their site of action, hence drugs are often withheld until the temperature rises.

Resuscitation should be continued until the patient's temperature has risen. Hypothermia has a protective effect on vital organs and prolonged CRP in hypothermic patients may still be successful. The patient is not dead until he is warm and dead.

51
Question on p.19.

Answer D
Left parietal lobe

Parietal lobe lesions produce a clinical picture that depends on which hemisphere is dominant. The majority of patients, including the majority of left-handed patients are left hemisphere dominant. In a **dominant parietal lobe lesion**, the following signs may be present:

- expressive or receptive dysphasia
- cortical sensory loss or sensory inattention
- attention hemianopia or full-blown hemianopia in a parietotemporal lesion
- mild contralateral upper motor neurone signs, e.g. upgoing plantar.

In a **non-dominant hemisphere parietal lesion**, patients exhibit dyspraxia instead of dysphasia. Patients lose the ability to do simple everyday tasks such as tying their shoelaces or having a shower. It can be tested clinically by asking the patient to do a simple task, such as taking a match out of a matchbox or asking the patient to copy a simple diagram.

A **frontal lobe lesion** produces the following physical signs:

- personality change
- intellectual decline
- loss of bladder control
- fits
  - focal motor (Jacksonian)
  - status epilepticus
- blindness in ipsilateral eye
- hemianosmia
- contralateral motor signs
  - These are often a late feature of a frontal lobe tumour.

A **temporal lobe lesion** produces the following clinical picture:

- psychomotor seizure
- hallucinations
  - auditory
  - visual
  - gustatory
- lip-smacking
- grimacing
- focal motor seizures.

---

52 Question on p.19.

Answer D
Amyotrophic lateral sclerosis

The most likely diagnosis is motor neurone disease. **Amyotrophic lateral sclerosis** is caused by degeneration of the lateral corticospinal tracts, which causes spastic tetraparesis/paraparesis with added lower motor neurone signs, including muscle fasciculation. Sensory signs are always absent. ➤

Syringomyelia is caused by a cyst in the cervical spinal cord. It causes damage to the corticospinal tracts and anterior horn cells, as these are most vulnerable to damage as the cyst expands from inside the cord. Typically, the patient has upper motor neurone signs in the legs and lower motor neurone signs in the arms, as in this case. However, sensory signs are common, owing to damage of the spinothalamic tracts, and the sensory disturbance is often dissociate. Neuropathic joints are also common.

Patients with **multiple sclerosis** (MS) usually have signs of patchy central and peripheral nervous system involvement. If this case was due to MS, it is inconceivable that the patient would not have any sensory symptoms or signs.

Subacute combined degeneration of the cord is caused by vitamin B_{12} deficiency. This condition seems to selectively affect the dorsal columns and corticospinal tracts. The classical combination of signs is a sensory neuropathy affecting the feet with loss of joint position sense, together with upper motor neurone signs in the lower limbs. This is one of the few causes of an absent ankle jerk and extensor plantars.

Patients with multiple cerebrovascular accidents (CVAs) present with bilateral upper motor neurone signs, rigidity, emotional lability and pseudobulbar palsy. The patient may be dysarthric. They do not have lower motor neurone signs.

53

Question on p.20.

Answer D
Clostridium perfringens

Food poisoning is most commonly caused by the consumption of food contaminated with bacteria or bacterial toxins. Food poisoning can also be due to parasites (e.g. trichinosis), viruses (e.g. hepatitis A) and other toxins (e.g. mushrooms). The most well-recognized causes of bacterial food poisoning are the following: *Clostridium perfringens, Staphylococcus aureus,* **Vibrio spp.** (including *V. cholerae* and *V. parahaemolyticus*), *Bacillus cereus, Salmonella* spp., *C. botulinum, Shigella* spp., toxigenic *E. coli* (ETEC and EHEC), and certain species of **Campylobacter**, *Yersinia, Listeria* and *Aeromonas*.

An enterotoxin elaborated by type A strains of **C. perfringens** is responsible for foodborne outbreaks with high attack rates but which are of short duration. *C. perfringens* food poisoning is characterized by severe, crampy abdominal pain and watery diarrhoea, usually without vomiting, beginning 8–24 hours after the incriminating meal. Fever, chills, headache or other signs of infection are usually absent. Strains of *C. perfringens* type C elaborate a similar enterotoxin that has been implicated in outbreaks of enteritis necroticans secondary to the consumption of rancid meat in Europe. This is a much more severe, necrotizing disease of the small intestine and carries a high mortality rate.

Staphylococcal food poisoning presents with severe vomiting, nausea and abdominal cramps, often followed by diarrhoea. Often the staphylococcus has been introduced by contamination from a small abscess, whitlow or other discharging lesion present during preparation of food, which is allowed to remain warm and not fully cooked before serving.

B. cereus is an aerobic, spore-forming, Gram-positive rod that has been associated with two clinical types of food poisoning, a diarrhoea syndrome and a vomiting syndrome. The latter has a short incubation period of about 2 hours, after which nearly all affected persons experience vomiting and abdominal cramps. In contrast, the diarrhoea syndrome has a median incubation period of 9 hours. The clinical illness is characterized by diarrhoea, abdominal cramps and vomiting. *B. cereus* is particularly associated with the ingestion of contaminated rice that has been kept for a long time in a warm or partially cooked state in takeaway food outlets.

Fevers are uncommon with all three of these bacterial toxin-mediated syndromes. Episodes of staphylococcal and *B. cereus* food poisoning are short-lived, usually resolving within 24 hours.

---

54 Question on p.20.

Answer B
Coeliac disease

This patient has a dimorphic blood picture, i.e. some of the cells are small (microcytes) and some of the cells are large (macrocytes). This is an uncommon combination. It is due either to a double deficiency of iron and folate or B_{12}, or is sometimes seen after a transfusion. Sideroblastic anaemia is a rare cause of a dimorphic blood film.

The patient has Howell Jolly bodies. These are red cells with small nuclear inclusions and are typically seen in patients following splenectomy or in patients with splenic atrophy (sickle cell disease and coeliac disease).

The most likely diagnosis, therefore, is coeliac disease. The commonest mode of presentation of coeliac disease is with iron-deficiency anaemia (>90%). Over 50% of patients have a concomitant folate deficiency. The reason for this is that the villous atrophy predominantly affects the proximal small gut, which is where folate and iron are mainly absorbed. Thirty per cent of patients will also have a B_{12} deficiency.

Splenic atrophy is a common finding in patients with coeliac disease. The spleen gradually shrinks with time. This can produce target cells and Howell Jolly bodies, but functionally has little clinical relevance. Patients with coeliac disease seem not to be more prone to infection with encapsulated organisms, unlike patients who have had a splenectomy.

Primary sideroblastic anaemia is usually a microcytic hypochromic anaemia. Ring sideroblasts (iron-laden premature cells) are found on bone marrow examination but not in the peripheral blood film. ➤

Sickle cell anaemia is usually a microcytic anaemia with sickle cells and a high reticulocyte count. Signs of splenic atrophy are present (target cells and Howell Jolly bodies). In a patient who has sickle cell disease who has recently received a blood transfusion, an identical blood picture to that described in the question is seen. This is not the correct answer to the question as the patient has not had a blood transfusion and appears to be presenting for the first time.

Hypothyroidism produces a macrocytosis without anaemia.

Myelodysplastic syndrome produces a macrocytic or normocytic anaemia.

55

Question on p.20.

Answer D
IgA nephropathy

A young male presenting with gross haematuria 2 days after the onset of a sore throat is IgA nephritis until proven otherwise.

IgA nephropathy is one of the most common types of glomerulonephritis. It tends to either present as macroscopic or asymptomatic microscopic haematuria. Children and young men seem most prone, characteristically presenting 1–2 days after the onset of symptoms of an upper respiratory infection. Diagnosis is usually clinical, biopsy being reserved for equivocal symptoms. Treatment is symptomatic, i.e. control of hypertension, if present. Steroids are of no benefit. Prognosis is generally good, especially if recurrent macroscopic haematuria is present, normal blood pressure and no proteinuria. However, up to 20% of patients develop renal failure.

Post-streptococcal GN is much less common than IgA nephropathy. Both present after an upper respiratory tract infection (URTI); however, in post-streptococcal GN, there is characteristically a 10–20-day lag between onset of upper respiratory tract symptoms and haematuria. This can be explained by the fact that the disease process is caused by immune complex deposition in the kidneys. These immune complexes are a reaction to the initial infection, but take 10–20 days to develop.

Urinary tract infections in young men are rare, but tend to present with classical lower urinary tract symptoms of frequency, burning and pain. Cystoscopy is always required after treatment.

Goodpasture's syndrome is a disease where autoantibodies are directed against the non-collagenous part of the α-3 chain of collagen type IV. This is found in both glomerular and alveolar basement membrane. Symptoms include recurrent haemoptysis and progressive glomerulonephritis. It is possible that this condition could present with one episode of haematuria; however, this condition is rare.

Minimal change GN is a common cause of adult nephrotic syndrome and, as the name describes, there are no changes to be seen on light microscopy and the only change present on electron microscopy is fusion of the podocytes. Haematuria is a very uncommon symptom.

Answer B
Gentamicin

Myaesthenia gravis is caused by autoantibodies against acetylcholine receptors in the post-synaptic membrane of the neuromuscular junction. There is a 2:1 preponderance amongst females. The most common presentation is ptosis, which is present in 70% of new diagnoses. Oropharyngeal weakness presents in 15% and limb weakness in 10%. It classically shows fatigability on repetitive testing. Thymomas are present in 15% and 60% having thymic hyperplasia.

The diagnosis of myasthenia gravis is by:

1. detecting IgG antibodies (present in 80%)
2. nerve conduction studies show characteristic gradual decrease in evoked action potentials
3. edrophonium test – this is now losing favour owing to its potentially lethal side effects, bronchial constriction and syncope.

Treatment is with:

1. oral anticholinesterases, e.g. pyridostigmine
2. thymectomy – 60% of patients without thymoma improve
3. immunosupressants, e.g. steroids and azathioprine
4. plasmaphoresis – acutely.

Many drugs are known to provoke myasthenia and patients should be carefully monitored when starting new drugs. Drugs commonly known to exacerbate myasthenia include the following:

Drugs that impair acetylcholine release
- Aminoglycosides, e.g. **gentamycin**
- Beta-blockers, e.g. propranolol, oxeprenolol
- Phenytoin
- Lignocaine
- Quinine
- Quinidine
- Procainamide

Formation of antibodies against acetylcholine (ACh) receptors
- Penicillamine

Impairing synaptic transmission
- Lithium

---

57 Question on p.21.

Answer D
20 mg

The breakthrough dose of morphine rises as the total 24-hour dose increases. To calculate the appropriate breakthrough dose you need to first work out the total 24-hour dose of morphine.
In this case it is
2×60 mg = 120 mg
The breakthrough dose is one-sixth of this.
Therefore, $120 \div 6 = 20$ mg

58 Question on p.21.

Answer E
Lead poisoning

This patient has abdominal pain, and signs and symptoms of a peripheral neuropathy. There are only a limited number of conditions that can cause this particular combination:

* alcohol-dependence syndrome
  – acute alcoholic pancreatitis
  – peripheral neuropathy
* diabetes
  – diabetic ketoacidosis
  – peripheral neuropathy
* intra-abdominal malignancy
* Guillain–Barré syndrome
* lead poisoning
* acute intermittent porphyria.

This patient has no other features of **alcohol abuse**. Her MCV is low, which is also against this diagnosis as in most alcoholics it will be over 100 fL.
It is possible that this patient is developing **Guillain–Barré syndrome**. Some patients with this syndrome may never develop an ascending neuropathy, and it is possible that she has presented before the onset of the ascending phase of the disease. Patients with Guillain–Barré syndrome often have abdominal pain (particularly when it is precipitated by a *Campylobacter* infection). Vomiting is uncommon: patients are more likely to have diarrhoea. Furthermore, a diagnosis of Guillain–Barré syndrome would not account for the hypochromic microcytic anaemia. This is an unlikely diagnosis in this case.
Bulimia is a very common problem. When severe it can lead to vitamin deficiencies, which could account for some of the clinical features in the

question. However, to produce the type of clinical picture presented, it would need to be very severe and there would be some other associated features, in particular profound weight loss. Furthermore, the urinary δ amino laevulinic acid is elevated. This is not a feature of bulimia.

Both **acute intermittent porphyria** and **lead poisoning** can produce abdominal pain and a peripheral neuropathy. In both conditions there is also a raised urinary δ amino laevulinic acid. Lead poisoning inhibits several enzymes in the haem biosynthetic pathway, including amino laevulinic acid dehydratase, coproporphyrin oxidase and ferrochetalase. This answer to this question is lead poisoning as, unlike acute intermittent porphyria, this causes a moderately severe hypochromic microcytic anaemia.

Features of lead poisoning
- Rare
- Anaemia
  - Hypochromic, microcytic
  - Basophilic stippling
  - Haemolytic
- Encephalopathy
- Proximal renal tubular acidosis
- Blue lines on the gums

---

59 Question on p.22.

Answer D
Selenium shampoo

Pityriasis versicolor is a dermatological infection caused by *Pityrosporum orbiculare*. It results in macules mainly on the upper trunk that do not pigment when exposed to the sun. For this reason, it commonly presents when patients return from a holiday.

Treatment is topically with **selenium shampoo** that needs to be left on overnight. Other accepted treatments include **topical clotrimazole** (not oral as in answer A), miconazole or ketoconazole.

Tioconazole is used for the treatment of fungal nail infections.

Benzyl benzoate is used topically for scabies.

Griseofulvin is an oral preparation for the treatment of dermatophyte infections of the skin where topical therapy has failed. However, pityriasis versicolor does not respond to griseofulvin.

60 Question on p.22.

Answer C
Hypercalcaemia

The QT interval is measured from the beginning of the QRS complex to the end of the T wave. It represents the time taken for the ventricles to depolarize and then repolarize. It is normally between 0.35 and 0.45 seconds (9–11 small squares), but should not be more than half the interval between adjacent R waves.

The QT interval varies according to heart rate (i.e. prolonged in bradycardia and decreased in tachycardia), so there is a formula to calculate the corrected QT interval (QTc):

$$QTc = \frac{QT}{\sqrt{R-R}} \text{ (seconds)}$$

Tachycardia is, therefore, not the correct answer, as the QTc is corrected for variations in heart rate.

Hypercalcaemia is associated with a shortened QTc.

Severe **subarachnoid haemorrhages** are associated with ST depression or elevation and T wave inversion; however, prolonged QTc can also be seen.

Cocaine and amitryptyline are both causes of prolonged QTc. Some non-cardiac conditions that prolong the QTc are:

- hypokalaemia
- hypocalcaemia
- hypothermia
- hypothyroidism
- hypoglycaemia.

61 Question on p.22.

Answer B
Sphincterotomy

Sphincter of Oddi dysfunction (SOD) is a motility abnormality of the biliary–pancreatic system characterized by abnormal biliary manometry studies. The patient complains of recurrent biliary pain in the absence of stones on ultrasound and endoscopic retrograde cholopancreatography (ERCP). SOD commonly presents as a post-cholecystectomy syndrome, where the patient complains of recurrent biliary pain following a cholecystectomy.

Classification of SOD

	Clinical features	Treatment
Type 1	Biliary pain Abnormal LFTs Dilated common bile duct	Sphincterotomy is successful in 60–80%
Type 2	Biliary pain Abnormal LFTs *or* dilated common bile duct	Sphincterotomy in patients with high sphincter pressures
Type 3	Biliary pain alone	Medical therapy ? sphincterotomy in patients with high sphincter pressures

Patients with type 1 SOD do not normally require confirmation of the diagnosis by biliary manometery. Such patients have a very good chance of responding to **sphincterotomy**, but there is a considerable risk of acute pancreatitis following this procedure (25%). This risk is reduced to 7% if a temporary pancreatic stent is placed at the time of ERCP and sphincterotomy.

Patients with type 2 and 3 SOD should be considered for a trial of medical therapy as the response to sphincterotomy is much lower and less predictable than in type 1. Some patients respond to a **fat-free diet**, calcium channel blockers or **antispasmodics**, or a combination of these therapies. Tricyclic antidepressants are sometimes helpful in this situation because of their anticholinergic properties. Sphincterotomy should be reserved for patients who fail medical therapy who have a dilated common bile duct on imaging or unequivocal evidence of a raised sphincter pressure on biliary manometry.

Pancreatic SOD

This is less common than biliary SOD, and presents usually with recurrent attacks of acute pancreatitis and a dilated pancreatic duct on imaging. Treatment is by pancreatic sphincterotomy.

A small number of patients have a combination of biliary and pancreatic SOD where there is dilatation of both the biliary and pancreatic ducts on imaging. These patients can be treated by performing a combined biliary and pancreatic duct sphincterotomy.

62
Question on p.22.

Answer C
Anaplastic carcinoma as part of a goitre

Thyroid carcinoma is responsible for about 400 deaths per year in the UK. Presentation tends to be with a thyroid nodule or cervical lymphadenopathy. Prognosis is highly dependent on cell type as shown below.

Cell type	Frequency	Aetiology	Spread	Prognosis
Papillary	70%	Slow growing Occurs in young people	Local Occasional lung and bone metastases	Good
Follicular	15%	Commoner in females	Lung and bone metastases	Good, if primary and/or secondary resectable
Anaplastic	5%	Occurs in older population Aggressive	Locally aggressive tumour	Very poor prognosis even with radical surgery and radiotherapy
Medullary cell	5%	20% part of multiple endocrine neoplasia	Local and distant spread	Good, if no metastases
Lymphoma	5%	History of thyroiditis		Some responsive to chemotherapy

63 Question on p.23.

Answer C
Non-Hodgkin's lymphoma

Sjögren's syndrome is an inflammatory condition affecting the salivary and lacrimal glands. It often occurs in association with other rheumatological conditions (secondary Sjögren's syndrome) but can occur *de novo* (primary Sjögren's syndrome). Patients complain of dry eyes and a dry mouth.

The following are associated with Sjögren's syndrome:

- Raynaud's
- organ-specific autoimmune diseases, e.g. thyroid
- vasculitis
- pulmonary fibrosis
- depression
- arthralgia
- dysphagia
- increased incidence of **non-Hodgkin's B-cell lymphoma**.

Disease associations for the other malignancies in the question are as follows.

- **Nasopharyngeal carcinoma**
  - Common in China
  - Increased incidence in carpenters
- **Adenocarcinoma of the parotid gland**
  - Presents as a rapidly growing mass
  - Can cause a VII cranial nerve palsy
  - No known disease associations

- **Oesophageal squamous cell carcinoma**
  - More common in men who smoke and drink
  - Associated with Plummer–Vinson, achalasia, coeliac disease and hereditary tylosis
- **Myeloma**
  - A disease of the elderly. Median age at presentation is 60 years

---

64 Question on p.23.

Answer D
Micropolyspora faeni

Farmer's lung is the most common type of extrinsic allergic alveolitis worldwide, effecting 1 in 10 farm workers. Extrinsic allergic alveolitis occurs due to inhalation of a number of different antigens, the most common being microbial spores contaminating vegetable matter. Classically, the patient experiences episodes of fever, chills, dry cough and dyspnoea 6 hours after exposure to the precipitating antigen.

Examples of disease are given below with relevant precipitating antigens.

Disease	Situation	Antigens
Farmer's lung	Forking mouldy hay or vegetable matter	Thermophilic *Actinomycetes* and *Micropolyspora faeni*
Bird fancier's lung	Handling pigeons, cleaning lofts or bird cages	Avian proteins present on the feathers and in faeces
Maltworker's lung	Turning germinating barley	*Aspergillus clavatus*
Mushroom worker's lung	Turning mushroom compost	Thermophilic *Actinomycetes* and *Micropolyspora faeni*
Bagassosis	Turning mouldy sugar cane	Thermophilic *Actinomycetes* and *Micropolyspora faeni*
Pandora's pneumonitis	Working in contaminated humidifying systems	*Naegleria gruberi*
Suberosis	Working with mouldy cork dust	*Penicillum frequentans*
Sequiosis	Sawmill workers with redwood dust	*Graphium* species

Chlamydia psittaci is a bacterium found in avian secretions. It causes pneumonia but is not associated with extrinsic allergic alveolitis. Treatment is with tetracycline or erythromycin.

Aspergillus clavatus is a fungus, one of the *Aspergillus* species. It is found particular in decaying leaves and trees, and is passed to humans by spore inhalation. The disease severity depends upon the dose of spores inhaled and the immune response of the host. There are three main forms recognized:

- **bronchopulmonary aspergillosis** – with symptoms similar to asthma
- **aspergilloma** or primary mycetoma
- **fulminant aspergillosis** – occurring in immunocompromised adults.

It is not a cause of extrinsic allergic alveolitis.

65   Question on p.23.

Answer D
Constrictive pericarditis

This patient has a very raised JVP, peripheral oedema and hepatomegaly in the face of a normal CXR, ECG and blood gases. There are very few conditions that could cause this combination.

This case is very unlikely to be due to **multiple pulmonary emboli** or cor pulmonale due to **pulmonary fibrosis**. In both these scenarios the resting arterial blood gases would show significant hypoxaemia. In patients with **Budd–Chiari** the JVP is not raised. **Tricuspid stenosis** is a possibility, but one should be able to hear a murmur and the ECG may show evidence of right atrial hypertrophy, with peaked P waves in lead II.

Constrictive pericarditis is a rare complication of rheumatoid arthritis. It occurs in patients with progressive seropositive disease, usually between 15 and 20 years from diagnosis. The diagnosis is often delayed as the patient usually presents with abdominal swelling owing to an expanding liver with or without ascites. This can be mistaken for a Budd–Chiari or other intrinsic liver problem. The key to such a case is the JVP. This will be raised in a patient with a constriction but not in patients with liver pathology or a Budd–Chiari.

In patients with a constriction, auscultation of the heart is usually normal, although a pericardial 'knock' can sometimes be heard. The ECG is often normal. The CXR shows a normal-sized heart. The lateral films do *not* show any evidence of calcification. This is in contrast to constriction caused by tuberculosis. The diagnosis is clinched by a combination of echocardiography and angiography.

Treatment is by surgical removal of the pericardium. This produces excellent results in the short to medium term. Another option, in non-surgical candidates, is high-dose corticosteroids, but the results are not as good.

Cardiovascular complications of rheumatoid arthritis

Pericarditis	Up to 10%
Endocarditis	Rarely a clinical problem
	Found in up to 10% at postmortem
Vasculitis	Common
	Causes end-organ damage in:
	• Skin – nailfold infarct
	• Nerves – mononeuritis multiplex
	• Gut – ischaemia
Ischaemic heart disease	RA is an independent risk factor for ischaemic heart disease, which increases the risk by a factor of 2
Constrictive pericarditis	Very rare
	Seropositive disease after 20 years
	Can be mistaken for Budd–Chiari

66 Question on p.24.

Answer E
None of the above

ARDS is a common clinical problem in an intensive care unit setting. The clinical features are refractory hypoxaemia and respiratory distress. There are diffuse pulmonary infiltrates and stiff lungs in the absence of cardiogenic pulmonary oedema.

ARDS usually occurs as a non-specific reaction to another serious medical problem.

Causes of ARDS
- Sepsis
- Trauma
- Aspiration
- Inhalation injury
- Disseminated intravascular coagulation
- Amniotic fluid embolism
- Drug overdose
- Acute pancreatitis
- Cardiopulmonary bypass
- Near drowning

There is generalized increase in microvascular permeability caused by the release of inflammatory mediators, associated with reduced surfactant production. This causes non-cardiogenic pulmonary oedema. This, together with up-regulation of systemic vasoactive peptides, causes ➤

pulmonary hypertension. A haemorrhagic, protein-rich, intra-alveolar exudate ensues and, after a week, pulmonary fibrosis begins to develop. The changes described above appear to be more severe in the dependent parts of the lung.

The management of ARDS is based on the treatment of the underlying medical condition together with appropriate ventilatory and circulatory support. Patients with ARDS almost invariably require ventilatory support (avoiding high levels of positive end expiratory pressure) and are kept in a negative fluid balance.

No specific treatment has been shown to improve survival in patients with ARDS. Inhaled **nitric oxide** improves oxygenation in patients with pulmonary hypertension by improving perfusion/ventilation mismatch. **Prostacyclin** given by aerosol has similar effects. There is no evidence that either of these treatments improve outcome in patients with ARDS.

There has been interest in the possible therapeutic benefit of **corticosteroids** in patients with ARDS for over 20 years. A meta-analysis of all the trials in this area has shown no survival benefit in patients with ARDS who are given corticosteroids. However, there has recently been renewed interest in this area.

---

67 Question on p.170.

Answer C
Oxytocin

Oxytocin and antidiuretic hormone are both produced in the hypothalamus. They pass along axonal nerve fibres via the pituitary stalk to the posterior pituitary. Here both hormones are stored in granules at the end of the axonal nerve fibres.

A list of hormones and their areas of production is given in the table below.

Hormone	Source	Target	Action
Prolactin	Anterior pituitary	Mammary glands	Milk production
Growth hormone	Anterior pituitary	Widespread	Modulates metabolism
Oxytocin	Produced in hypothalamus Secreted from posterior pituitary	Uterus Mammary glands	Uterine contraction Milk production
FSH	Anterior pituitary	Ovaries, testes	Spermatogenesis Oogenesis Menstrual cycle
MSH	Anterior pituitary	Varied	Of dubious significance in adults[a]

[a] MSH causes hyperpigmentation in patients with Cushing's disease who have had a bilateral adrenalectomy (Nelson's syndrome).

68　　Question on p.171.

Answer B
Penicillin

Many drugs have unwanted side effects but on the whole it is the adverse reactions, contraindications and 'with caution' section that we look at in the BNF. Skin rashes are of utmost concern to patients taking drugs and it is the most frequent way of presenting with a drug allergy. Some drugs are more likely to cause allergy than others and some present with characteristic rashes.

Presentation	Common causes
Maculopapular	Penicillins
Urticaria	Aspirin and non-steroidal anti-inflammatory drugs (NSAIDs)
Angioedema	NSAIDs
Angioneurotic oedema	ACE-I
Erythema multiforme	NSAIDs, barbiturates, sulphonamides, phenytoin
Erythema nodosum	Sulphonamides, oral contraceptive pill
Allergic vasculitis	NSAIDs, sulphonamides, thiazides, phenytoin
Photosensitivity	Amiodarone, chlorpromazine, sulphonamides
Lupus erythematosus	Hydralazine, penicillamine, isoniazid
Pemphigus	Penicillamine, penicillin, captopril
Pemphigoid	Frusemide, penicillin
Hair loss	Cytotoxics, acitretin, oral contraceptive, heparin, gold, sodium valproate

69　　Question on p.171.

Answer D
Spirometry

Guillain–Barré is a potentially life-threatening condition of unknown aetiology. It usually follows a trivial infection 1–3 weeks previously. *Campylobacter* is a common precipitating cause; however, in 40% of cases no preceding cause can be identified. Symptoms are those of a sensory, motor and occasionally autonomic polyneuritis. In most cases the disease is mild and self-limiting, but in 20% there is progressive proximal neurological involvement including the respiratory muscles. This results in hypoventilation and respiratory failure that occasionally necessitates admission to ITU for intubation and ventilation.

　The onset of respiratory failure can be insidious and thus regular monitoring of the patient is essential. This is best achieved by 4-hourly **spirometry** and forced vital capacity (FVC) assessment. If the FVC falls below 1.5 L, the intensive care team should be asked to review the patient. **Peak flows and blood gases** are a relatively insensitive method of monitoring respiratory impairment in such patients. ➤

Patients with progressive Guillain–Barré syndrome also often have involvement of the autonomic nervous system. This is manifest by tachyarrhythmias and large swings in blood pressure. It is important to monitor both **blood pressure** and the **ECG** on a regular basis. However, the correct answer is D, as respiratory muscle impairment is common and can be difficult to spot.

Poor prognostic indicators in Guillain–Barré syndrome
- FVC < 1.5 L
- $PO_2 < 8$ kPa
- $PCO_2 > 6$ kPa
- Bulbar muscle involvement
- Tachyarrhythmias
- Sustained and progressive hypertension

Treatment is a 5-day course of immunoglobulins and/or plasmaphoresis. The role of corticosteroids remains controversial. Eighty-five per cent of patients make a full recovery. The mortality approaches 10%.

70
Question on p.25.

Answer E
Ursodeoxycholate

This patient has primary biliary cirrhosis. This characteristically causes a raised alkaline phosphatase and IgM, and has a male to female ratio of 1:10. Patients are often diagnosed on routine testing of the LFTs for another reason and most are asymptomatic. As the disease progresses the symptoms are very non-specific with tiredness and general malaise. Itching, owing to bile acid deposition in the skin, can be a major problem. This will often respond to cholestyramine. In some patients it does not. This can cause a major management problem, particularly if severe. Resistant cases sometimes respond to naloxone, rifampicin or Temgesic.

None of the above measures will alter median survival, which is 16 years in asymptomatic and 8 years in symptomatic patients. The liver function gradually deteriorates and eventually, unless liver transplantation is performed, the patient will develop end-stage liver disease and die.

The only treatment that has been shown to improve survival is **ursodeoxycholic acid** given at high doses (13–15 mg/kg per day). This has been shown to improve liver biochemistry and slow down the progression of the disease, and so delay the time at which a transplant is required. However, a recent meta-analysis has cast doubt on the efficacy of ursodeoxycholic acid in this situation. Having said this it is still widely used.

Prednisolone, azathioprine and penicillamine have all been tried in patients with primary biliary cirrhosis. They are all ineffective.
Cyclosporin, colchicine and methotrexate all improve liver biochemistry, but do not improve survival.

---

71 Question on p.25.

Answer D
Mycoplasma

The blistering target lesions described are most likely erythema multiforme. All the possible answers may cause this, although it is commonest in *Mycoplasma*, tuberculosis and *Varicella*.

The most likely answer is **Mycoplasma**. It is a common cause of pneumonia and often occurs in teenagers, especially those living in boarding schools. Chest symptoms are usually preceded by a few days flu-like illness with the chest X-ray showing involvement in one of the lower lobes. Treatment is with tetracycline or erythromycin. Of all the options, erythema multiforme is most commonly seen in *Mycoplasma*.

Tuberculosis is unlikely for several reasons:

- he is not immunocompromised
- he will have been immunized as a child
- the presentation and radiological findings do not suggest tuberculosis.

Varicella is also unlikely. *Varicella* pneumonia usually occurs 5–6 days after the appearance of skin lesions and the chest X-ray is more likely to show diffuse changes throughout both lung fields.

Legionella **pneumonia** may occur in previously fit individuals frequenting places that have showers contaminated with the organism. It is spread by the aerosol route and has an incubation of 2–10 days. Males are more commonly affected than females. The characteristic picture is of malaise, myalgia, headache and fever with rigors. Pyrexia of 40°C is usual. Chest X-ray usually shows lobar and then multilobar shadowing. The organism is sensitive to Clarithromycin.

Psittacosis is usually seen in people in contact with infected birds, especially parrots and budgies. When birds are infected, they become listless and develop a runny beak. The incubation period is 1–2 weeks and the disease may follow a low-grade protracted course over several months. Cases of pneumonia are often reported without any history of bird contact and their presentation is similar to *Mycoplasma*. Chest X-ray shows a segmental pneumonia. The skin lesions are more commonly seen on the abdomen. Treatment is with erythromycin or tetracycline. ➤

Causes of erythema multiforme
- Viruses
  - *Herpes simplex* I and II
  - Epstein–Barr
  - *Varicella*
  - Adenovirus
  - Mumps
- Bacteria
  - *Mycoplasma pneumoniae*
  - *Proteus* species
  - Tuberculosis
  - Psittacosis
  - *Yersinia enterocolitica*
- Multisystem diseases
  - SLE
  - Polyarteritis nodosa
  - Wegener's granulomatosis
- Carcinoma, lymphoma
- HIV infection
- Drugs
  - Sulphonamides
  - NSAIDs
  - Anticonvulsants
  - Barbiturates
  - Antituberculous drugs

72 Question on p.25.

Answer C
Intravenous urography

Radiological investigations in the presence of recurrent urinary tract infections are used to exclude structural abnormalities or urolithiasis. This woman is describing symptoms of upper urinary tract involvement in that she has fevers and back pain. It would, therefore, be pointless just investigating the lower tract.

Excretion urography provides detailed visualization of the calyces, pelvis and ureters. It also gives a functional view of the kidneys. Hence this investigation is able to assess the presence of functional abnormalities, such as reflux nephropathy as well as identify structural abnormalities, e.g. the presence of calculi. It can also determine how the kidneys are affected by these abnormalities.

Ultrasound is unable to detect ureteric anatomy or calyceal detail.

KUB X-rays are able to identify calculi but are not 100% reliable. They also have no ability to detect functional or anatomic abnormalities.

Micturating cystourethrography is used to evaluate bladder emptying, thus is unable to evaluate the upper renal tract.

---

73 Question on p.26.

Answer E
Becker muscular dystrophy

Becker muscular dystrophy (BMD) is an X-linked neuromuscular disorder caused by mutations at the same locus as Duchenne muscular dystrophy (DMD). There are some important differences between the two conditions, however; in particular, the age of onset of symptoms and the course of the disease.

In BMD, symptoms usually develop in adolescence but affected males remain ambulant into adulthood albeit with increasing disability.

The DMD gene, the largest known human gene with approximately 2 million base pairs, codes for a protein called dystrophin. In DMD, dystrophin is usually absent, which can be demonstrated by immunohistochemical staining of muscle tissue, whereas in BMD dystrophin is usually present but altered either in structure or amount.

In recent years, it has become apparent that patients with BMD have an increased risk of developing cardiomyopathy and an annual ECG is recommended.

Marfan syndrome is a connective tissue disorder inherited in an autosomal dominant pattern. Clinical features include a characteristic body habitus with variable skeletal, cardiac and ophthalmological involvement. The major cardiac complication is aortic root dilatation and dissection, so routine follow-up of these patients includes echocardiography and aortic root measurement.

Polycystic kidney disease (PKD) is another autosomal dominant condition with an incidence of around 1 in 1000. It is characterized by renal cysts that are detectable by ultrasound. Clinically the condition may present as end-stage renal failure, or with hypertension or haematuria. Since one of the major complications of the condition is hypertension, regular blood pressure monitoring is essential for any patient with PKD and those family members at risk.

Huntington's disease is a neurodegenerative disorder comprising variable degrees of movement disorder, cognitive impairment and psychiatric illness. There is no cardiac involvement and no cardiological investigations are indicated as part of routine follow-up.

Di George's syndrome is a microdeletion syndrome caused by the loss of chromosomal material on the long arm of chromosome 22. Clinical features are extremely variable and include characteristic facies, cleft palate, mental retardation or learning difficulties, hypocalcaemia in infancy and heart defects. The heart defects are structural, most commonly tetralogy of Fallot, and are usually picked up clinically or by echocardiography. ECG monitoring is not helpful.

74 Question on p.26.

Answer D
Theophylline

This is a tough question because it specifically asks about haemoperfusion and *not* haemodialysis.

Haemodialysis involves blood from the patient being pumped through an array of semipermeable membranes in close contact with dialysate, which flows countercurrent to the blood. It is considered in severe poisoning from:

- lithium
- salycilates
- phenobarbital (a long-acting barbiturate)
- methyl alcohol (methanol)
- ethylene glycol.

Haemoperfusion involves heparinized blood passing through devices containing absorbant particles, such as activated charcoal, to which the drugs are adsorbed. It is recommended for the treatment of severe poisoning by:

- medium- and short-acting barbiturates
- chloral hydrate
- mepobromate
- theophylline.

This sort of question is much easier if it just asks about 'dialysis' without differentiating between haemodialysis and haemoperfusion, since all the drugs listed above are 'dialysable'.

75 Question on p.26.

Answer C
283.6 mOsm/L

The plasma osmolality is calculated by the formula:

$$2([Na] + [K]) + [Urea] + [Glucose]$$

Simple once you know how and certainly not worth losing marks over!

76 Question on p.27.

Answer B
Schistosomiasis

There is a well-documented association between chronic **schistosomiasis** and recurrent *Salmonella* septicaemia. The parasite is thought to bind to bacteria and makes eradication attempts difficult. Chronic urinary carriers are infected with S*chistosomia haemotobium* and chronic bowel carriage by those infected with *Schistosomia mansoni*.

Arguably any person from sub-Saharan Africa with recurrent infectious disease should also receive counselling for HIV screening.

African trypanosomiasis is caused by *Trypanosoma brucei* species. The Rhodesian variety was responsible for an outbreak around Lake Victoria, which caused the death of over a quarter of a million people and was transmitted by the vector *Glossina fuscipes*.

Lissa virus is endemic to bat colonies and in humans causes fatal encephalitis very similar to rabies. It is transmitted by the bite of infected bats and is considered an occupational hazard in bat-keepers. Post-exposure treatment should include use of rabies vaccine as prophylaxis and the disease is endemic to bat colonies of Australia.

Entamoeba histolytica is the most important cause of amoebiasis in humans, causing colitis, dysentery and liver abscesses. It occurs worldwide but commonly in the Tropics. Treatment is with metronidazole. Complications that can occur include colonic perforation, haemorrhage, stricture formation and amoeboma.

Histoplasma capsulatum is the fungus responsible for histoplasmosis. Transmission is via spores that travel in the air or are carried in bird droppings. It occurs worldwide but is particularly common in Mississippi. Primary lung infection is mostly asymptomatic; however, chest X-ray changes at this time are similar to those of tuberculosis (TB). Chronic lung infection is mostly seen in those over 50 and is remarkably similar to TB – persistent cough, fever, bronchiectasis etc. Treatment is with amphotericin or ketoconazole.

---

77 Question on p.27.

Answer A
Metformin

Metformin-induced lactic acidosis is a serious complication of its use and tends to occur in patients with renal impairment. Therefore, it should be stopped in this patient whilst his renal function improves. Other situations where it should be avoided include dehydration, respiratory failure, hepatic impairment, CCF and post-contrast media (for 3 days). These can all predispose to lactic acidosis.

Doxazosin is an alpha-blocker used in the control of both hypertension and BPH. It is safe in renal failure.

Amlodipine is a dihydropyridine calcium-channel blocker used to treat hypertension and angina. It is safe to use in renal failure.

Atorvastatin is a Hydroxymethyl glutaryl-coenzyme A (HMG-CoA) reductase inhibitor, which lowers cholesterol. The most common adverse effect being a transient rise in LFTs. This does not preclude its use. Other side effects include raised muscles enzymes and rarely myositis. It is safe to use in renal failure. ➤

Aspirin is used as an antiplatelet agent to lower the risk of thrombotic cerebrovascular or cardiovascular disease. It is safe to use at this lower dose; however, at higher doses, it can restrict renal blood flow by decreasing the formation of protaglandins, which some renal arteries rely on to maintain blood flow.

78
Question on p.27.

Answer B
Hand-washing by staff in between each patient

MRSA is an increasing problem in the hospitals in which we work. MRSA may be part of the normal flora in a healthy individual but sometimes causes overwhelming sepsis in those with poor immunity.

There is no one thing that will prevent the spread of this bacterium in the hospital setting. Many processes need to be implemented and all of the potential answers each have a role to play. However, the one that has been shown to be of most benefit is **hand-washing**. This decreases patient to patient spread: it is a simple and easy task that should be part of everyday life in hospital.

Isolation of the infected patient also decreases infection and is current practice.

Washing of all rooms after an MRSA-positive patient is current practice.

Treatment of MRSA-positive patients with antibiotics for MRSA is only indicated if they are symptomatic from that infection.

Staff who are found to be MRSA positive should be sent home with eradication therapy. This policy has not been implemented in a rigorous fashion in the UK.

79
Question on p.28.

Answer D
Coronary vasospasm

There are an increasing number of patients presenting to casualty with cardiac complications related to cocaine use. It can cause acute cardiac ischaemia due to coronary vasospasm. It is known to cause cardiomyopathy after prolonged use.

The effect of cocaine on cardiac muscle and coronary vessels remains poorly understood. In acute cocaine exposure, the vasoconstrictive action of the drug seems to be the predominant effect and **coronary vasospasm** is the most likely cause of the chest pain in this question. Both coronary vasoconstriction resulting in myocardial ischaemia or infarction, and systemic vasoconstriction resulting in hypertension or organ ischaemia (particularly cerebral) may be observed.

Cocaine is known to block the reuptake of noradrenaline and dopamine at pre-ganglionic sympathetic nerve endings, and this action of cocaine is presumed responsible for the increase in heart rate and blood pressure, and the acute vasospastic syndromes observed in individuals who use cocaine. Pathological similarities between cocaine cardiomyopathy and those seen in phaeochromocytomas suggest that chronic adrenergic stimulation may play a role in the development of **cocaine cardiomyopathy**.

Pericarditis is a recognized phenomenon in young adults frequently taking recreational drugs. It is usually viral in origin following episodes of sustained partying and little rest. The chest pain associated with pericarditis tends to be substernal and sharp, relieved by leaning forward and made worse by lying down.

Intercostal muscle pain is likely to be focal, sharp and associated with breathing. The pain described by the patient sounds cardiac in nature and should be considered as such until proven otherwise.

---

80 Question on p.28.

Answer C
Dysequilibrium syndrome

Emergency dialysis can cause grand mal seizures owing to a rapid osmotic flux across the blood–brain barrier. This causes cerebral oedema. This is known as **dysequilibrium syndrome** and is the most likely cause of the seizure in this case. In order to prevent this from occurring, most patients who require acute dialysis are only initially treated for 1 hour.

There are a number of other diagnostic possibilities in a patient who has a seizure on dialysis.

Because of the anticoagulation necessary for dialysis, there is an increased incidence of intracerebral haemorrhage and, in particular, **subdural haematoma**. This effect is compounded by the anticoagulant effect of uraemia, which impairs platelet function. Subdural haematomas seem to be more common in patients on chronic dialysis, and this is not the most likely diagnosis in this case.

Dialysis encephalopathy is an uncommon problem found in long-term dialysis patients. It is characterized by a progressive deterioration in mental health. Symptoms include dysarthria, hyperreflexia and a tendency to seizures. It is thought to be due to aluminium toxicity. It is not a complication of acute dialysis.

This man's seizure is not due to **uraemia**, as the fit occurs after 2 hours of dialysis by which time levels of urea have dramatically decreased.

Hypovolaemia is a common problem in patients requiring haemodialysis. The loss of blood into the filter system is poorly tolerated, particularly by patients with coexisting ischaemic heart disease. It is rare for hypovolaemia to cause a grand mal seizure.

Question on p.28.

Answer B
Strict isolation of the patient

This patient could still have malaria, but this would be unlikely in view of three negative thick films and a normal platelet count. It is important to take the blood at the time of a peak in temperature or rigor, as this is the time of the maximum parasitaemia, and to take further **thick films** for up to 3 days to exclude malaria for certain. A negative antigen enzyme-linked immunosorbant assay (ELISA) or PCR is also helpful in this situation, but a negative test does not exclude the disease.

Acute schistosomiasis can present in this fashion, and usually follows swimming in infected waters. In this case, the River Nile runs through this area and schistosomiasis is endemic in this part of Africa. Patients with acute schistosomiasis often have generalized lymphadenopathy and hepatosplenomegaly. Some patients develop an inflammatory response at the site of the invading cercariae (swimmers itch). Nausea, diarrhoea and respiratory symptoms are common. The diagnosis is confirmed by assays of antibodies to the gut-associated polysaccharide antigen by ELISA or immunofluorescence. Treatment is by oral **praziquentel**.

It is possible that this patient has *Ebola* virus disease. This is a viral haemorrhagic fever, which occurs in outbreaks in sub-Saharan Africa. It is transmitted from animal hosts, such as rats or monkeys, and the human is the secondary host. The incubation period is 2–21 days, and the illness is characterized by myalgia and fever. From day 5, patients develop a bleeding diathesis. There is no known treatment and the patient should receive appropriate supportive therapy in an area with **strict isolation** in a tertiary referral centre, which is used to dealing with such cases.

In 1995 there was an outbreak in Zaire with over 300 cases. The mortality rate was 65%. There was a significant incidence of disease in healthcare workers looking after patients with the disease. *Ebola* virus is highly infectious and is spread by close bodily contact and by body fluids. Healthcare workers looking after patients with suspected *Ebola* virus disease should, therefore, take full barrier precautions and the patient should be isolated until the diagnosis is clear.

Over the last year or two there has been a further small outbreak of *Ebola* virus disease in western Uganda. It is possible that this patient could have this disease. This patient should be strictly isolated. A tertiary referral centre should be contacted and blood sent for ***Ebola* virus PCR**.

Answer D
Antihistone antibodies

Drug-induced SLE is usually mild and resolves once the offending drug is withdrawn. It presents with a rash on the face (butterfly) together with arthralgia, myalgia and pleurocarditis/pericarditis. Neurological or renal involvement in drug-induced LES is extremely rare. Ninety-five per cent of patients are antinuclear antibody positive but are usually anti-double-stranded DNA antibody negative. Over 50% of patients are antihistone antibody positive.

The causes of drug-induced SLE are listed on p. 255.

Anti-Ro antibodies are found in SLE and in Sjögren's syndrome.

Anti-smooth muscle antibodies are found in patients with autoimmune chronic active hepatitis.

Anticentromere antibodies are found in patients with limited cutaneous systemic sclerosis (CREST syndrome).

Answer B
Insulin

Gestational diabetes refers to diabetes that develops during pregnancy. Patients tend to have a family history and it normally remits after delivery. It can pave the way for development of type II diabetes later on in life. It is picked up during routine screening random glucose levels in antenatal clinics. If these are raised, two fasting glucose tests are performed, which confirm diabetes if levels are greater than 7.0 mmol/L. The diagnosis can also be confirmed by oral glucose tolerance test.

Complications from diabetes during pregnancy occur for both fetus and mother. Fetal malformation is four times increased, sacral agenesis is almost exclusively seen in babies of diabetic mothers. Macrosomia is common as is neonatal respiratory distress and post-natal hypoglycaemia. Maternal complications include an increased risk of pre-eclampsia, polyhydramnios and pre-term labour. It is essential to maintain good glycaemic control, as it has been shown to decrease the risk of the complications, both maternal and fetal.

Treatment initially consists of **diet alone**; however, more often than not, **insulin therapy** is needed if BMs are not strictly controlled on diet alone.

Oral hypoglycaemics should be avoided because they cross the placenta and lead to fetal hypoglycaemia.

This lady has already tried a diabetic diet and this has failed to control blood glucose; therefore, the next step in management is initiation of insulin therapy.

84   Question on p.29.

Answer C
Check spirometry

This is a tricky question and catches many people out.

According to the British Thoracic Society's recommendations for the management of chronic asthma, this patient is currently on 'Step 3'. She is taking regular inhaled steroid, long acting β2-agonists and still requiring large doses of salbutamol. The guidelines recommend that the next step would be either a **leukotriene receptor antagonist** or modified release **oral theophylline**. However, there are other things to consider.

The question establishes that she is taking all her medicines but we do not have evidence that she is taking them correctly. In any asthma clinic, it is vital that **inhaler technique** is assessed to ensure that she is actually receiving her medicines.

The other trick to this question is that, we have not been told that this girl has asthma. We have assumed this because the patient is attending an asthma clinic. However, she may have been given this diagnosis without confirmation. Asthma is frequently misdiagnosed and the patient should not be labelled asthmatic until objective testing has been carried out. Therefore, the best answer is C.

This may seem an unfair question. We agree. It is extremely unfair but likewise this answer would constitute best practice in the real world. Assuming for one moment that this 17-year-old does not have asthma, there is a very strong possibility that she will find herself on theophylline and steroids within a short period of time. Without clear objective reasons for starting these, she is likely to spend considerable time on unnecessary drugs, which will cause many harmful long-term effects.

85   Question on p.29.

Answer E
Leave and call for an ambulance immediately

This is a question that will continue to cause debate and is often a source of confusion for candidates on advanced life support courses.

On assessing any collapsed patient, having established that it is safe to approach, the following should be done:

- check responsiveness
- head tilt and chin lift to open airway
- look, listen and feel for breathing for 10 seconds.

In the absence of trauma or drowning, the cause of the person's arrest is almost certainly a primary cardiac event, i.e. the heart will have stopped first and the breathing shortly after. Therefore, in the absence of anything to suggest a primary respiratory event, it is 'odds on' that the person's heart has stopped.

In this situation, the only arrest scenario that the patient has any likelihood of surviving is a reversible arrhythmia, i.e. ventricular fibrillation (VF) or pulseless ventricular tachycardia (VT), and the definitive treatment for this is immediate defibrillation. Evidence shows that the likelihood of successful defibrillation falls rapidly with time and the most important management is to call for an ambulance so that defibrillation can occur as soon as possible.

Giving **two rescue breaths** and checking the pulse will waste vital time. Likewise, **starting BLS** will not defibrillate the patient and will increase the delay in defibrillation. If there were a suggestion that there was a primary respiratory cause of the arrest, then D would be the correct answer as **1 minute of BLS** is recommended for this.

A **pre-cordial thump** delivers approximately 8 Joules of electricity but has no place in the management of a non-witnessed arrest.

If the arrest is not due to VF or pulseless VT, the likely cause is either electromechanical dissociation (EMD), also known as pulseless electrical activity (PEA) or asystole. Causes of EMD/PEA include:

- hypovolaemia
- hypothermia
- hypoxia
- hyperkalaemia/hypokalaemia
- tamponade
- thromboembolism
- tension pneumothorax
- toxins.

The chances of surviving an out-of-hospital arrest from any of these causes is minimal and none of them will have an improved prognosis, if definitive treatment is delayed by giving CPR before calling an ambulance.

It is important to note that, with the wide availability of mobile phones, the likelihood of a lone person having to leave a patient to call for help is less common now. However, this question not only tests knowledge of ALS protocols but also an appreciation of the causes of cardiac arrest.

---

86 Question on p.30.

Answer A
Alzheimer's disease

The relevant clinical features are:

- gradual onset
- dyspraxia
- deterioration of executive dysfunction and self-care
- low mood. ➤

It is also important to note that the history does not report any change in personality, unsociable behaviour or mood swings.

Alzheimer's disease is the most common cause of dementia, accounting for 50% of cases. It presents with gradual decline in memory and mood. Families may report lack of spontaneity and deterioration in self-care. Formal examination may demonstrate dysphasia, agnosia, apraxia and decline in executive function.

It is unlikely to be **frontal lobe dementia**, which usually demonstrates personality changes, antisocial behaviour and deterioration in social skills.

Lewy body dementia accounts for up to 25% of cases and sometimes presents with parkinsonian features. Level of cognition tends to fluctuate and patients often experience hallucinations and delusions. They are very sensitive to neuroleptics.

Up to 20% of dementias are vascular in aetiology and are associated with the presence of vascular disease elsewhere. The presentation of **vascular dementia** is often difficult to distinguish from Alzheimer's and the main clues are that it often has a fluctuating course with stepwise deterioration. The presence of localizing signs is also highly suggestive.

The patient is too old for **Huntingdon's disease** to be likely. It usually presents between the age of 30 and 40, although cases have been reported up to the age of 80. It may present with low mood and other features include irritability, anxiety, choreoathetosis and memory impairment.

87

Question on p.30.

Answer C
The maxillary division of the trigeminal nerve (cranial nerve V$_2$)

The trochlear nerve (cranial nerve IV), ophthalmic division of the trigeminal nerve (cranial nerve V$_1$) and the abducens nerve (cranial nerve VI) all exit the skull via the orbital fissure. The mandibular division of the trigeminal nerve (cranial nerve V$_3$) exits the skull via the foramen ovale.

88

Question on p.30.

Answer D
Turner's syndrome

To answer this question, it is necessary to know that genetic disorders are classified into three main categories:
a. single gene disorders
b. chromosomal disorders
c. multifactorial disorders.

Each single-gene disorder is caused by mutations in one particular gene and shows a characteristic inheritance pattern, e.g. autosomal dominant, autosomal recessive, X-linked or mitochondrial. Most are rare but, as a group, they are responsible for a significant proportion of deaths and disease, and affect 2% of the population during their lifetime. **Marfan's syndrome** and **NF1** are single-gene disorders due to mutations of the fibrillin-1 (FBN1) and NF1 genes, respectively. In most cases, the diagnosis can be made clinically and mutation analysis of these genes is not routinely undertaken. However, as molecular techniques advance and become more automated, this may change.

Fragile X syndrome is caused by an unstable trinucleotide (CGG) repeat sequence in the FMR1 gene on the long arm of the X chromosome. In some cases, a visible 'fragile site' or non-staining gap can be seen on routine chromosomal analysis and, before the molecular basis of the condition was understood, this was the standard method of diagnosis. However, it is not reliably present in all cases of fragile X and diagnosis of this condition is now routinely carried out using a molecular approach.

In chromosomal disorders, there is not a single mistake in the genetic code or DNA sequence. The problems occur because of an excess or deficiency of the genes contained in whole chromosomes or chromosome segments. For example, **Down's syndrome** is due to an extra copy of chromosome 21 even though none of the genes on that chromosome are abnormal. Chromosome disorders are quite common, affecting about 1% of liveborn infants and accounting for about half of all spontaneous first trimester miscarriages.

Chromosome analysis requires cells capable of growth and rapid division in culture, and the most readily accessible cells that meet these requirements are white blood cells, specifically T lymphocytes. The dividing cells are examined in metaphase after being fixed, spread on slides and stained, most commonly using a technique called G-banding. They are then viewed under a microscope allowing the number, structure and arrangement of the chromosomes in each cell to be recorded.

Chromosomal abnormalities fall into two main categories – numerical and structural. Structural abnormalities include deletions, duplications, inversions and translocations. **Williams' syndrome** is a microdeletion syndrome caused by the loss of a small region of the long arm of chromosome 7 around the elastin (ELN) gene. The characteristic clinical features of the condition include typical facies, heart defects, such as supravalvular aortic stenosis, hypercalcaemia in infancy and mental retardation with an outgoing personality. It is not visible on routine chromosome analysis, so diagnosis is by fluorescence *in situ* hybridization (FISH), which involves the use of specific DNA probes labelled non-radioactively with compounds that can be visualized by fluorescence microscopy. The DNA probes can be designed to recognize individual whole chromosomes, particular chromosome regions or individual genes. The technique can be carried out on chromosomes arrested in metaphase, as described above, or on cells in interphase. ➤

The number of fluorescent signals corresponds to the number of copies of the region of interest. In Williams' syndrome, one copy of the elastin gene is deleted so only one signal is seen.

Numerical abnormalities are more common and almost inevitably associated with some degree of abnormal physical or mental development. The normal somatic cell chromosome complement is diploid (2n), but both triploid (3n) and tetraploid (4n) chromosome complements have been reported. The term 'aneuploidy' refers to any other disturbance of chromosome number, most commonly trisomy (three copies instead of the usual two of a particular chromosome) or monosomy (only one copy of a particular chromosome). Although the exact causes of aneuploidies are not well understood, the commonest mechanism is non-disjunction during one of the two meiotic cell divisions.

Some of the most common numerical abnormalities involve the sex chromosomes (see table) and one of these is **Turner's syndrome**, where the classical chromosome constitution is 45,X sometimes written as 45,XO. Females with Turner's syndrome can often be identified at birth or in childhood because of the characteristic phenotypic features including short stature, characteristic facies, lymphoedema, webbed neck, low posterior hairline and a broad chest with widely spaced nipples. Other features include gonadal dysgenesis (streak ovaries), and an increased incidence of renal and cardiovascular abnormalities, such as coarctation of the aorta. Turner's syndrome is less common than other sex chromosome aneuploidies with an incidence of 1 in 4000 female live births.

	Chromosome constitution	Phenotypic sex	Gonads	Fertile	Intelligence	Behavioural problems	Other features
Klinefelter's syndrome	47,XYY	Male	Atrophic testes	No	Normal or slightly reduced	May occur	Hypogonadal features
XYY syndrome	47,XYY	Male	Normal	Yes	Usually normal	May occur	Tall, severe acne
Turner's syndrome	45,X	Female	Streak ovaries	No	Usually normal	Minimal	Several (see text)
Triple X syndrome	47, XXX	Female	Often normal	Yes	Usually reduced	May occur	Few

Multifactorial disorders include congenital malformations and many common disorders of adult life, e.g. cleft palate, diabetes mellitus and multiple sclerosis.

---

89 Question on p.30.

Answer B
Renal stone disease

In a man of this age with loin pain and dipstick haematuria, the diagnosis is a renal stone until proven otherwise. Renal stone disease has a prevalence of 1–2% in most Western countries and is more common in men (M:F = 2:1). Most commonly, the stones contain calcium (80%).

Seven per cent of men have idiopathic hypercalciuria and a significant proportion of these individuals will form calcium-containing renal stones at some time in their life.

The other alternatives presented are far more rare and do not usually present with both loin pain and haematuria. Common presentations of the other diseases are shown below.

Disease	Common presentation
Acute tubular necrosis	Acute deterioration of renal function in the presence of direct toxin (e.g. gentamycin, myoglobin) or prolonged renal ischaemia (e.g. septic shock)
IgA nephropathy	Asymptomatic microscopic or macroscopic haematuria
Renal artery stenosis	Deteriorating renal function in a vasculopath
Minimal change glomerulonephritis	Nephrotic syndrome

90
Question on p.31.

Answer E
Augmentin

It is possible that this lady could have encountered all of these drugs and all of them can cause jaundice. The blood results demonstrate a *high alkaline phosphatase* indicating a cholestatic jaundice. Many drugs can cause jaundice but the key is to knowing which cause hepatotoxicity and which cholestasis. For the purposes of the exam, it is also worth learning which of these are idiosyncratic and which are dose related. Augmentin is a very common cause of drug-induced cholestasis. This appears to be most common in men over the age of 65 years.

Interpretation of liver function tests

Test	Acute hepatitis	Chronic hepatitis	Cirrhosis	Cholestasis	Malignancy and infiltration
Bilirubin	N to ↑↑	N to ↑	N to ↑	↑ to ↑↑↑	N
Aminotransferases	↑↑↑	↑	N to ↑	N to ↑	N to ↑
Alkaline phosphatase	N to ↑	N	N to ↑↑↑	↑↑↑	↑↑
Albumin	N	N to ↓	N to ↓	N	N to ↓
γ-Globulins	N	↑	↑	N	N
Prothrombin time	N to ↑	N to ↑	N to ↑	N to ↑	N

N, normal; ↓, decreased; ↑, increased; ↑↑, high; ↑↑↑, very high.

➤

Drugs and liver disease

Hepatotoxicity		Cholestasis	
Dose-dependent	Idiosyncratic	Idiosyncratic	Dose-dependent
Paracetamol (overdose) Salicylates (high doses) Tetracyclines Azathioprine Methotrexate	Isoniazid Halothane Methyldopa Rifampicin Dantrolene	Chlorpromazine Erythromycin Flucloxacillin Augmentin Anticonvulsants Chlorpropamide Tolbutamide Tricyclics Monoamine oxidase inhibitors (MAOIs)	Methyltestosterone

91 Question on p.32.

Answer C
RBC cell mass measurement

This patient has a polycythaemia, with slightly raised WCC and platelet count. The first step in investigating this kind of patient is to determine whether the polycythaemia is a true polycythaemia or just a reflection of a decrease in plasma volume (pseudopolycythaemia). This is best achieved by a red blood cell (RBC) cell mass measurement. In patients with a true polycythaemia, the RBC cell mass measurement will be elevated and, in patients with pseudopolycythaemia, it will be normal.

Causes of polycythaemia
- Pseudopolycythaemia
  - Diuretic use
  - Dehydration
  - Burns
  - Gaissbock's syndrome
- Primary
  - Polycythaemia rubra vera
- Secondary
  - Chronic hypoxia
    - COPD
    - Cyanotic heart disease
    - Smoking
    - High altitudes
  - Inappropriate erythropoietin production
    - Hypernephroma
    - Hepatocellular carcinoma
    - Phaeochromocytoma
    - Cerebellar haemangioblastoma

Notes:

- pseudopolycythaemia is a common finding in middle-aged men who smoke (Gaissbock's syndrome)
- erythropoietin levels are usually raised in all causes of secondary polycythaemia.

The next step in the diagnostic work-up is arterial blood gases. Hypoxaemia is strongly suggestive of secondary polycythaemia, the most common cause being heavy smoking and COPD.

The diagnosis of polycythaemia rubra vera is based on the following criteria in a patient with polycythaemia and a raised PCV.

Major criteria	Minor criteria
Raised red cell mass	Platelets $> 400 \times 10^9$/L
Normal blood gases	WCC $> 12 \times 10^9$/L
Splenomegaly	Increased leukocyte alkaline phosphatase
	Increased B_{12} binding capacity

If all three major criteria are present, this is diagnostic of polycythaemia rubra vera. If the patient has an increased red cell mass and a normal PO_2, then two additional minor criteria need to be present to establish the diagnosis.

Polycythaemia rubra vera is a clonal expansion of red cell, white cell and platelet progenitor cells. It is very uncommon before the age of 50 years and is more common in men. It presents with non-specific symptoms such as tiredness, headaches, depression and visual disturbances. On examination the patient is plethoric and in 70% the spleen is palpable. Treatment is with regular venesection. Chemotherapy with busulphan or hydroxyurea helps control the stem cell proliferation. Allopurinol is often used to prevent acute gout, which is common in these patients. Thirty per cent develop myelofibrosis and up to 10% develop acute myeloid leukaemia.

92 Question on p.32.

Answer B
Haemolysis

Ribavarin is a purine analogue and is most commonly used in the treatment of chronic hepatitis C, in combination with pegylated interferon. Viral clearance, as defined by PCR negativity, depends on the genotype of the virus: ➤

Genotype	Viral clearance at 12 months
I	45%
II	70%
III	70%

Haemolysis is a common side effect and patients receiving therapy need to have their FBC measured regularly. The haemolysis is often low grade and responds to dose reduction, but occasionally it is severe and the ribavarin needs to be stopped. The exact mechanism of action of ribavarin, and the way it produces haemolysis is not understood. Ribavarin is teratogenic and should be avoided in pregnancy. Female patients taking this drug should use a safe method of contraception. Ribavarin can cause cardiac problems including chest pain, tachycardia, syncope and dyspnoea, and should be used with caution in patients with established cardiac disease. The other side effects are:

- Nausea
- Vomiting
- Stomatitis
- Glossitis
- Taste disturbance
- Bowel disturbance
- Pancreatitis
- Anorexia/weight loss
- Cough
- Rhinitis
- Pharyngitis
- Psychiatric disturbance
- Tinnitus
- Thrombocytopenia
- Neutropenia
- Aplastic anaemia
- Hyperuricaemia
- Myalgia
- Paraesthesia
- Photosensitivity

93

Question on p.32.

Answer C
Pyoderma gangrenosum

There are several aetiological factors underlying ulcer formation, and the description and characteristics will virtually define the type of ulcer present.

Pyoderma gangrenosum (PG) is a rapidly forming ulcer, often at the site of minor trauma. It typically has a violacious undetermined edge and a purulent surface. It is associated with underlying diseases:

- inflammatory bowel disease
- rheumatoid arthritis
- chronic active hepatitis
- myeloid blood dyscrasias.

The diagnosis is a clinical one. Treatment consists of powerful topical steroids, silver dressings and oral anti-inflammatory antibiotics, such as dapsone or minocycline. If severe, second-line therapy includes oral steroids, cyclosporin, methotrexate, cyclophosphamide or topical tacrolimus. The underlying cause should be treated but often improvement of this condition does not reflect in the prognosis of PG.

The diagnosis of an **ischaemic leg ulcer** is impossible with the presence of foot pulses. Typically the patient presents with a very painful, 'punched out' ulcer on the toes or heel. Normally the ankle–brachial pressure index is reduced. Patients will have an arteriopathic history.

Venous ulcers are common. They are the result of venous hypertension caused by incompetent valves in the legs. Other signs include venous eczema, heamosiderin deposition and lipodermatosclerosis. Treatment consists of compression stockings and dressings, as well as elevation. They present in a chronic, slowly expanding fashion.

Basal cell carcinomas are the most common cancer in humans. The aetiology is related to sun exposure and the effect is cumulative, hence they are more common in later life. Typically they present on the face and upper trunk as nodules with overlying telangiectasia. They are slow growing and almost never metastasize. Surgical excision is the treatment of choice. They tend not to present on the legs and rarely ulcerate.

Squamous cell carcinomas also form on areas that have been exposed to sun. They present as rapidly growing nodules that ulcerate with 'rolled edges'. They have the propensity to metastasize. Treatment is surgical excision.

| 94 | Question on p.32. |

Answer C
Long thoracic nerve

The long thoracic nerve (of Bell) supplies serratus anterior. It arises from the posterior aspect of the ventral rami of the brachial plexus. Serratus anterior rotates the scapula. ➤

Nerve	Roots	Muscle	Action
Long thoracic	C 5,6,7	Serratus anterior	Rotates scapula and holds it against thoracic wall
Dorsal scapular	C 4,5	Rhomboids	Rotates scapula
Suprascapular	C5, 6	Supraspinatus Infraspinatus	Abduction of arm Lateral rotation of humerus
Thoracodorsal	C 6,7, 8	Latissimus dorsi	Adducts, extends and medially rotates the humerus
Subscapular	C5, 6	Subscapularis	Adducts arm/humerus Medial rotation of arm/humerus

95

Question on p.32.

Answer E
Blind-loop syndrome

Blind-loop syndrome is caused by an overgrowth of bacteria that consume vitamin B_{12}. Blind loops formed by surgical procedures can become colonized by these bacteria that compete for the vitamin. This can occur in non-surgical patients who have small bowel diverticulae or decreased motility. Treatment is with antibiotics.

Malabsorption from lack of intrinsic factor would become apparent after 2 years.

Post-partial gastrectomy patients are at increased risk of developing **carcinoma**. The absence of weight loss, anorexia or abdominal pain makes this less likely. In addition a microcytic blood film from blood loss would be expected.

Post-gastrectomy hypergastrinaemia is an overproduction of gastrin from G-cells in the pancreas but does not cause a macrocytic anaemia.

Folic acid occurs in vegetables and yeast. Absorption takes place in the jejunum not the stomach. Diseases affected by jejunal malabsorption include Crohn's and coeliac disease.

96

Question on p.33.

Answer E
Transphenoidal hypophysectomy

The symptoms are suggestive of acromegaly and this is confirmed by an oral glucose tolerance test. Acromegalics fail to suppress growth hormone (GH) in response to a glucose bolus. This is diagnostic of this disorder.

Acromegaly is caused by an excess of GH. The principal cause is almost exclusively a primary pituitary tumour. It carries a considerable mortality predominantly related to ischaemic heart disease and diabetes. Therefore, the aim is to attempt to cure all patients. In a young fit man, **surgery** is considered the most appropriate treatment, resulting in a remission in 60% of cases.

Octreotide is a somatostatin analogue used in refractory cases. It has to be given subcutaneously up to three times per day and thus tends to be unsuitable for outpatient treatment. However, long-acting somatostatin analogues are now available which can be given every 2–4 weeks. These are well tolerated in the outpatient setting.

Prednisolone is a corticosteroid and is not used in the treatment of acromegaly.

Bromocriptine is a dopamine antagonist that is used to suppress growth hormone secretion. It is often used to shrink tumours just prior to surgery. It may be appropriate to use it in this patient, but not for 6 months and only as an adjunct to surgery

---

97 Question on p.33.

Answer A
Sporadic amyotrophic lateral sclerosis

Motor neurone disease (MND) is a progressive neurological disease for which there is no cure. It most commonly presents in adults aged 40–70 with males more likely affected at a ratio of 3:2. Its incidence is 2 per 100 000 with a prevalence of 7 per 100 000. Diagnosis is made on the basis of meticulous neurological assessment, progressive history and appropriate tests to rule out other possible diagnoses. There are several subtypes of MND, which are as follows.

- **Amyotrophic lateral sclerosis (ALS)** is the classical subgroup of MND. It is the most common, affecting 60–65% of MND patients. It has a mixture of upper motor neurone (UMN) and lower motor neurone (LMN) signs, and affects the limb, trunk and bulbar muscles.
- **Progressive muscular atrophy (PMA)** is rare, affecting 7.5–10% of patients. It demonstrates LMN signs only, affecting limb and trunk muscles only. It rarely affects the brainstem.
- **Progressive bulbar palsy (PBP)** affects 20–25% of patients and is commoner in females. Patients have UMN and LMN signs and symptoms, but it affects bulbar muscles only.
- **Primary lateral sclerosis (PLS)** is very rare, affecting 5–7.5% of patients. Patients have UMN signs and symptoms only. Limb, trunk and bulbar muscles are affected.

The patient in the question has UMN and LMN signs affecting limbs and bulbar muscles. It is likely that, of the choices given, he has a form of ALS. The question is whether he has the sporadic form (SALS) or familial form (FALS). The sporadic form is seen in 90% of ALS cases, with 5–10% having the familial form. Statistically he is more likely to have SALS and, in the absence of any family history in the question, answer A is correct.

It is now known that 10% of familial cases (1% of all ALS cases) are caused by a mutation of the SOD-1 gene.

98 Question on p.33.

Answer E
Neovascularization of the optic disc

Diabetic changes in the eye include the following.

- **Background retinopathy** – does not require ophthalmology referral or treatment
  - microaneurysms
  - blot haemorrhages
  - hard exudates.
- **Pre-proliferative retinopathy** – non-urgent referral to ophthalmology:
  - venous beading
  - cotton wool spots (due to retinal infarcts)
  - large blot haemorrhages
  - intraretinal microvascular abnormalities.
- **Proliferative retinopathy** – urgent referral to ophthalmology:
  - Neovascularization.
- **Diabetic maculopathy**
  - Hard exudates.
- **Cataracts**

Neovascularization is the formation of new blood vessels as a result of retinal ischaemia. They can form at the optic disc or anywhere along the vascular arcades. The new abnormal vessels tend to be fragile and likely to rupture causing vitreous haemorrhage. This requires an urgent referral to ophthalmology with a view to laser photocoagulation treatment.

Microaneurysms, a feature of background retinopathy, do not cause vitreous haemorrhages.

99 Question on p.34.

Answer B
Haematopoietic stem cell transplantation

Multiple myeloma is a neoplastic disease of plasma cells. It is more common in men and rarely occurs before the age of 60 years. It is characterized by clonal proliferation of plasma cells with the production of a paraprotein. In addition there is an associated humoral immunodeficiency, anaemia, lytic bony lesions and renal impairment. Treatment of patients with myeloma has advanced considerably in recent years, and median survival has improved from 6 months to 5 years.

Conventional treatment is with corticosteroids and melphalan. Other combinations of chemotherapeutic regimens show very good response rates in myeloma, and these include vincristine, doxorubicin, and cyclophosphamide. Patients are given initial chemotherapy with one of the above combinations and then **receive haematopoietic stem cell**

transplantation. Stem cell transplantation has been shown to increase the median survival by 12 months, and can be used in the very elderly and in patients with renal failure.

Prednisolone and/or **alpha-interferon** are used to maintain remission, but it is not clear whether they improve overall survival.

Bisphosphonates are commonly given to patients with myeloma to improve bone density and to try to minimize the skeletal complications of the disease. They do not improve overall survival.

Radiotherapy is used in patients with painful bony lytic lesions, and in patients who develop vertebral collapse and cord compression. It is not used prior to stem cell transplantation and it does not improve overall survival.

Thalidomide has considerable antimyeloma activity. It is effective in 30% of patients with advanced disease and is synergistic with the other agents listed above. It is increasingly used in maintenance therapy. **CC5013** is a recently synthesized derivative of thalidomide. It has greater biological effects and fewer adverse effects than the parent compound. Early data suggest that up to 50% of patients with myeloma are sensitive to this drug. Its effect on overall survival remains to be established.

| **100** | Question on p.34. |

Answer C
Carcinoma of the breast

This patient has a spastic paraparesis with a lesion at L1 together with hypercalcaemia and a raised alkaline phosphatase. The commonest cause for this is metastatic involvement of the vertebral column. In this patient, given her age and sex, the most likely diagnosis is metastatic breast carcinoma. The other causes of malignant cord compression are given below.

Frequency of tumour types causing spinal cord compression:

Breast	29%
Lung	17%
Prostate	14%
Lymphoma	5%
Thyroid	4%
Kidney	4%
Myeloma	4%
Other	23%

Myeloma is very uncommon in a patient of this age, unlike breast cancer.

Sarcoidosis causes hypercalcaemia by producing an endogenous hypervitaminosis D via sarcoid tissue hydroxylating endogenous 25-hydroxyvitamin D to 1-25-dihydroxycholecalciferol. The alkaline phosphatase is usually normal. Sarcoid can cause neurological involvement with cranial nerve palsies, especially in the VIIth cranial ➤

nerve. It can also cause diffuse cerebral involvement with granuloma deposition in the white matter.

The other causes of a spastic paraparesis are not associated with hypercalcaemia.

Causes of spastic paraparesis
- Cord compression
  - Extrinsic
    - Trauma
    - Tumour
    - Prolapsed intervertebral disc
  - Intrinsic
    - Cord glioma
    - Meningioma
    - Syrinx
- Transverse myelitis
  - MS
  - Viral
  - Anterior spinal artery occlusion
  - Radiation myelopathy
- Subacute combined degeneration of the cord – B_{12} deficiency
- Parasagittal meningioma
- Friedreich's ataxia

101
Question on p.34.

Answer A
Collagen

The commonest form of osteogenesis imperfecta is type I. This produces relatively mild bony abnormalities and the patients often have a virtually normal life expectancy. The defective **collagen** genes produce a number of abnormalities in addition to the bony deformities including:

- hypermobile joints
- blue sclera
- deafness
- defective teeth
- aortic and mitral incompetence.

Disease	Clinical subtypes	Genetic abnormality
Osteogenesis imperfecta	I. Mild bony deformity. Normal life span II. Death as infant III. Very severe bone deformity IV. Severe bone deformity. Normal life span	Defect in **collagen** genes COL1A1 and COL1A2
Ehlers–Danlos	At least 10 different subtypes. Commonest are autosomal dominant. Clinical features include hypermobile joints and bruising	Defect in **collagen** genes in some subtypes
Marfan's syndrome	Autosomal dominant. Incidence 1 in 15 000	Defect in **fibronectin** gene on long arm of chromosome 15
Pseudoxanthomia elasticum	Plucked-chicken skin appearance. Recurrent gastrointestinal (GI) bleeds, angioid streaks in retina, early myocardial infarction (MI) and vascular disease	Defect in **collagen** and **elastin** genes

102 Question on p.35.

Answer D
Intravenous teicoplanin and gentamycin

In any patient, the combination of fever with new or flitting murmur is infective endocarditis until proven otherwise (regardless of the absence of splenomegaly, splinter haemorrhages or haematuria). This is even truer of a young intravenous drug user (IVDU) who is unlikely to have any pre-existing valve pathology to explain the murmur. IVDUs commonly get right-sided endocarditis, hence the murmur of tricuspid regurgitation. The shortness of breath is caused by embolic phenomena from the right side of the heart travelling to the lungs. The chest X-ray can show multiple cavitating lesions due to abscess formation.

A normal transthoracic echo does not rule out infective endocarditis, as vegetations will be missed in 20% of cases. Transoesophageal echo is the investigation of choice, although this is still not 100% accurate. Clinical acumen is essential. The diagnosis of endocarditis must be considered and treated empirically, since a missed diagnosis could be fatal.

The most likely organisms in this group are *Staphylococcus aureus* (50%) and *Pseudomonas* (15%), so treatment needs to cover both. Teicoplanin tends to be similar to vancomycin, having activity against Gram-negative anaerobes, including *Staphylococcus* and *Pseudomonas*.

Choice of antibiotics in infective endocarditis

Causative organism	Antibiotics of choice
Streptococci	Benzylpenicillin (vancomycin or teicoplanin) + low-dose gentamycin
Enterococci	Amoxicillin (vancomycin or teicoplanin) + low-dose gentamycin
Staphylococci	Flucloxacillin (vancomycin or teicoplanin) + gentamycin or fusidic acid

103 Question on p.35.

Answer C
Renal angiogram

This man has asymmetrical kidneys, hypertension and mild proteinuria, all suggestive of atherosclerotic **renal artery stenosis**. Unilateral ischaemia of the kidney causes an increase in production of renin and hence angiotensin II. This is the cause of the hypertension, which is an almost invariable finding in these patients. ACE inhibitors should be avoided as it can lead to a rapid deterioration in renal function by reducing the blood flow to the affected kidney. Investigations of choice in patients with suspected renal artery stenosis include **angiography** and magnetic resonance MR angiogram, the latter of these being less invasive. Treatment options include transluminal angioplasty and insertion of stents across the stenosis. The response rate is about 50%. Most patients have other evidence of vascular disease and ischaemic heart disease is a particularly common concomitant finding.

An **intravenous urogram (IVU)** is able to delineate the anatomy of not only the kidneys but also the renal tract. It is particularly useful in stone disease. In patients with renal artery stenosis, the IVU sometimes shows a delayed nephrogram and the affected kidney often avidly takes up contrast after the initial delay. The affected kidney may, therefore, appear 'brighter' and smaller than the unaffected kidney. These findings are not universal and in many patients with renal artery stenosis the IVU is normal. For this reason, the IVU is not a particularly helpful test in suspected renal artery stenosis.

Renal biopsy is not without risk and should be undertaken only if the diagnosis is going to alter management, e.g. nephrotic syndrome (although not in children because the diagnosis is nearly always minimal change). Renal biopsy is indicated for intrinsic renal disease, e.g. glomerulonephritis. Complications of the procedure include perirenal haematoma, haematuria (requiring transfusion 2%, or embolization/nephrectomy 0.25%).

Dimercaptosuccinic acid (DMSA) scans are performed to assess the relative function of each kidney and are able to show areas of scar formation.

Retrograde urography is performed by passing a catheter into the ureter. Contrast is passed up the catheter into the lower urinary tract. Its main use is in suspected lower urinary tract disease.

<hr>

104 Question on p.35.

Answer E
Keratoacanthoma

Keratoacanthomata are benign epidermal tumours. They occur on sun-exposed skin causing ulceration with central necrosis. The natural history is that they resolve with time; however, they are frequently excised for cosmetic benefit and to exclude malignancy, which occasionally they can mimic.

Lentigo maligna, as the name suggests, has the potential to become malignant. It is a slow growing area of pigmentation seen mostly on the face. The border can be indistinct. Excision is recommended, as there is an increased incidence of invasive melanoma in these areas.

Bowen's disease presents as scaly red plaques similar to psoriasis. It is intraepidermal carcinoma *in situ* and can become invasive. Treatment is with 5-fluorouracil, cryotherapy or excision.

Xeroderma pigmentosa is an autosomal recessive disease characterized by abnormalities in the repair of DNA in response to damage by ultraviolet (UV) light. The incidence of skin cancer in these patients is particularly high. ➤

Actinic keratoses or solar keratoses are very common. They present in later life and on sun-exposed skin. Patches are erythematous scaly papules. Sometimes these areas progress to squamous cell carcinoma. Treatment is with 5-fluorouracil, cryotherapy or excision.

105

Question on p.35.

Answer B
QRS complexes with duration of < 0.16 seconds

Distinguishing VT from SVT with aberrant conduction is a common clinical problem. It can be very difficult to do so, and sometimes impossible using a standard 12-lead ECG. The following ECG criteria can be helpful in making the distinction between VT and SVT with bundle branch block.

	VT	SVT with LBBB
Axis deviation	Yes, often extreme	No
QRS duration	> 0.16 seconds (4 small sq)	0.12–0.16 seconds (3–4 small sq)
V6	Predominantly negative	Predominantly positive
V1	rS	—
Concordance in chest leads	Yes, negative deflection	No

Making the distinction between VT and SVT is clinically important, as the treatments are very different. If you are completely unsure how to proceed and the patient is haemodynamically stable, iv amiodarone would be a good choice of drug, as it is very quick and effective at treating both types of arrhythmia.

106

Question on p.36.

Answer B
Onset of symptoms before the age of 14

Fifteen per cent of patients will die from anorexia nervosa, 15% will develop bulimia, 33% will have long-term psychological impairment and 62% will make a moderate to good recovery.
Factors suggesting a poor prognosis are as follows:

- older age at onset
- premorbid obesity
- illness duration of > 6 years
- personality disturbance
- bulimic behaviour
- male gender.

There is a higher prevalence in higher social classes and a high rate in certain occupational groups, e.g. ballet students and nurses, and in cultures where there is value placed on thinness.

Questions about anorexia nervosa often focus on the medical effects of the disease and they are outlined below.

- **Endocrine**
  ↑Growth hormone, ↑ cortisol
  ↓ Gonadotrophin, ↓ oestrogens, ↓ testosterone
  ↓T_3 (sick euthyroid syndrome)
- **Gastrointestinal**
  Swollen salivary glands, dental caries, erosion of enamel
  Constipation, acute pancreatitis, delayed gastric emptying
- **Musculoskeletal**
  Osteoporosis, stress fractures, stunted growth, muscle cramps
- **Metabolic**
  ↓ Glucose, ↓ K^+, ↓Mg^{2+}, ↓Ca^{2+}, ↓PO_4^-
  ↑ Plasma amylase, ↑ liver function tests, ↓ plasma proteins
- **Haematological**
  Relative lymphocytosis, hypocellular marrow, leucopenia
  Normochromic, monocytic or iron-deficiency anaemia
- **Cardiovascular**
  Bradycardia, QT prolongation, arrhythmias, pulmonary oedema
  Hypotension, decreased heart size
- **Neurological**
  'Pseudoatrophy' on imaging, EEG abnormalities, seizures
  Peripheral neuritis, autonomic dysfunction
- **Others**
  Hypothermia, lanugo hair, normal secondary sexual hair pattern

↑, increased; ↓, decreased.

107
Question on p.36.

Answer D
Bleomycin-induced pulmonary fibrosis

The arterial blood gases demonstrate hypoxia with a normal PCO_2. The lung function tests suggest a restrictive lung defect with a low transfer factor.

He will have been treated for his previous Hodgkin's with **chemotherapy rather than radiotherapy,** as his disease was stage 2b. Stages 1a and 2a can be treated with radiotherapy (and pulmonary fibrosis is a recognized complication). The most widely used **chemotherapy** regimen is ABVD (Adriamycin, bleomycin, vinblastine and dacarbazine). Although patients are more prone to get infections, this regimen does not induce the ➤

profound immunosuppression required for a ***Pneumocystis*** pneumonia. Besides, he is no longer having chemotherapy.

Adriamycin can cause a cardiomyopathy but this rarely occurs with the doses used in Hodgkin's therapy. The pulmonary function tests may not show such a restrictive lung defect, although a reduced transfer factor would occur in pulmonary oedema.

Relapse of his disease is unlikely to present with the respiratory symptoms and pulmonary function tests outlined above. Patients tend to relapse with symptoms similar to the ones they presented with. If he had relapsed with significant pulmonary disease, it would have shown an obstructive picture and his transfer factor would be normal.

Bleomycin can cause **pulmonary fibrosis**, and his pulmonary function tests show a restrictive defect and reduced lung capacity in keeping with this.

Long-term complications of Hodgkin's therapy

Radiotherapy	Chemotherapy
Pulmonary fibrosis	Adriamycin – cardiomyopathy
Ischaemic heart disease	Bleomycin – pulmonary fibrosis
Cardiomyopathy	Vinblastine – peripheral neuropathy
Hypothyroidism	

Reduced transfer factor	Raised transfer factor
Pulmonary fibrosis	Polycythaemia
Anaemia	Pulmonary haemorrhage
Pulmonary oedema	Left to right shunts
Lymphangitis	Asthma
Emphysema	

108 Question on p.37.

Answer C
All adverse reactions to drugs marked with a black triangle in the BNF should be reported to the CSM

Any drug may produce unwanted or unexpected adverse reactions. Suspected adverse reactions to any therapeutic agent should be reported including:

- drugs (prescribed and self-medicated)
- blood products
- vaccines
- radiographic contrast media
- herbal products.

It is not just doctors who are encouraged to report adverse reactions. Nurses, pharmacists, dentists and coroners are also urged to report. It is not compulsory and there is almost certainly an under-reporting within the UK. We are, therefore, unlikely to get an accurate picture of all adverse drug reactions, as only 10% are currently reported.

The British National Formulary (BNF) contains yellow cards for reporting adverse reactions. They can also be reported online at the Medicines and Healthcare products Regulatory Agency (MRHA) website.

Newer drugs and vaccines will only have limited information available from clinical trials on their safety. The black triangle symbol (▼) identifies newly licensed medicines that are monitored intensely by the MHRA/CSM. Therefore, **any suspected adverse reaction** (including non-serious reactions) should be reported, even if it is not certain that the drug has caused it.

Regarding established drugs, professionals are requested to report **all serious** suspected reactions including those that are life-threatening, disabling or require hospitalization. Such examples include:

- anaphylaxis
- haemorrhage
- infertility
- endocrine disturbances
- reactions in pregnant woman.

109   Question on p.37.

Answer A
Pulmonary embolus

This question demonstrates beautifully the differences between the old-style 'true/false' questions and the newer 'best of five'. A few years ago, candidates were tested on their knowledge of rare and esoteric conditions, and clinical cases appeared several times as one of the old-style 'grey cases' in the Part 2 written exam. In the old days, the correct answer would be **SLE pericarditis**, although it is extremely rare. The exam now calls for more clinically applied answers and the important thing here is not to miss potentially life-threatening diagnoses.

Without a history of trauma, a **fractured rib** is less likely and, although an **apical pneumothorax** is not out of the question, a **pulmonary embolus** is more likely. A recent study suggests the annual risk of venous thromboembolism (VTE) increases by 12% if one long-haul flight is taken yearly. The risk of VTE is greatest up to 2 weeks after the flight. Pulmonary embolism presents in many ways and should always be considered in a young adult presenting with sudden-onset dyspnoea, tachycardia and chest pain.

The patient took no **malaria** prophylaxis for good reason: it is not required in Thailand unless travelling to the Cambodia border. A diagnosis of malaria is very unlikely and the presentation described uncharacteristic.

110 Question on p.38.

Answer C
Antiphospholipid syndrome

Antiphospholipid syndrome is characterized by recurrent abortions, and arterial and venous thromboses caused by antiphospholipid antibodies. These are circulating IgG and IgM immunoglobulins directed against phospholipid molecules. Other features include:

- thrombocytopenia
- migraine
- livedo reticularis
- TIAs
- pulmonary hypertension
- chorea
- valvular heart disease.

Twenty per cent of strokes occurring under the age of 45 are thought to be due to this syndrome.

Investigations demonstrate the presence of anticardiolipin antibodies, which are diagnostic. Clotting studies reveal a paradoxical increase in APTT, indicating an anticoagulant effect *in vitro*. This fails to correct with the addition of plasma, suggesting the presence of a coagulation inhibitor.

A minority of patients have **SLE**. A total of 15–40% of patients with SLE have anticardiolipin antibodies.

Treatment is by anticoagulation.

Protein S deficiency and protein C deficiency are not associated with an increase in APPT.

Christmas disease is not associated with DVT.

111 Question on p.38.

Answer C
Aminoaciduria

Mitochondial DNA is carried in ova and not sperm hence all mitochondrial DNA disease is maternally inherited. It is compact DNA and so any mutation has a high probability of having an effect. Fortunately, cells have hundreds of mitochondria, so the chance of a total effect is low.

Mitochondrial DNA mutations tend to produce neurodegenerative and metabolic abnormalities. Several patterns of disease have been described;

- **MERRF** – **m**yoclonic **e**pilepsy with **r**agged **r**ed **f**ibres (on muscle microscopy)
- **MELAS** – **m**itochondrial **e**ncephalomyopathy, **l**actic **a**cidosis and stroke-like episodes
- Leber's optic atrophy – late-onset bilateral loss of central vision
- Kearns–Sayre – progressive external ophthalmoplegia, cardiomyopathy, retinitis pigmentosa.

Aminoaciduria is not a feature of mitochondrial cytopathies.
Causes of aminoaciduria include:

1. abnormally high plasma amino acid levels, e.g. PKU;
2. inherited disorder causing damage to renal tubules, e.g. galactosaemia;
3. tubular reabsorption defects, e.g. cystinuria;
4. defects of amino acid transport.

112   Question on p.38.

Answer E
Thymoma

The mediastinum is divided into three compartments: anterior, middle
and posterior.

Causes of mediastinal masses

Anterior mediastinum	Middle mediastinum	Posterior mediastinum
Retrosternal thyroid	Aortic arch aneurysm	Pharyngeal pouch
Ascending aortic aneurysm	Bronchogenic cyst	Neurogenic tumour
Thymoma	Enlarged pulmonary	Dilated oesophagus
Teratodermoid tumour	artery	Descending aortic
Pericardial cyst	Lymph nodes	aneurysm
Lymph-node enlargement		Paravertebral mass
		Hiatus hernia

Fifty per cent of thymomas are asymptomatic and picked up as
incidental findings. The other 50% are associated with myasthenia gravis.
They are most commonly located behind the manubrium sterni.

113   Question on p.39.

Answer C
Serum lactate of 20 mmol/L

The best indicator of outcome from cerebral malaria is the degree of
acidosis. In patients with severe malaria, 70% are acidotic. The acidosis is
usually caused by a combination of renal and lactic acidosis. The lactic
acidosis is caused by a combination of factors including microvascular
obstruction, resulting in anaerobic glycolysis, reduced hepatic clearance
of lactate and anaerobic glycolysis in the splanchnic bed.

The most accurate method of determining the degree of acidosis in a
patient with severe malaria is by calculating the standard base deficit. This
can be calculated by employing the following formula:

$$\text{Standard base deficit} = 1.56\ \text{lactate} + 1.34\ \text{creatinine} - 3.5$$

➤

Research has shown that, in patients with severe malaria, the higher the standard base deficit, the poorer the prognosis. This is the best indicator of outcome in this situation. This formula is, however, slightly cumbersome to use and, in practice, the serum lactate is often used as a surrogate marker. In this case, the serum lactate is very raised, indicating that this patient has a poor prognosis. Alternatively, the base excess can be used to determine the degree of acidosis.

Indicators of a poor prognosis in patients with severe malaria

Indicator	Effect on prognosis
Standard base deficit (SBD)	Raised levels are best indicator of poor prognosis
Bilirubin	Raised levels indicate a poorer outcome but not as accurately as SBD
Creatinine	Raised levels indicate a poorer outcome but not as accurately as SBD
Glasgow coma scale	A low GCS may indicate a poor outcome but this is not very reliable, and an inferior way of predicting outcome
Degree of parasitaemia	A high level of parasitaemia is usually seen in patients with severe malaria, but is of no use in predicting outcome

114

Question on p.39.

Answer D
Polymyalgia rheumatica

Polymyalgia rheumatica (PMR) is rare before the age of 50, and most commonly starts between 60 and 70 years of age. Usually both limb girdles are affected with pain and stiffness, and there may be associated temporal headache and/or visual symptoms, if there is an associated temporal arteritis. Women are more commonly affected than men (3:1). Characteristically, the ESR is raised, but a mild elevation of the alkaline phosphatase is also seen in a minority.

This case is unlikely to be due to **carcinoma of the prostate with bony metastases**. In patients with this diagnosis, with symptoms in both limb girdles, there is a large tumour burden in skeletal tissue. This would cause a much larger increases in the alkaline phosphatase and the serum calcium would also probably be raised.

Polymyositis can present with discomfort in both limb girdles. The pain is usually in the proximal limb muscles. Polymyositis can present at any age, but most commonly presents between 30 and 60 years of age. The creatine phosphokinase is invariably raised.

Hypothyroidism can cause a proximal myopathy that is occasionally painful. This is sometimes associated with a raised ALT. The cause of this is unclear, and the alkaline phosphatase is normal.

Common causes of a raised alkaline phosphatase
• Paget's disease
• Bony metastases
• Malabsorption
• Hyperparathyroidism
• PMR
• Primary biliary cirrhosis (PBC)[a]
• Biliary disease[a]

[a]ALT is usually elevated as well

115
Question on p.39.

Answer B
High-dose alternate day steroids

This is a difficult question as focal segmental glomerulosclerosis is difficult to treat and a consensus regarding the optimal management is only just emerging.

Focal segmental glomerulosclerosis is diagnosed at renal biopsy with the typical appearances. Most patients with primary focal segmental glomerulosclerosis present with a nephrotic syndrome with heavy proteinuria often greater than 5 g/24 hours. It is often resistant to treatment but some patients benefit **from high-dose alternate day steroids**. If the patient shows no response after 4–6 months, second-line therapy is with **cyclosporin.**

Focal segmental glomerulosclerosis can occasionally be secondary to other disorders, the two most common being HIV disease and obesity. These patients have less heavy proteinuria (< 3 g/24 hours) and often respond much better to treatment.

Finally, there is a collapsing form of focal segmental glomerulosclerosis, which also carries a much better prognosis.

116
Question on p.40.

Answer C
Von Willebrand's disease

This man has not presented until the age of 30, which immediately makes you think whether he has got an acquired bleeding disorder or low platelets. Leukaemia needs to be ruled out in any adult who presents with new onset of bleeding or easy bruising. This is usually done simply with a full blood count and film examination. In this case, the FBC is normal. We are thus looking for underlying bleeding conditions, most of which are congenital. ➤

This man has a normal prothrombin time, indicating normal function of Factors II, V, VII and X, and normal liver function. His activated partial thromboplastin time (APTT) is raised, indicating a defective functioning or lack of Factor I, II, V, VIII, IX, X or XI. This means it must be a problem with Factor I, VIII, IX or XI.

As the bleeding time is slightly prolonged, there must be a defect of platelet function. The condition that best fits this picture and is common is **von Willebrand's disease**. It is an autosomal dominant condition resulting from a defective von Willebrand's factor. This factor aids platelet aggregation *in vivo* as well as stabilizing Factor VIIIc and helping to prevent its breakdown.

Haemophilia A is caused by a reduction in Factor VIII:C. It is an X-linked condition. There is an increase in APTT but bleeding time is normal. It can be mild, moderate or severe, depending on the levels of factor VIII:C.

Haemophilia B or Christmas disease is caused by a lack of Factor IX. It is almost identical to haemophilia A but it is rare, occurring in 1:30 000 males.

Alcoholism can cause defects of clotting in several ways.

- There is a decrease clotting factors because of impaired hepatic synthetic function. This is the most sensitive mechanism of calibrating liver dysfunction in a patient whose liver biochemistry is abnormal.
- Thrombocytopenia is the result of splenomegaly.
- Vitamin K deficiency is a result of poor diet, malabsorption and liver disease. All of these put together would cause abnormalities of all clotting pathways and not just APTT and bleeding time.

Aspirin causes a prolongation of bleeding time as it interferes with platelet adhesion however there would be no effect on APTT.

117 Question on p.40.

Answer E
Sarcoidosis

Immune-mediated hypersensitivity reactions

Type	Antigens	Mediators	Response time	Disease examples
I. Immediate	Pollen Mites Drugs	IgE Mast cells	5 minutes or less	Atopic asthma Anaphylaxis
II. Cytotoxic	Cell surface Tissue bound	IgG IgM Complement	6–36 hours	Autoimmune haemolytic anaemia Goodpasture's
III. Immune-complex	Autoantigens Viral proteins Exogenous antigens	IgG IgA IgM Complement	4–12 hours	SLE Rheumatoid Hepatitis C/B Farmer's lung
IV. Delayed	Cell/tissue bound	T cells	2–3 days	TB Sarcoid
V. Stimulating/blocking	Cell surface receptors	IgG	Variable	Grave's disease

Answer C
Dermatitis herpetiformis

Dermatitis herpetiformis is commonly associated with coeliac disease and other autoimmune disorders. It is more common in males and can occur at any age, but most commonly presents in young adults with small itchy blisters. They usually occur at the elbows, forearms and back/buttocks. At the time of presentation, blisters are often not seen as the lesions are very itchy and have been scratched off.

Ninety per cent of patients are HLA B8-DR3DQ2-positive. Skin biopsy is diagnostic and shows IgA in the dermal papillae and patchy IgA in the basement membrane. The duodenal biopsy is abnormal in approximately 50% but full-blown villous atrophy is uncommon. Treatment is by gluten-free diet that heals the enteropathy. It also helps the skin lesions in a proportion of patients. However, most patients will also require oral dapsone or sulphonamides to control the dermatological manifestations fully.

The skin biopsy in **pemphigus** shows interepidermal staining of IgG in the epidermis.

In **pemphigoid** the skin biopsy shows deposition of IgM along the basement membrane.

Linear IgA disease occurs in adults and children causing circular clusters, which may mimic pemphigoid or dermatitis herpetiformis. Involvement of the mouth, eyes and vulva also occurs. Skin biopsy is diagnostic showing IgA autoantibodies deposited along the basement membrane. Treatment is with oral dapsone or sulphonamides.

Epidermolysis bullosa is a rare genetically determined group of blistering disorders. It can be autosomal dominant or recessive depending on clinical subtype. The clinical spectrum of disease is wide, from minor blistering to severely disabling or even fatal. The blistering tends to arise following trauma and is frequently associated with scarring.

Answer E
PR3-ANCA

Wegener's granulomatosis is a necrotizing granulomatous vasculitis that affects the respiratory tract, kidneys and other organs to a lesser degree. Any disease that involves these two organs should suggest the diagnosis.

Initial symptoms of Wegener's granulomatosis include rhinitis, nasal ulceration, cough and haemoptysis. The CXR shows single or multiple nodular masses with cavitating infiltrates. The X-ray changes often fluctuate rapidly. Renal involvement can ensue, although not always.

Most patients (85%) are **PR3-ANCA** (cANCA) positive, which seems to be specific for Wegener's. Tissue diagnosis is usually best achieved by renal biopsy.

Involvement of other systems is rare but can occur. These include skin, nervous system (mononeuritis multiplex and cranial nerve palsies), cardiovascular system (pericarditis and tachyarrhythmias/bradyarrhythmias) and the eye (scleritis and retro-orbital granulomata). Treatment is with cyclophosphamide and steroids initially and then azathioprine.

The other granulomatous vasculitis that is worth considering is Churg–Strauss. This is a small vessel vasculitis occurring in young men. They present with rhinitis, asthma-like symptoms, a skin rash and occasionally neuropathies. There is a marked **eosinophilia**. The organs affected are lungs, peripheral nerves and skin. It tends not to affect the kidneys. There are patchy X-ray changes, which again are flitting.

Goodpasture's syndrome also affects the lung and renal tract. It is an autoimmune disease characterized by circulating autoantibodies to the antibasement membrane. ANCA can be positive.

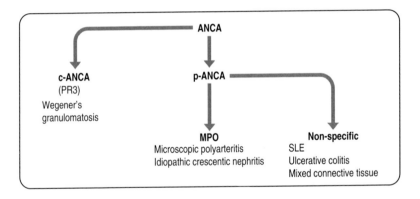

120   Question on p.41.

Answer A
Nevirapine

The management of HIV infection involves combination therapy of different classes of antiretroviral drugs. They target two key HIV enzymes:

• reverse transcriptase
• proteases.

At the time of writing, there are three main classes of drugs for the treatment of HIV. ➤

Nucleoside reverse transcriptase inhibitors (NRTI)	Non-nucleoside reverse transcriptase inhibitors (NNRTI)	Protease inhibitors
Zidovudine (AZT)	Nevirapine	Ritonavir
Lamivudine (3TC)	Efavirenz	Indinavir
Didanosine (DDI)	Delavirdine	Amprenavir
Stavudine (D4T)		Nelfinavir
		Sanguinavir

Therapy requires a combination of at least three different drugs.

All protease inhibitor drugs **inhibit** the cytochrome P450 enzymes and this can lead to many drug interactions. Of the non-nucleosides:

- Delavirdine inhibits
- Efavirnez can inhibit and induce
- Nevirapine induces.

Drugs that commonly induce the cytochrome P450 enzyme are:

- alcohol
- carbamazepine
- griseofulvin
- phenobarbitone
- phenytoin
- prednisolone
- rifampicin.

121 Question on p.41.

Answer E
Cluster headache

The patient describes a classical presentation of cluster headache. Characteristic features are as the following list.

- Severe unilateral orbital, supraorbital and/or temporal headache.
- Constant, intense, boring pain.
- Typical attacks last 15 minutes to 3 hours, occur 1–3 times daily for 4–8 weeks. Clusters occur once or twice a year.
- 80–90% have recurrent attacks at the same time each day.
- Often occurs in early hours of morning ('alarm clock headache').
- Alcohol is a potent trigger.
- Examination is usually normal between attacks (in the chronic form a permanent Horner's may develop).
- In addition there are several associated features as outlined below.

Associated features
- Conjunctival injection
- Lacrimation
- Nasal congestion
- Rhinorrhoea
- Ptosis
- Meiosis
- Eyelid oedema

Treatment is as follows:

- 100% oxygen relieves 80% of attacks within 15 minutes.
- sumatriptan 50–100 mg po
- ergotamine po or pr used the night before alarm clock headaches
- verapamil, lithium and sodium valproate have all been used with some benefit.

Tension-type headache is described as a tight or band-like sensation around the head, which is non-pulsatile. It is bilateral in 80–90% of cases and not aggravated by physical activity.

Trigeminal neuralgia occurs in patients over 40 years old. Patients describe severe paroxysmal pain in the distribution of the trigeminal nerve (usually mandibular or maxillary). Pain is lancinating or electric shock-like lasting a few seconds. Triggers are common, e.g. chewing, shaving, washing or talking. Pain is unilateral in 95% of cases. Bilateral trigeminal neuralgia should raise suspicion of multiple sclerosis. Examination is usually normal.

122 Question on p.41.

Answer E
Nifedipine po

This gentleman has malignant hypertension as diagnosed by the WHO criteria (severe hypertension with bilateral retinal haemorrhages and exudates). Malignant hypertension is now divided into 'emergency' and 'urgency'.

Emergencies are those in which, if the increase in arterial pressure persists over hours, there would irreversible organ damage, e.g. hypertensive encephalopathy. Encephalopathy presents with symptoms of headache, nausea, vomiting, decreasing consciousness, seizures and visual loss.

This is in contrast to urgency, where there is risk of end-organ damage if untreated. Common presenting symptoms in this group are headaches and visual upset, but not visual loss. ➤

Emergencies are treated in ITU with **parenteral compounds** and continuous monitoring as sudden drops in blood pressure can cause watershed infarcts. For this reason, oral treatment is preferred in all but the few who present with encephalopathy. This gentleman does have evidence of end-organ damage, but his headaches have been present for 1 month and he has little evidence of encephalopathy.

Several trials have been carried out using **oral atenolol** and **nifedipine** for the treatment of hypertensive urgency, both of which are equally effective and with few side effects. Thus from the list above, oral nifedipine would be the drug of choice.

Captopril has been known to cause unpredictable first-dose hypotension and therefore would not be used in this situation.

There has been no consistent evidence for the use of **sublingual nifedipine** in this clinical scenario and there is, therefore, a large risk of unpredictability of response. This drug should not be used in this situation.

123

Question on p.42.

Answer A
Oral propranolol

This patient has bled from some gastric erosions and it is entirely reasonable to put him on a **proton pump inhibitor** at this stage to heal the gastric mucosa. The proton pump inhibitor will, however, not reduce the chance of this patient subsequently bleeding from his oesophageal varices.

This is really a question about what is the best treatment for primary prophylaxis for patients with oesophageal varices, i.e. in a patient who has not bled from the varices, which therapeutic intervention is most likely to prevent a subsequent variceal haemorrhage? The correct answer is a non-selective β-blocker such as **propranolol**. Several meta-analyses have shown that non-selective β-blockers significantly reduce the risk of bleeding from oesophageal varices in patients who have never bled from them.

Care needs to be taken with the dose of propranolol in this situation, as patients with chronic liver disease are often very sensitive to small doses of this drug. The reason for this is that propranolol has a very high first-pass metabolism and, when there is significant liver disease, this effect is partially lost. This results in very high systemic concentrations of propranolol when given at normal doses in patients with chronic liver disease. In practice, propranolol is started at a dose of 10 mg bd and the dose carefully titrated upwards. The aim is to achieve a reduction in the resting pulse rate of 25%. This is a surrogate marker for a significant reduction in portal pressure. Portal pressures are difficult to measure and are rarely used in clinical practice outside of the setting of a clinical trial.

Variceal banding is the treatment of choice for secondary prophylaxis, i.e. it reduces the chances of rebleeding in patients who have already bled. In practice, it is often difficult to apply the bands at endosopy in a patient having a very major active haemorrhage. In these patients it is often easier to inject the varices with a sclerosant and, if this fails, a **Sengstaken–Blakemore tube** would be a reasonable next step. The patient should be given intravenous terlipressin for 72 hours to reduce the portal pressure. A further attempt at sclerotherapy or banding should be attempted and, if this fails and the patient continues to bleed, the patient should be considered for a transjugular intrahepatic portosystemic shunt (TIPSS). This is a means of decompressing the portal circulation by the radiological placement of a metal stent between the portal and hepatic veins. This procedure is performed by an interventional radiologist via a transjugular approach.

124   Question on p.42.

Answer E
COPD with PO_2 7.5 kPa

The commonest indication for the use of long-term domiciliary oxygen therapy is chronic obstructive pulmonary disease (COPD). Such patients need careful clinical evaluation before long-term oxygen therapy is prescribed.

It is essential that patients have stopped smoking and, if there is any doubt, the **carboxyhaemoglobin** levels should be checked. Levels of carboxyhaemoglobin in non-smokers are < 3%. Carboxyhaemoglobin levels > 3% are thus an absolute contraindication to long-term domiciliary oxygen therapy.

Assessment for long-term oxygen therapy needs to be performed when the patient is stable and at least 4 weeks after the most recent exacerbation of their disease. Blood gases should be performed at least 3 weeks apart and taken with the patient breathing room air. The PCO_2 is of no relevance in assessing the need for domiciliary oxygen. ➤

Criteria for the use of long-term domiciliary oxygen therapy

Disease	PO$_2$ (kPa) on air	Associated findings
COPD	< 7.3	—
	7.3–7.8	Plus polycythaemia, nocturnal hypoxia, peripheral oedema or pulmonary hypertension
Interstitial lung disease	< 8	—
	> 8	With disabling dyspnoea
Cystic fibrosis	< 7.3	—
	7.3–7.8	Plus polycythaemia, nocturnal hypoxia, peripheral oedema or pulmonary hypertension
Pulmonary hypertension	< 8	
Obstructive sleep apnoea		After failure of continuous positive airways pressure (CPAP) and further assessment by a respiratory physician
Pulmonary malignancy		Used in patients with terminal disease and disabling dyspnoea
Heart failure	< 7.3	Or in patients with nocturnal hypoxia
Paediatrics		Only after specialist assessment

Patients with COPD treated with long-term continuous oxygen therapy using the above criteria have improved survival rates. The oxygen needs to be used for at least 15 hours per day and preferably for at least 19 hours per day for a survival benefit to be achieved. When oxygen is used in this way, it is cheapest and most practical for it to be delivered via an oxygen concentrator rather than cylinders.

125

Question on p.42.

Answer A
Intravenous clonazepam

Seizures may occur as a manifestation of acute porphyria, secondary to the hyponatraemia, which develops in up to 35% of acute attacks or due to a cause unrelated to porphyria. Treatment firstly involves terminating the seizure, and then assessing the likely cause and planning the most appropriate therapy. In the case of hyponatraemia, this involves slow correction of the electrolyte imbalance by fluid restriction and isotonic or hypertonic saline where necessary. For this question it is reasonable to assume that the seizure is related to the acute porphyria.

Infection, dieting, alcohol pregnancy, periods and certain drugs may precipitate acute attacks.

Clinical features of an attack may include:

- gastrointestinal (95%) abdominal pain, vomiting and constipation
- peripheral neuropathy (66%)
- psychiatric symptoms (50%) – depression, hysteria, psychosis
- seizures (35%)
- other features include hypertension, tachycardia, fever and hyponatraemia due to SIADH.

One of the problems in treating seizures in acute porphyria is that many of the anticonvulsant medicines will make the attack worse. **Phenytoin, carbamazepine** and **phenobarbitone** must be avoided at all costs.

Benzodiazepines are not without their risks but best clinical practice recommends their use for a single intravenous injection. **Clonazepam** has been reported to be safer than diazepam in these patients.

If seizures continue, **paraldehyde** or intravenous magnesium is recommended.

The BNF lists over 100 drugs to avoid in porphyria. Those that seem to come up most often in the exam are:

- sulphonamides
- barbiturates
- anticonvulsants
  - phenytoin
  - carbamazepine
  - phenobarbitone
- antifungals
- oral contraceptive pill
- diclofenac
- metoclopramide
- lignocaine
- alcohol

126 Question on p.43.

Answer A
Ibuprofen

Recent research has shown that non-steroidal anti-inflammatory drugs (NSAIDs) such as ibuprofen may interfere with the cardioprotective effects of aspirin.

Non-steroidal anti-inflammatory drugs work by interfering with both COX 1 and COX 2 enzyme systems. When aspirin and NSAIDs are taken together they both bind to the same place on the COX 1 enzyme. The binding of NSAIDs to this enzyme seems to occur first, thereby inhibiting the effect of aspirin.

The clinical importance of this interaction, particularly for the millions of patients who take aspirin for its cardioprotective actions, remains to be elucidated.

Answer A
ST segment elevation > 1 mm in a non-Q wave lead

ST elevation of > 1 mm in the absence of Q waves is an abnormal response to exercise. This finding suggests severe coronary artery disease and is a poor prognostic indicator.

Inverted **U waves** are a specific sign of cardiac ischaemia. U waves are often difficult to identify at high heart rates, so this finding is not a sensitive indicator of ischaemia. Inverted U waves are not a reason to stop the exercise ECG.

This patient has not reached his **maximum predicted heart rate** (168 beats/minute), which is calculated as 220 (210 for women) minus the patient's age. A satisfactory heart rate response is achieved by reaching 85% of the maximum predicted heart rate, but achieving this heart rate is not in itself a reason to stop the exercise test. Attainment of the maximum heart rate is a good prognostic sign.

As the exercise test progresses, the patient's **blood pressure** rises. A level of up to 225 mmHg is normal in adults, although athletes can have higher levels.

ST segment depression of 2 mmHg is highly suggestive of coronary artery disease, but is not a reason for stopping the test.

Indications for stopping an exercise ECG

ECG criteria	Symptoms/signs
VT/VF	Severe chest pain/dyspnoea
ST depression > 3 mm	Fatigue
ST elevation > 1 mm in non-Q wave lead	Fall in systolic BP > 20 mmHg
Frequent ventricular ectopics	Rise in systolic BP > 300 mmHg
New onset AF or SVT	Rise in diastolic BP > 130 mmHg
Cardiac arrest	
New bundle branch block	
New second- or third-degree heart block	

Normal ECG changes during an exercise ECG
- Depression of J point
- R wave decreases in height
- P wave increases in height
- Up-sloping ST segment
- QT interval shortens
- T wave decreases in height

Question on p.43.

Answer B
Chromosome 15

The unifying diagnosis here is Marfan's syndrome. It is a disease causing a defect in connective tissue. There is a mutation in the gene encoding the protein fibrillin, located on chromosome 15. It is inherited as an autosomal dominant.

The disease affects several systems as listed below.

- Skeletal:
  - tall
  - kyphoscoliosis
  - arachnodactly
  - high arched palate
  - pectus excavatum
  - flat feet
  - hyper-extensible joints
  - increased incidence of pneumothorax.
- Ocular:
  - weakened suspensory ligaments of the lens causing dislocation, normally upwards
  - retinal detachment.
- Cardiovascular:
  - mitral valve prolapse
  - aortic regurgitation
  - aortic root dilatation
  - aortic dissection.

Those with Marfan's syndrome have to be distinguished from those with homocystinuria, a condition phenotypically similar. Those with homocystinuria have the same skeletal and ocular problems (although the lens dislocation tends to be downwards) as well as an increased thrombotic tendency and neurological involvement (50% mental handicap, 20% epilepsy). They do not have the cardiovascular complications that are associated with Marfan's. Homocystinuria is due to a deficiency of cystathionine. This results in an increase in homocystine. It is inherited as an autosomal recessive, the defect being located on chromosome 21.

Neurofibromatosis type I is an autosomal dominant single gene disorder located on chromosome 17.

Cystic fibrosis is an autosomal recessive single gene disorder located on chromosome 7.

Answer D
Nephrotic syndrome

The differential diagnosis of a pleural effusion is a commonly encountered problem in medicine. The causes are differentiated by the protein content of the aspirated fluid. An exudate is characterized by a protein content greater than 30 g/L. Transudates have less than 30 g/L. The causes of each are shown in the table below.

Transudate	Exudate
Congestive cardiac failure	Pulmonary infarction
Hypoproteinaemic states, e.g. nephrotic syndrome	Pneumonia
Constrictive pericarditis	Malignancy
Hypothyroidism	TB
Meig's syndrome	Connective tissue disease
	Pancreatitis
	Mesothelioma
	Subphrenic abscess

As this lady has a transudate, it is not therefore **carcinoma of the bronchus** or **secondary to rheumatoid**.

Meig's syndrome (ascites, effusion and ovarian fibroma) is a rare cause of a transudate and unlikely here.

Constrictive pericarditis does occur as a complication of rheumatoid arthritis, particularly those who are strongly seropositive. However, it is very rare and would present with symptoms and signs of right heart failure i.e. ascites, hepatomegaly and an increased JVP.

Nephrotic syndrome occurs secondary to amyloidosis. It is caused by a deposition of serum amyloid A protein in the kidneys. It occurs in chronic inflammatory conditions, such as rheumatoid arthritis and inflammatory bowel disease. Nephrotic syndrome is the most likely to produce the clinical picture above.

There is often considerable overlap between the cause of pleural effusion, i.e. causes of an exudate can cause a transudate and vice versa but, when the protein is this low, it is largely suggestive of a hypoproteinaemic state.

Pulmonary complications of RA	Pleural effusion in RA
• Nodules – may cavitate	• ↑White cells
• Pleural effusions	• ↑ Lactate dehydrogenase (LDH)
• Pulmonary fibrosis	• ↓ Glucose
• Bronchiolitis obliterans	• ↑ Rheumatoid factor
• Haemorrhage	• ↓ Complement
• Caplan's syndrome	

130   Question on p.44.

Answer C
Poor response to sodium valproate

It is important to know about juvenile myoclonic epilepsy (JME) as it is common and has a good response to treatment. Features include:

- cause of 5–10% of all epilepsy
- myoclonic jerks, generalized tonic clonic seizures +/− absences
- attacks precipitated by alcohol and sleep deprivation
- diurnal variation – attacks occur within an hour of waking
- early morning twitching
- 90% become seizure free on sodium valproate
- linked to chromosome 6.

> **Side effects of sodium valproate therapy** (*Mnemonic:VALPROATE*)
> - Valproate
> - Ataxia
> - Liver failure
> - Pancreatitis
> - Reversible alopecia
> - Obesity/ oedema
> - Amenorrhoea
> - Thrombocytopenia
> - Epilim

131   Question on p.44.

Answer C
Polymyositis

This patient has pain and weakness in his proximal muscles and a raised creatinine phosphokinase (CK).

Polymyalgia rheumatica can present with similar symptoms. However, the patient is usually over the age of 60 and the CK is normal. Therefore, this is not the most likely diagnosis.

Hyperthyroidism can sometimes present with a proximal myopathy in the absence of any other symptoms or signs. This presentation is more common in males. Pain is not usually a major feature and the CK is not elevated.

There are two ways in which **alcohol** can cause a myopathy. In acute alcoholic myopathy, owing to acute alcohol intoxication, there is a painful myositis with a very high CK. In the chronic variety there is a non-painful proximal myopathy with a normal CK. It is possible, but unlikely, that this patient has an acute alcoholic myopathy on the background of chronic alcohol abuse. This is not, however, the most likely diagnosis. ➤

The most likely diagnosis is **polymyositis**. This is an uncommon disorder with inflammatory infiltrate in muscle of unknown cause. It predominantly affects the limb girdle but oesophageal involvement causing dysphagia is seen in 50%. Polymyositis usually presents in men in their 40s and 50s. A small minority of patients have an underlying malignancy.

The diagnosis is suggested by the history. The ESR is raised in 60%. The CK is always elevated and sometimes very markedly so. Anti-Jo-1 antibodies and rheumatoid factor are present in up to 50%. The diagnosis is confirmed by electromyography and muscle biopsy, but these may not be necessary. The condition responds well to high-dose oral corticosteroids. Some patients require corticosteroid therapy for several years to keep the disease under control.

The clinical features of **dermatomyositis** are identical to those of polymyositis, except that in addition there are dermatological features. These include a purple 'heliotrope' rash around the eyes and a vasculitic rash (colloidon patches) over the joints of the fingers.

---

132 Question on p.44.

Answer A
Reduce isoniazid dose

Certain drugs are metabolized by acetylation in the liver by the enzyme **N-acetyltransferase**. Fast acetylators have more of this enzyme in the liver than slow acetylators and this feature is inherited as an **autosomal dominant** trait.

Drugs affected by acetylator status are listed below and can be remembered by the mnemonic **'DHIPS'**:

- dapsone
- hydralazine
- isoniazid
- procainamide/phenelzine
- sulphonamides.

In clinical practice, slow acetylators require lower doses of these drugs and the patient in question will require lower dosage of isoniazid.

These patients are more likely to develop the lupus erythematosus-like syndrome caused by isoniazid, procainamide and hydralazine, and the peripheral neuropathy due to isoniazid.

Drugs that cause a lupus erythematosus-like syndrome
- Antibiotics
  - Isoniazid
  - Penicillin
  - Tetracyclines
  - Sulphonamides
- Antihypertensives
  - β-Blockers
  - Clonidine
  - Hydralazine
  - Methyldopa
- Others
  - Phenytoin
  - Procainamide
  - Lithium

133 Question on p.45.

Answer E
Admit to hospital

This gentleman has erythroderma, which is a dermatological emergency. Treatment is carried out in the **hospital setting**. Erythroderma is the term used to describe global (> 90%) extreme reddening of the skin. It is usually hot to touch. There are a variety of underlying causes, as listed below, but in up to 30% no cause can be found.

It is more common with age and onset can be very rapid.

Causes of erythroderma
- Pre-existing dermatoses
  - Atopic eczema
  - Psoriais
  - Cutaneous T-cell lymphoma
  - Pemphigus
- Systemic disease
  - Internal malignancy, e.g. colorectal, lung
  - Drugs, e.g. sulphonamides, gold, zopiclone (in this case)
  - Haematological malignancy, e.g. leukaemia
  - HIV
  - Graft versus host disease

Investigation of the underlying diagnosis is necessary if it is not clear from the history. ➤

Complications that can occur include:

1. hypothermia, from loss of heat over a large surface area.
2. high-output cardiac failure from the increased blood flow
3. hypotension and its consequences from vascular dilatation
4. hypoalbuminaemia secondary to protein loss and an increased metabolic rate
5. 'capillary leak syndrome' caused by a general increase in vascular permeability, leading to ARDS.

Treatment is supportive, i.e. fluid balance, keep warm, correct metabolic abnormalities. All unnecessary drugs must be stopped. Topical emollients and **mild topical steroids** are used to treat the skin.

Paste bandaging is used in resistant eczema as an overnight preparation to aid absorption.

---

134 Question on p.45.

Answer B
Raise in temperature

A 'shift' to the right or the left refers to the oxygen dissociation curve that illustrates the haemoglobin saturation against PaO_2. It shows a sigmoid curve and nicely demonstrates the fact that the binding is not a linear relationship and in fact oxygen is freely released at the lower ranges of PaO_2. However, at a higher concentration, haemoglobin and oxygen are tightly associated. As the curve shows, once saturation falls below 90–92%, there is a sharp decline in saturation for a relatively small change in PaO_2.

A shift to the left means that there is an increased affinity between haemoglobin and oxygen so the oxygen molecule is less easily released. However, a shift to the right means the two have a decreased affinity and oxygen is readily released. This means that, for any given saturation of haemoglobin, the partial pressure of oxygen will be that much higher.

Haemoglobin F (HbF) has an increased affinity for oxygen.
Polycythaemia should have no effect on the curve.

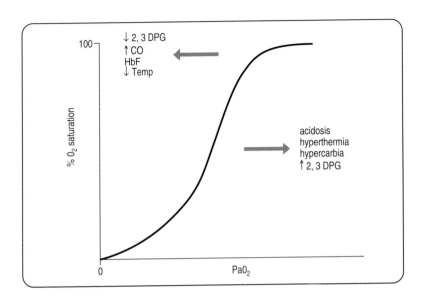

Question on p.45.

135

Answer D
Peak flow monitoring diary

The diagnosis of asthma can be made if there is greater than 15% improvement in the patients FEV_1 or peak flow (PEFR) following the inhalation of the bronchodilator.

None of the options given will diagnose asthma in isolation but a **peak flow monitoring diary** may demonstrate the variable airflow limitation that is characteristic of asthma. Patients should be asked to record peak flows on waking, during the afternoon and before bed. Asthmatics demonstrate a diurnal variation in airflow, with morning dips and improvement during the day. Peak flow monitoring is a simple, cheap and non-invasive test. In addition, it may provide an objective assessment of treatment response.

Prescribing **salbutamol** without objective assessment of response is of no use in diagnosing asthma. Even patients with no reversibility seem to feel subjectively better after an inhaler and will quickly become dependent on them. Likewise, prescribing **steroids** without objective response assessment is likely to cause problems in the future. Many causes of dyspnoea will be improved by steroid and symptomatic benefit merely suggests that steroids improve the cause of dyspnoea. It does not diagnose asthma. If this young man is started on steroid without proper assessment it will be very difficult to convince him to come off them if he has a symptomatic response. ➤

Spirometry, via a vitalograph, measures the FEV_1 and forced vital capacity (FVC). The FEV_1 expressed as a percentage of the FVC is a good measure of airflow limitation. In healthy adults it is in the region of 75%. This patient may demonstrate airflow limitation, with a reduced FEV_1/FVC ratio but this is not specific to asthma.

Arterial blood gas analysis is of little use in the diagnosis of asthma in this patient and is unnecessarily invasive. Unless the patient is acutely unwell, the results are likely to be normal. Abnormal results will not demonstrate changes specific to asthma.

136
Question on p.45.

Answer D
Plasma electrophoresis

This man has anaemia and renal failure with a high normal total protein and low albumin, suggesting the presence of another, undetectable protein (paraprotein). This all points towards multiple myeloma.

Myeloma is characterized by the presence of a paraprotein that is present in the serum and is detected by **protein electrophoresis**. A paraprotein is an abnormal proliferation of plasma cells producing either IgG, A or D. Features include the following.

1. Bony destruction – this results in hypercalcaemia, pathological fractures, spinal cord compression.
2. Marrow infiltration – this results in anaemia, neutropenia, thrombocytopenia and hyperviscosity syndrome.
3. Renal impairment – secondary to:
   - tubular obstruction by light chains
   - infiltration of plasma cells into the kidney
   - hypercalcaemia
   - hyperuricaemia
   - amyloidosis
   - recurrent pyelonephritis
   - renal vein thrombosis with hyperviscosity

137
Question on p.46.

Answer C
Recombinant activated protein C

Disseminated intravascular coagulation is an abnormality of the clotting system that manifests clinically as bleeding, haemorrhagic tissue necrosis and thrombosis alone or in combination. There are a number of important aspects in the pathophysiology of disseminated intravascular coagulation which include the following.

- Thrombin generation. The normal protein C related homeostatic mechanism of thrombin generation is lost
- Dissemination. The extrinsic pathway normally plays a major role in the initiation and generation of thrombin. In disseminated intravascular coagulation, thrombin production is also driven by activation of the intrinsic pathway leading to consumption of protein C, protein S and antithrombin. Increased exposure of negatively charged phospholipid surfaces and cell damage also drives this abnormal clotting cascade.
- Cytokine release. Tissue ischaemia and inflammation cause a release of cytokines and inflammatory mediators that further induce coagulation.
- Endothelial cell activation. There is a maladaptive response in disseminated intravascular coagulation leading to generalized intravascular coagulopathy.

Causes of disseminated intravascular coagulation
- Sepsis
- Major trauma
- Severe acute pancreatitis
- Malignancy (especially acute promyelocytic leukaemia)
- Fat embolism
- Amniotic fluid embolism
- Placental abruption
- Transfusion reaction
- Snake bite
- Acute transplant rejection

Diagnosis of disseminated intravascular coagulation

Test	Result
Prothrombin time	Raised
Platelets	Low
APTT	Raised
Fibrin degradation products	Raised
Fibrinogen	Low
Protein C	Low

The treatment of disseminated intravascular coagulation is firstly to treat the underlying cause aggressively. In a patient with sepsis, this means high-dose intravenous antibiotics. Secondly, appropriate supportive care should be provided. This may include circulatory and ventilatory support in an intensive care unit setting. Thirdly, specific therapy for the coagulopathy should be considered.

Treatment for the coagulopathy in disseminated intravascular coagulation has been a contentious issue. Patients with clinically ➤

significant bleeding are often treated with **fresh-frozen plasma, cryoprecipitate** or **platelets**, or a combination of all three. These therapies have never been shown to improve mortality in randomized trials. Furthermore, the use of these products in an attempt to reduce or stop bleeding may make the coagulopathy worse by 'stoking the fire' (i.e. increase the production of fibrin and hence the risk of thrombosis).

The use of **unfractionated heparin** in patients with disseminated intravascular coagulation has not been shown to improve outcome, and is potentially hazardous as it may increase the risk of bleeding.

A recent study has shown that the use of **human recombinant protein C** in patients with disseminated intravascular coagulation secondary to sepsis improves mortality from 31% to 25%. It is given by infusion over 4 days. Its efficacy in this situation may be related to its anti-inflammatory properties in addition to its anticoagulant action. Human recombinant protein C needs to be given with caution in patients with a platelet count of $< 30 \times 10^9$, as such patients have an increased risk of intracerebral haemorrhage.

138

Question on p.46.

Answer E
Giardiasis

Giardia lamblia is a waterborne protozoan parasite. Found worldwide, it occurs particularly in areas with poor water supplies or hilly areas where streams and rivers may become contaminated. It adheres to the jejunum and ileum causing malabsorption, diarrhoea and villous atrophy. Diagnosis is by demonstrating cysts in the faeces. However, as there may be irregular excretion, one negative stool sample does not rule out the diagnosis. Treatment is with metronidazole.

Inflammatory bowel disease could present with an 8-week history of watery diarrhoea and weight loss even in the absence of abdominal pain (i.e. Crohn's) or blood in the stool (ulcerative colitis). The history of foreign travel strongly suggests an infective cause.

Although **Schistosomiasis mansoni** is found in parts of South America (predominantly the East), it is not found in Peru.

Tropical sprue is a condition of unknown aetiology occurring in most of Asia and Central America. It causes persistent diarrhoea after an initial gastrointestinal infection. It can progress to weight loss, anaemia and folate deficiency in particular. It often presents years after the patient has lived in the tropics and usually responds to therapy with tetracycline, but this may need to be given for up to one year.

Answer C
61-year-old with ischaemic heart disease (BP 90/70 mmHg, pulse 60 beats/minute)

The mortality from upper gastrointestinal haemorrhage is approximately 8%. Mortality risk is directly related to the age of the patient and coexisting disease, and is particularly high in patients who have a gastrointestinal haemorrhage in hospital after being admitted for another cause, e.g. fractured neck of femur.

In the mid-1990s a large prospective audit of upper gastrointestinal haemorrhage was performed in the UK, involving several thousand patients. This work has led to the development of a simple scoring system (Rockall score) which allows the mortality risk of an individual to be calculated prior to endoscopy. These criteria use simple clinical parameters, are easily applied in the clinical setting and are robust.

Rockall score

Clinical parameter	Score
Age	
< 60	0
60–79	1
> 80	2
Shock	
None	0
Pulse > 100	1
BP < 100	2
Comorbidity	
None	0
Ischaemic heart disease, CCF and other major conditions	2
Renal/liver failure or disseminated malignancy	3

Patients with a Rockall score of 0 have a < 1% in-hospital mortality. The mortality risk then rises linearly from this point and, in patients with a Rockall score of 7, the in-hospital mortality is approximately 40%. This scoring system is useful clinically, as patients with a high Rockall score should be looked after in a high dependency unit setting with early aggressive therapeutic endoscopy. Ideally, such patients should be managed jointly by GI physicians and surgeons. Patients with a Rockall score of zero may possibly be managed in the outpatient setting, but there are currently no prospective data confirming that this is a safe practice. ➤

Applying the Rockall scoring system to our five patients gives the following result:

Patient	Rockall score
A	3
B	4
C	5
D	2
E	1

Patient C has the highest Rockall score and hence the highest predicted in-hospital mortality (approximately 12%).

140

Question on p.47.

Answer E
Henoch–Schonlein purpura

This young girl has a combination of:

- abdominal pain
- bloody diarrhoea
- purpuric rash
- arthropathy
- renal involvement – nephritis (haematuria, proteinuria, hypertension, oedema).

This combination of symptoms in any young person should make you think of **Henoch–Schonlein purpura**. It is a small-vessel vasculitis that mostly affects children and occasionally adults. Symptoms are of abdominal pain, diarrhoea, rectal bleeding, flitting arthralgia of large joints, nephritis and a purpuric rash on the buttocks and legs. Diagnosis in children is normally clinical; however, in adults, most have a biopsy to confirm the diagnosis. This can be either skin or renal and shows deposition of IgA.

IgA nephropathy is a common cause of asymptomatic dipstick haematuria in young men. Macroscopic haematuria tends to affects younger patients. Paradoxically the occurrence of macroscopic haematuria is a good prognostic sign. The pathological basis is mesangial deposition of IgA and a focal proliferative glomerulonephritis. IgA nephropathy does not cause a systemic illness as detailed in the case in question.

Polyarteritis nodosa is a rare medium-sized vessel vasculitis. It tends to affect middle aged men and has many possible presenting symptoms. The mode of presentation depends on which system is predominantly involved. However, systemic symptoms e.g. fever malaise and weight loss, are almost universally present. It could present with the symptoms above but it would be very uncommon in a young girl.

Systemic lupus erythematosus is a rare autoimmune disease with autoantibodies directed against double-stranded DNA. It has a plethora of presenting symptoms and could account for all the symptoms listed above. There is a male to female ration of 1:9. The answer is unlikely to be this as bloody diarrhoea is not characteristic.

This is not **haemolytic uraemic syndrome** (HUS). The characteristic features of HUS are microangiopathic haemolysis, renal failure and thrombocytopenia. It is precipitated by infection with the toxin-producing *E. coli* 0157. This seems to set in motion a cascade of events, which results in damage to the endothelial surface. Patients who have HUS have anaemia, profound thrombocytopenia and nephritis. Usually there is no joint involvement.

---

141 Question on p.47.

Answer B
Half-life

Digoxin exhibits first-order kinetics. Excreted renally, it has a **half-life** of 40 hours.

Regarding **bioavailability**, 67% of orally administered digoxin is absorbed (80% if given as an elixir) and two-thirds of the absorbed drug will remain in the system after 1 day. It requires several subsequent administrations of the drug before reaching a steady state and this is achieved after 4–5 days.

Digoxin is less than 50% **protein bound** and has a very high **volume of distribution** (> 200 L) indicating that it distributes extensively in the body tissues. It accumulates in renal failure but this occurs after continued administration of the drug. In this question, one is assuming that the patient has normal **creatinine clearance** and estimation of time to steady state will be made according to this.

It is important to be aware that quinidine, spironolactone and verapamil inhibit tubular secretion of digoxin. Concomitant administration of these drugs may lead to a rise in plasma digoxin concentrations (usually twofold).

---

142 Question on p.48.

Answer E
Aspirin

A tender thyroid gland suggests thyroiditis. There are several causes of thyroiditis as follows. ➤

- Hashimoto's:
  - autoimmune
  - more common in women
  - thyroid microsomal antibodies normally present
  - euthyroid/hypothyroid.
- Postpartum:
  - hyperthyroidism or hypothyroidism
  - transient
  - can precede clinical disease.
- Reidel's:
  - hard 'woody' thyroid
  - fibrotic
  - associated with midline fibrosis.
- De Quervain's:
  - inflammatory, probably viral
  - transient hyperthyroidism
  - raised ESR
  - subsequent hypothyroidism
  - treat acutely with **aspirin**.

Severe symptomatic cases can be treated in the short term with **prednisolone**. As this woman's only symptom is the painful neck, initial treatment should be with aspirin. If this fails to settle the condition a trial of prednisolone would be the next step. There is no role for **carbimazole** in this setting as the hyperthyroidism is transient and often followed by a period of hypothyroidism.

143
Question on p.48.

Answer B
Left ventricular hypertrophy

Restrictive cardiomyopathy and constrictive pericarditis may present similarly (with signs of right heart failure, raised JVP, ascites and oedema). Whereas surgery is necessary for pericardial constriction, it is of no benefit and possibly harmful to patients with restrictive cardiomyopathy.

Causes of restrictive cardiomyopathy can be divided into myocardial causes (mnemonic: GI-SHAGS) and endomyocardial causes (mnemonic: M-TECH)

Myocardial causes	Endomyocardial causes
Glycogen storage disorders	**M**alignancy or radiotherapy
Idiopathic	**T**oxin-related
Sarcoid	**E**ndomyocardial fibrosis
Haemochromatosis	**C**arcinoid
Amyloid	**H**yper-eosinophilic syndrome (including Loeffler's
Gaucher's disease	syndrome)
Scleroderma	

Signs common to both conditions include:

- atrial fibrillation
- raised JVP with prominent x and y descents
- non-pulsatile hepatomegaly
- normal systolic function
- LVEDV < 110 mL/m^2.

Constrictive pericarditis is unlikely to have evidence of left ventricular hypertrophy, although this is not unheard of.

Features of restrictive cardiomyopathy not found in constrictive pericarditis include

- prominent apical impulse
- conduction abnormalities on ECG.

Causes of constrictive pericarditis include:

- iatrogenic
  - drugs, e.g. hydralazine
  - post-cardiac surgery
  - post-mediastinal radiotherapy
- infective
  - tuberculosis
  - post-viral or bacterial pericarditis
- others
  - connective tissue disease, e.g. longstanding seropositive rheumatoid arthritis
  - post-uraemic pericarditis
  - pericardial malignancy.

144 Question on p.48.

Answer C
Oral metronidazole

The most likely diagnosis is giardiasis, given the relatively short duration of symptoms and the recent history of travel to an endemic area. Giardiasis can be quite difficult to diagnose, as stool cultures are not infrequently negative, as shedding of the organism into the intestinal lumen can be sporadic. Giardiasis is one of the causes of partial villous atrophy (see box). *Giardia lamblia* can frequently be seen on duodenal biopsy but are not always present and can frequently be overlooked by an unwary histopathologist.

The main differential diagnosis in this case, in a patient of this age is coeliac disease. Such patients frequently have a history of recurrent anaemia and many have other suggestive symptoms, such as recurrent mouth ulceration, delayed menarche or a family history.

To complicate things further, occasionally coeliac disease presents as a case of giardiasis and it is possible that patients with coeliac disease are more prone to this infection. ➤

The correct treatment is, therefore, oral **metronidazole**. Ideally this should be started after taking several stool samples, rechecking the duodenal biopsies for *Giardia lamblia* organisms and checking the antiendomysial antibodies. Treatment is usually continued for up to a week and the patient's symptoms will rapidly improve. Should the patient not improve on the above therapy, the diagnosis needs to be reconsidered in light of the additional tests outlined above.

Causes of subtotal villous atrophy
- Coeliac disease
- Giardiasis
- Erosive jejunitis
- Lymphoma
- HIV enteropathy
- Graft versus host disease
- IgA deficiency
- Tropical sprue

---

145 Question on p.49.

Answer D
Streptococcus bovis

Infective endocarditis is an infection of the endocardial surface. There are a wide variety of organisms, including fungi and rickettsiae, that are capable of causing it. Previously there were a limited number of organisms implicated, such as *Staphylococcus aureus* and *Streptococcus viridans*. However, in recent years more unusual pathogens are featuring. This is in part due to the increase in valvular heart surgery and the increase in number of intravenous drug users.

Occasionally the identification of the causative organism gives an idea to a possible related condition. This is the case with *Streptococcus bovis*. It is a Gram-positive coccus that has been strongly associated with GI neoplasms, in particular colorectal carcinoma. Some studies have suggested that up to 84% of sepsis caused by *Streptococcus bovis* is secondary to a GI source.

Several recommendations have thus been drawn up as follows.

- Colonoscopy is performed on all those with endocarditis caused by *Streptococcus bovis* whilst an inpatient, even if no symptoms are present.
- Colonoscopy should be performed as part of follow-up. Malignancies have been detected up to 2 years after the initial sepsis.

Endocarditis secondary to **Pseudomonas** is most frequently seen in iv drug abusers. It tends to come from the contaminated water that is mixed with the drug before injection. Usually the tricuspid valve is affected.

The most common way **S. pyogenes** affects the heart is through rheumatic fever. It is a complication of infection. During the initial infection antibodies are produced that cross-react with valvular heart tissue, producing valvular scarring.

Coxiella burnetii or Q fever characteristically is a chronic infection of a damaged or prosthetic heart valve. Diagnosis is often delayed as symptoms are vague. Prognosis is poor.

E. coli is a Gram-negative bacillus. It is a commensal organism capable of causing bateraemia and hence endocarditis. Sepsis caused by this organism tends to involve either bowel (perforation) or the urinary tract. There is no association to colorectal conditions.

---

146 Question on p.49.

Answer E
Patient whose sister had breast cancer at 42 and mother had ovarian cancer at 49

The aim of this question is to examine whether you know which types of cancer can be familial. It also tests whether you know which types of cancers are associated with each other in familial cancer syndromes.

The main factors in a family history of cancer that suggest the possibility of a familial (Mendelian) cancer syndrome are:

1. the presence of multiple affected family members
2. an unusually early age of onset of the cancers in the family
3. a characteristic pattern of different cancer types within one family, such as breast with ovarian cancer, or bowel with endometrial cancer.

The commonest familial cancers are breast and bowel. Familial breast cancer accounts for no more than 5% of all breast cancers and the majority of familial breast cancers are due to mutations in the BRCA1 and BRCA2 genes. These cancer syndromes follow autosomal dominant inheritance with reduced penetrance (i.e. not all mutation carriers develop cancer). A BRCA1 mutation carrier has an up to 80% chance of developing breast cancer and a 20–40% chance of developing ovarian cancer. A BRCA2 mutation carrier has a similar risk of developing breast cancer but the ovarian cancer risk is lower at 10–20%. BRCA2 mutations are also associated with an increased risk of male breast cancer.

Isolated cases of breast cancer or ovarian cancer, particularly those that do not occur at an unusually young age, are unlikely to be genetic in origin and, in the absence of any other family history of breast or ovarian cancer, would not warrant a genetics referral. A combination of young onset breast cancer and young onset ovarian cancer in first-degree relatives is suggestive and should be referred.

Familial bowel cancer again only accounts for a small percentage of all bowel cancers but there is a well-recognized familial bowel cancer syndrome called hereditary non-polyposis colon cancer (HNPCC) in which ➤

there is an association between early-onset bowel cancer and endometrial cancer.

Uterine cancer is known to occur more frequently in those breast cancer patients who have been treated previously with tamoxifen and this combination does not suggest a familial cancer syndrome.

Both lung cancer and cervical cancer are almost exclusively environmental in origin and, even when they occur at a young age, there is no indication for a referral to the clinical genetics service.

In most cases, the regional clinical genetics service will have developed guidelines to clarify which patients with a family history of cancer are eligible for referral.

147 Question on p.49.

Answer C
6 mg

There are many different corticosteroids on the market with different anti-inflammatory potencies. It should be remembered that corticosteroids have glucocorticoid and mineralocorticoid effects. The anti-inflammatory effects are due to the glucocorticoids, but high glucocorticoid activity is of little use unless it is accompanied by low mineralocorticoid activity.

The table below summarizes the principal side effects of steroids according to activity.

Glucocorticoid effects	Mineralocorticoid effects
Diabetes	Hypertension
Osteoporosis	Sodium/water retention
Avascular necrosis	Hypokalaemia
Proximal myopathy	
Peptic ulceration	
Psychiatric disturbance	
Paranoia	
Depression	
Euphoria	

Long-term corticosteroid use may lead to Cushing's syndrome, with moon face, striae, acne, buffalo hump and central body fat redistribution.

Fludrocortisone has such high mineralocorticoid activity that its anti-inflammatory activity is of little relevance. Likewise, the relatively high mineralocorticoid activity of **cortisone** and **hydrocortisone**, resulting in marked fluid retention, make them unsuitable in the longterm. They are useful in long-term adrenal replacement therapy. Hydrocortisone is also used short term for some emergencies.

Prednisolone is the most commonly used corticosteroid for long-term disease suppression and has predominantly glucocorticoid activity.

Betamethasone and **dexamathasone** have very high glucocorticoid activity and insignificant mineralcorticoid effects. In addition, they have a long duration of action and are very useful in high-dose therapy where fluid retention would be a disadvantage.

The anti-inflammatory effect of 5 mg of prednisolone is equivalent to:

- 0.75 mg dexamethasone
- 20 mg hydrocortisone
- 4 mg methylprednisolone.

Hence,

$$40 \text{ mg} \div 5 \text{ mg} \times 0.75 \text{ mg} = 6 \text{ mg (answer C)}$$

---

148 Question on p.49.

Answer D
Intravenous iron sulphate

Anaemia is one of the major complications of renal failure and it has several causes which all tend to exert an influence at any one time, making the diagnosis complex.

This lady is anaemic, we assume asymptomatic because we are not told. She has recently started synthetic **erythropoietin** (EPO) injections that should help to stimulate her bone marrow. The haemoglobin should, therefore, be coming up and not going down. Therefore, there must some other rate-limiting factor.

Note that the MCV is on the low side of normal, possibly indicating an iron deficiency. The reticulocyte count is low, indicating a low turnover in the marrow. We know that EPO is not the rate-limiting step because she has been on it now for 2 weeks, so there must be another problem. When EPO is first given, there is a huge demand for iron by the bone marrow and it can induce an iron-deficient state. Iron should be started at the same time as EPO therapy, suggesting the best answer is either C or D.

Parenteral iron should be used in patients on long-term haemodialysis. **Oral iron** is poorly absorbed, especially in renal failure, and unpleasant to take. The parenteral route is preferred because it produces a faster haemoglobin response (only in renal patients). It is also used because the patients attend units three times a week to have a large needle put in their arm so it seems a good opportunity to give them iron.

Transfusions should be avoided because blood product antibodies may prejudice successful subsequent renal transplant.

It would be futile increasing the EPO injections, because this is not the limiting step in red cell formation in this patient.

Referral to a haematologist for a bone marrow would be correct if we were questioning a haematological malignancy or myeloproliferative disorder.

Question on p.50.

Answer A
Discoid lupus

Alopecia or hair loss has to be divided into non-scarring and scarring. Non-scarring alopecia is a complaint of the hair follicle itself and the underlying scalp is normal. Scarring alopecia is a complaint of the scalp whereby there is loss of the follicle and hence hair loss.
   Some causes of alopecia are listed below.

Scarring alopecia	Non-scarring alopecia
Discoid lupus erythematosus	Androgenic alopecia
Lichen planus	Telogen effluvium
Dissecting cellulitis	Alopecia areata
Tinea capitis	Trichotillomania (self-hair pulling)
	Metabolic, e.g. hypothyroidism
	Drugs

   Discoid lupus erythematosus has an autoimmune basis and occurs in light-exposed areas, particularly on the face, ears and scalp. The rash is erythematous and can occur in plaques. Frequently, the rash is scaly and shows follicular plugging. Scarring alopecia is common. The disease progresses over many years but in up to 50% eventually burns itself out. It can sometimes be difficult to differentiate clinically from **psoriasis** as both produce scaly plaques on the face and scalp. However, discoid lupus produces scarring and alopecia, features that are usually absent in psoriasis.
   The diagnosis is based on clinical suspicion and a skin biopsy that characteristically shows deposits of IgG, IgM, IgA and C3 in the basement membrane zone. Discoid lupus rarely progresses to full-blown systemic lupus erythematosus.
   Treatment is by potent topical corticosteroids and sunscreens/avoidance. Resistant cases sometimes respond to intralesional injections of triamcinolone or oral hydroxychloroquine.
   Lichen planus is an itchy inflammatory condition characterized by papules that are purple with fine white lines (Wickham's striae) on the surface. Lesions are normally seen on the arm and leg flexures, and mucosal involvement is frequent. Facial involvement is very uncommon. It is associated with nail dystrophy and, rarely, scarring alopecia. It affects 1% of the population. Treatment is with potent topical steroids, PUVA or azathioprine.
   Trichotillomania can cause alopecia. It does not produce scarring and the alopecia is usually patchy. **Pemphigus** can occasionally cause blisters on the scalp and face. Scarring alopecia is not a feature.

Answer E
Acoustic neuroma

This woman has sensorineural deafness on the left indicating involvement of the VIIIth cranial nerve. This is implied by the presence of deafness and proved by Weber's test. Weber's test involves placing a vibrating tuning fork on the forehead of the patient. Sound is localized to the affected ear in conductive deafness and the unaffected ear in sensorineural deafness.

Loss of the corneal reflex implies involvement of the Vth cranial nerve. This lady also has ipsilateral ataxia implying involvement of the cerebellum. Therefore, if both Vth and VIIIth cranial nerves are involved as well as the cerebellum, this must be a question about a cerebellopontine angle (CPA) lesion.

The CPA is a shallow triangle lying between cerebellum, lateral pons and the petrous ridge. It contains the Vth to the VIIIth cranial nerves. Any lesion here can produce a variety of symptoms caused by damage to vestibular, sensory, auditory and motor pathways.

The most common cause of a cerebellopontine angle lesion is an **acoustic neuroma** (VIIth nerve neurofibroma). Initial symptoms and signs are hearing loss and loss of the corneal reflex. Signs are often then limited to this for a considerable time because of the ability of the cranial nerves to 'stretch' as the tumour grows. As the tumour grows medially, it starts to cause distortion of the cerebellum and midbrain giving rise to vertigo, ipsilateral ataxia and a mild spastic paraparesis.

Ramsey–Hunt syndrome or *Herpes zoster* of the VIIth cranial nerve first presents with intense pain in and around the affected ear and then the subsequent outbreak of vesicles. There is a facial nerve palsy, but there can also be loss of the corneal reflex and importance has to be paid to the protection of the cornea during this period. There is no involvement of the cerebellum.

Otosclerosis is a common cause of conductive deafness. The normal healthy bone of the stapes is substituted by spongy bone that adheres to the oval window.

Paget's disease causes deafness by compression of the nerve. The remodelling associated with this disease squashes the nerve as it comes out of the internal auditory canal.

A **vertebrobasilar stroke** would not fit this clinical scenario, as in this condition there is a mixture on ipsilateral cranial signs and contralateral limb signs. The signs would not be all ipsilateral as in this case.

151 Question on p.50.

Answer B
Gout

Acute **gout** presents as an acute onset monoarthropathy with tenderness, swelling and erythema. In 50% of cases, the first metatarsophalangeal joint is affected, although any joint may be affected. The diagnosis is confirmed by joint fluid microscopy, which shows negatively bifringent urate crystals when viewed under polarized light.

The serum urate is usually raised, but it may be normal as the serum urate sometimes falls following an acute attack. If the urate is normal, it is best to recheck it several weeks after the acute attack. Attacks typically last for a week and treatment is by high-dose NSAIDs or colchicine.

Allopurinol is used in patients who get recurrent attacks, with the uricosuric agent probenecid reserved for patients who are intolerant of allopurinol. In patients with renal impairment the dose of allopurinol should be reduced and probenecid should not be used.

Allopurinol should not be used during acute attacks as it may precipitate attacks when first introduced.

152 Question on p.51.

Answer A
Acute hepatitis C

The picture in the question suggests previous exposure or immunization against hepatitis B, but this would not give a clinical picture of jaundice and so another cause needs to be considered. The history of needle sharing is significant and suggests **hepatitis C** may be the cause of her jaundice. The reported prevalence of hepatitis C amongst intravenous drug users is up to 90%.

This patient is hepatitis C antibody negative. In a patient with acute hepatitis C, the antibody response is often delayed for up to 3 months following infection. This patient is at significant risk of acquiring the disease through parenteral spread. The only way of reliably making the diagnosis of acute hepatitis C in the acute phase is by PCR testing.

This is not acute **hepatitis B** as the patient is anti-HBs positive. Anti-HBs antibodies typically rise several months after an attack of acute hepatitis and are usually taken to indicate recovery from acute hepatitis B. This patient has, therefore, either had a previous attack of hepatitis B or has been immunized. Moreover, the patient is negative for HBsAg. This in itself makes the diagnosis of acute hepatitis B extremely unlikely, as 95% of patients with acute hepatitis B are HBsAg positive during the icteric phase. Rarely, patients with acute hepatitis B are HBsAg negative, as occasionally the HbsAg is cleared early or not produced at all (hepatitis B mutant).

Anti-HBc typically starts to rise during an acute infection. It remains elevated for many months afterwards but eventually returns to normal. Anti-HBc IgM levels are often taken to indicate an acute attack of hepatitis B but, in the context of the other serological markers given, this is a very unlikely diagnosis.

Hepatitis E is an RNA virus closely related to the *Calicivirus* species. It is mainly confined to developing areas of the world, such as south east Asia, north Africa and central America, where it is endemic. It is probably transmitted by the orofaecal route and is found in areas of poor sanitation. Animal reservoirs have been described including rats and pigs. It causes an acute self-limiting hepatitis similar to acute hepatitis A, except in pregnant women where it carries a 20–25% mortality. Chronic infection is unknown. Diagnosis is by demonstrating a raised hepatitis E IgM, a rise in IgG and confirmed by PCR.

Hepatitis E was thought to be very rare in the UK, except in patients returning from travel to endemic areas. However, evidence is starting to emerge that this may not be the case. Several case studies have reported that hepatitis E does occur *de novo* in the developed world in patients who have not travelled. These patients are typically over the age of 50 years. PCR evidence indicates that the source of the virus is probably porcine, as part of the hepatitis E viral genome isolated from some of the human cases carries 100% sequence homology with hepatitis E virus isolated from UK pigs.

153

Question on p.51.

Answer D
Daily production is 550 mL

Cerebrospinal fluid (CSF) has a composition identical to that of the brain extracellular fluid. It differs from plasma in several ways:

- PCO_2 is higher resulting in a lower CSF pH (7.33)
- very low cholesterol content
- very low protein content (0.2 g/L) leaving a low buffering potential
- lower glucose concentration

CSF is present in the ventricles and subarachnoid space, cushioning the brain and spinal cord. It is formed by the choroid plexus (50%) and walls of the ventricles (50%). Total volume is 150 mL and daily production is approximately 550 mL. It flows from the 3rd and 4th ventricles into the subarachnoid space.

154 Question on p.51.

Answer B
Normal grief reaction

This man is showing features of a **normal grief reaction**. Bereaved people often believe they have seen their loved one. This is a normal part of the reaction and not evidence of a **psychosis.**

Immediately following the loss of someone close, it is normal for adults to experience a sense of shock and numbness. A week or two after the loss, the sense of shock is replaced by intense pining, preoccupation with the deceased and mild symptoms of depression. It is quite common for there to be illusions that the deceased is coming in or walking about in the house, and to see him or her. There will also be symptoms of anxiety, restlessness and feelings of hostility towards other people for allowing the loved one to die.

Most of these symptoms should have mostly cleared up by around 6 months after the death. In abnormal grief reactions, symptoms are prolonged for more than a year. Abnormal grief is also characterized by very marked social withdrawal, inability to concentrate and work, and by suicidal thoughts. The mortality from physical illnesses is raised.

Abnormal grief is more likely to occur when the death is sudden and unexpected, when there was an ambivalent relationship with the deceased, when the loss involves a grown-up child, and when the person has been unable to view the body or to express their grief. Abnormal grief is also more likely to occur in people who are unsupported by relatives or friends.

155 Question on p.52.

Answer A
Nicotine replacement patches plus counselling

Many studies have been done to investigate the effectiveness of smoking cessation techniques. **Advice alone** in the form of a 3-minute consultation will result in 3% of patients still not smoking at 6 months. Face to face support from a behavioural specialist will be effective in 7%.

It is now recognized that medicines to relieve the nicotine craving combined with support from a smoking cessation specialist have the best results. Some trials quote up to 20% success with **nicotine replacement patches** or **buproprion.**

Acupuncture has success in between 5% and 15% depending upon the studies. There is insufficient robust evidence on the success of **hypnotherapy.**

Buproprion has been previously used as an antidepressant. It is indicated as an aid to smoking cessation in those smoking more than 10 cigarettes a day in combination with motivational support. It is contraindicated in patients with a history of seizures or eating disorders. In addition, it should be avoided in drugs that may lower the seizure threshold, e.g.

- antidepressants
- antimalarials
- theophyllines
- corticosteroids
- tramadol.

The patient in question is likely to be taking corticosteroids and perhaps theophylline. Therefore, buproprion should be avoided. The best choice would be **nicotine replacement** therapy in the form of a patch.

156 Question on p.52.

Answer B
Hereditary spherocytosis

This patient has a Coombe's negative extravascular haemolytic anaemia. The most likely diagnosis in a patient this age is hereditary spherocytosis.

Hereditary spherocytosis is an autosomal dominant condition and is the most common inherited haemolytic anaemia. Spontaneous mutation is common and 20% of patients may have no family history at all. Hereditary spherocytosis is caused by a defect in the red cell membrane, resulting in excessive destruction of the red cells in the spleen.

Patients often present in childhood, but there is a spectrum of disease severity and it is not uncommon for patients to present in adult life. The clinical features are anaemia, jaundice and splenomegaly. Aplastic and haemolytic crises can occur. Pigment gallstones are more common, as is the case in all causes of haemolytic anaemia. Treatment is by splenectomy.

Hereditary eliptocytosis is a very similar condition to hereditary spherocytosis. However, the disease is less common and milder. Splenectomy is rarely required.

Warm agglutinin disease is an acquired autoimmune haemolytic anaemia caused by a 'warm' IgG immunoglobulin. It can occur at any age but is most common in women in their 30s or 40s. The Coomb's test is positive. Causes include SLE, lymphoma, chronic lymphocytic leukaemia, metastatic carcinoma and drugs, such as methyldopa. In the majority of patients, no cause can be found. Treatment is by immunosuppression with corticosteroids or azathioprine. Splenectomy is sometimes necessary.

Paroxysmal nocturnal haemaglobinuria is a very rare cause of intravascular haemolysis. The condition gets its name from the fact the urine voided on waking is very dark. The reason for this is not entirely clear. However, in severe cases the urine is dark all the time.

The primary defect lies in the red cell membrane that renders red cells liable to destruction by activated complement. It is more common in women and presents with haemolysis. This is often precipitated by a ➤

stressor, such as surgery or an intercurrent infection. Patients are more prone to thromboembolic disease, which may be severe and life threatening. Patients presenting with Budd–Chiari syndrome (thrombosis of the hepatic veins) should always have a prothrombotic screen including exclusion of paroxysmal nocturnal haemaglobinuria.

Long-term anticoagulation may be required in patients who develop thromboembolic disease. There is no other specific treatment for this condition.

157
Question on p.53.

Answer C
Salicylate overdose

The arterial blood gases show a mixed picture of metabolic acidosis and respiratory alkalosis.

Salicylate overdose results in a complex acid–base disturbance. Initially the drug causes centrally stimulated hyperventilation, which results in a respiratory alkalosis and is then followed by a metabolic acidosis as shown in the question.

Asthma is unlikely since it will not produce a metabolic acidosis. The hyperventilation caused by dyspnoea will result in a low CO_2 and a mild alkalosis, but the bicarbonate is too low for this to be asthma.

Chronic pulmonary emboli would not give this blood gas picture. The PO_2 will be much lower on air and hyperventilation from pulmonary emboli tends not to be seen after the acute event. An **acute pulmonary embolus** may result in a low CO_2, but one would expect the PO_2 to be lower and the low bicarbonate would not be usual.

Diabetic ketoacidosis is unlikely, as this would demonstrate a predominantly metabolic acidosis. The patient may hyperventilate and have a low CO_2 but the pH would be much lower.

158
Question on p.53.

Answer B
10%

The incidence of meningococcal septicaemia and meningitis in the UK has increased significantly in the past few decades. The incidence has increased by nearly tenfold since the early 1960s. The reasons for this are unknown.

The case fatality rate from meningococcal disease has not altered significantly during this time period and remains at just over 10%. This is despite an increased awareness of the condition by both the general public and GPs. Furthermore, in cases of suspected meningococcal disease it is now standard practice for the patient to receive parenteral antibiotics as soon as the diagnosis is suspected. This practice became established in the early 1980s but appears not to have made a major impact on the case fatality rate.

In patients with meningococcal disease, the time period from onset of symptoms to death is usually very rapid. Of the patients that die from meningococcal disease, up to 30% die on the day of admission to hospital. A total of 25% of patients who die, do so on the day following admission. A significant proportion (15–20%) of patients who die do so in the community, without ever reaching hospital. Death in the community is more common in adults than in children. This may reflect the misconception that meningococcal disease is a condition that affects children and adolescents. In fact, over 20% of cases occur in patients who are over the age of 20 years.

159
Question on p.53.

Answer E
Rheumatoid arthritis

The American College of Rheumatology have devised the following criteria for the diagnosis of **rheumatoid arthritis**:

Morning stiffness	>6 weeks
Arthritis of three or more joints	>6 weeks
Arthritis of hands and wrists	>6 weeks
Symmetrical arthritis	>6 weeks
Subcutaneous nodules	
Positive rheumatoid factor	
Erosions and or perarticular osteopenia on X-ray	

The diagnosis of rheumatoid arthritis is based on four or more of the above criteria being present.

Remember that 30% of patients will be rheumatoid factor negative.

The patient in question has four of the above criteria and, therefore, has rheumatoid arthritis.

160
Question on p.54.

Answer E
Poverty of speech on admission

The prognosis in schizophrenia is variable. On average, 20–30% of patients have a good prognosis, 20–30% continue to have mild symptoms and 40–60% are significantly affected for all of their life.

Predictors of poor outcome are:

- male
- low IQ
- abnormal pre-morbid personality
- single status
- early age of onset
➤

- insidious onset
- substance abuse
- family history of schizophrenia
- absence of obvious precipitant
- presence of negative symptoms at presentation
  - blunted affect
  - apathy
  - poverty of speech
  - attentional impairment
  - poor motivation.

The relatively young age of this patient will also be a poor prognostic feature.

161

Question on p.54.

Answer D
Multiple myeloma

Cryoglobulins are immunoglobulins that reversibly precipitate in the cold. There are three main types. Identification of the type of cryoglobulin helps allude to the underlying diagnosis.

Type I

- Monoclonal immunoglobulin – can be any but commonly IgM or IgG.
- Tends to present with acrocyonosis, Raynaud's and arterial thrombosis.
- Clinical associations – **myeloma**, Waldenstrom's macroglobulinaemia and CLL

Type II

- Polyclonal antigen + monoclonal immunoglobulin.
- Associated with lymphoproliferative disease, rheumatic disease and chronic infection.

Type III

- Polyclonal antigen + polyclonal immunoglobulin.
- Associated with rheumatic disease and chronic infection.

Type II and type III are often grouped together as 'mixed cryoglobulins' as they have similar symptomatology including arthralgia, renal disease and a purpuric rash. Currently the vast proportion of those being diagnosed as having mixed cryoglobulins are found have **chronic hepatitis C infection** and it is thought that cryoglobulins are formed as part of the immune response.

Treatment depends on the type of cryoglobulins, associations and severity of disease. Those suffering hyperviscosity and renal failure would benefit from plasmaphoresis and treatment of the underlying disease, whether this may be chemotherapy or immunosuppression.

The diagnosis here is **myeloma** as he has a monoclonal cryoglobulin.

162 Question on p.54.

Answer B
Acute inferior myocardial infarction

The key clinical findings are:

- bradycardia
- cannon waves
- hypotension
- recent history of chest pain relieved with GTN.

Cannon waves are seen in the jugular venous pulse when atrial contractions occur against a closed tricuspid valve. Causes include:

- nodal rhythm
- ventricular tachycardia
- ventricular paced rhythm
- complete heart block
- ventricular asystoles.

The right coronary artery supplies the atrioventricular node in up to 90% of people. Occlusion of this vessel will result in ischaemia of the inferior territory of the myocardium as indicated by changes in leads II, III and aVF. This may result in ischaemia of the AV node, leading to bradycardia or complete heart block.

In theory, an **overdose of β-blocker** could cause hypotension and complete heart block, but this is much less likely and would not explain the acute deterioration with chest pain.

Likewise, an acute proximal **thoracic dissection** may present in a similar way but this would be very rare. Five per cent of thoracic dissections extend down to the coronary ostia, impinging on coronary blood flow.

163 Question on p.55.

Answer E
Benign positional vertigo

All of the answers could cause nystagmus as described in the question. It is important to note that examination is normal, suggesting that the clinical signs as well as symptoms may be transient.

Benign positional vertigo (BPV) is characterized by brief attacks of rotational vertigo, precipitated by rapid head–trunk tilt toward the affected ear or by neck extension from various positions. Rotatory nystagmus may be seen during an acute attack. Symptoms usually occur a few seconds ➤

after head tilt and will last less than 40 seconds. It is the most common cause of vestibular vertigo and can occur at any time throughout life.

Menière's disease should be considered in a patient with tinnitus, fluctuating hearing loss and a feeling of fullness in the ear. Episodes of vertigo/nystagmus occur and are associated with nausea. Unlike BPV, symptoms tend to be prolonged. It tends to occur between the ages of 30 and 50.

Vestibular neuritis involves an acute onset of sustained rotatory vertigo with postural imbalance, falling towards the affected ear. Patients will have horizontal-rotatory nystagmus toward the unaffected ear and commonly feel nauseated. It is the third commonest cause of vestibular vertigo and affects patients aged 30–60 years.

Vestibular migraine is also known as basilar migraine with episodic vertigo lasting a few minutes to several hours. There is an increased tendency to motion sickness during and after the attack. A total of 66% of cases are associated with headache; 33% may experience dysarthria, tinnitus, decreased hearing, diplopia, ataxia, bilateral paraesthesia or decreased level of conscious. It occurs in up to 8% of migraine sufferers with a mean age of presentation at 40 years of age.

A **cerebello-pontine angle lesion** is unlikely to be the cause of this patient's dizziness. CPA lesions are likely to have several hard neurological signs on cranial nerve examination, including absent corneal reflex, diminished hearing and facial nerve palsy.

164

Question on p.55.

Answer D
Send stool for immediate microscopy and, if negative for amoebic cysts, start intravenous hydrocortisone

The differential diagnosis in this patient lies between acute severe ulcerative colitis presenting for the first time and infective colitis. It is often not possible to be sure which of these two that you are dealing with until the results of the rectal biopsies and stool cultures are known.

Clinical features, which favour a diagnosis of ulcerative colitis (UC), rather than an infective cause are:

• Onset – gradual in UC
• Pain – usually absent in UC
• Fever – low-grade or absent in UC
• Infectious contacts – usually none in UC

It is important to start treatment as soon as possible because, if this patient has UC, any delay in treatment may be hazardous. This patient is opening her bowels 15 times per day and, if this is due to UC, this makes the diagnosis that of acute severe ulcerative colitis. This condition can rapidly progress to toxic dilatation and perforation and needs to be treated promptly with high-dose intravenous corticosteroids. It is, therefore, inappropriate to delay treatment until the **biopsy and culture results** are available.

Intravenous corticosteroids can be hazardous when given to patients with infective colitis. However, it seems to be safe to use this drug in patients with this kind of presentation whilst awaiting biopsy and culture results, providing the colitis is not caused by amoebic dysentery. The best answer is therefore D.

165	Question on p.56.

Answer B
Squamous cell carcinoma

There is nothing to suggest that this man is at risk of **tuberculosis** and this is unlikely to be the best answer. Although tuberculosis is a cause of dyspnoea, weight loss and cavitation on a chest X-ray, lung cancer is much more likely. A total of 33 000 adults are diagnosed annually in the UK with lung cancer compared to 7000 new cases of tuberculosis. This question is really asking which histological type of lung cancer causes cavitation on the chest X-ray.

Lung cancer is divided into small cell carcinoma or non small-cell carcinoma.

Small-cell carcinoma (also known as oat cell) accounts for 20–30% of all lung cancers. It arises from Kulchitsky cells, which are endocrine cells that make up part of the amine precursor uptake and decarboxylation (APUD) system. This explains why small-cell carcinomas frequently have endocrine-related non-metastatic complications, such as SIADH, gynaecomastia etc. This is a rapidly growing, highly malignant tumour, although it is the most responsive, of all the lung cancers, to chemotherapy.

The non-small-cell carcinomas include squamous, large-cell, adenocarcinoma and alveolar cell carcinoma.

Squamous or **epidermoid carcinoma** is the most common histology and accounts for 40% of lung cancers. Situated centrally it may cause bronchial obstruction, which leads to infection. This explains why so many lung cancers are diagnosed after presenting as pneumonia. Widespread metastases tend to occur late and its main symptoms are related to local spread. Ten per cent of cases demonstrate cavitation at presentation.

Large-cell carcinoma accounts for 25% of all lung cancers. It tends to metastasize early.

Adenocarcinomas arise peripherally from mucous glands in the small bronchi. Their incidence has increased over recent years and this is attributed to smokers converting to low-tar cigarettes. People tend to inhale more deeply with low-tar brands and this will disperse carcinogens more peripherally. They account for 10% of lung cancers and commonly metastasize to brain and bone. Owing to their peripheral position, invasion of the pleural wall is common. It is the most likely of the lung cancers to develop following asbestos exposure. ➤

Alveolar cell carcinoma accounts for 1–2% of lung cancers. It occurs as a solitary nodule or as diffuse nodular lesions. Patients may produce large quantities of mucoid sputum.

Causes of a cavitating lung lesion on X-ray
- Abscess
- Squamous carcinoma
- Tuberculosis
- Wegener's granulomatosis
- Fungal infection
- Pulmonary infarction
- Hydatid cyst

166
Question on p.56.

Answer B
Subthalamic nucleus

Hemiballismus is characterized by the sudden flinging movement of a limb. It usually occurs in elderly hypertensive and/or diabetic patients as a result of a stroke. The vascular lesion usually affects the **subthalamic nucleus**, although lesions at other anatomical sites may be responsible. It often appears as the hemiplegic weakness improves and may be accompanied by thalamic pain. In other patients the hemiballism appears abruptly without weakness or sensory deficit.

The **caudate nucleus** along with the putamen is the main area affected in patients with Huntington's disease.

The **basal ganglia** and **substantia nigra** are involved in Parkinson's disease. Parkinson's disease classically demonstrates degeneration of the dopaminergic nigrostriatal pathway. In particular, the ventral tier of the zona compacta of the substantia nigra undergoes degeneration, and there is a reduction of dopamine in the striatum. The loss is predominantly posterior in the putamen, extending forward into the anterior putamen and the caudate. In most cases of Parkinson's disease, Lewy bodies can be found in the substantia nigra.

Recent functional imaging studies have implicated the **red nucleus** in the pathophysiology of benign essential tremor along with the cerebellum and the thalamus.

167
Question on p.56

Answer D
1 in 18

The lifetime risk of asymptomatic individuals with a family history of colorectal cancer is given below.

Family history	Lifetime risk
None	1 in 25
One first-degree relative > 45 years	1 in 18
One first-degree relative < 45 years	1 in 10
Two first-degree relatives	1 in 6

Screening colonoscopy is currently recommended for patients who have a first-degree relative affected < 45 years or two first-degree relatives of any age. The screening should start at age 40 years or 10 years before the index case, whichever is sooner.

Colonoscopic screening is also recommended in patients with the following.

A family history of hereditary non-polyposis colon cancer

This causes mainly right-sided tumours, which often occur at a relatively young age (30–40 years). First-degree relatives should be offered screening colonoscopy from the age of 25 years or 10 years younger than the index case, whichever is sooner. Colonoscopy should be repeated at least every 3 years and possibly yearly in patients who are perceived to be at highest risk. Family members should also be tested for microsatellite instability and germline mutations of the DNA mismatch repair genes.

A family history of familial adenomatous polyposis

Patients should be offered genetic testing at puberty to identify gene carriers. Carriers and indeterminate carriers should be offered an annual screening flexible sigmoidoscopy beginning at puberty. Patients who are found to have multiple adenomas are offered panproctocolectomy, as the lifetime risk of colorectal cancer in such patients is 100%.

Patients with familial adenomatous polyposis are at increased risk of developing upper gastrointestinal malignancies. They are particularly prone to develop carcinoma of the duodenum as adenomas grow in the second part of the duodenum and the ampulla of Vater. Such patients should, therefore, also have screening upper gastrointestinal endoscopies to detect early malignant change.

Inflammatory bowel disease

Patients with ulcerative colitis and Crohn's colitis are at increased risk of colorectal cancer. The risk in patients with Crohn's colitis is of a similar magnitude to that in patients with ulcerative colitis. The risk in ulcerative colitis depends on the extent of the disease. Patients with panulcerative colitis have a lifetime risk approaching 1 in 10. Patients with limited left-sided disease have a risk similar to that in the general population. Patients with extensive UC and Crohn's colitis are offered screening colonoscopy every 3 years after 8 years from diagnosis and every 2 years after 20 years. Multiple biopsies are taken to check for dysplastic change.

168   Question on p.56.

Answer E
Glomerulonephritis

This is a difficult question and is best approached by excluding answers that are incorrect.

The answer is not **essential hypertension,** as one would not expect significant proteinuria in this condition. It would also be very uncommon in someone of this age.

The answer is not **gestational hypertension**, as this can only be diagnosed from 20 weeks of pregnancy onwards.

The answer is not **pre-eclampsia**, as this can only be diagnosed in the second or third trimester.

The **blood pressure** falls in normal pregnancy and a reading of 148/90 mmHg is abnormal.

By exclusion, the correct answer, therefore, is **glomerulonephritis**. This condition is not more common in pregnancy.

169   Question on p.57.

Answer D
Clinical features worsen in subsequent generations

The **worsening of clinical features in subsequent generations** is a characteristic feature of this group of disorders and is known as anticipation. The phenomenon has been recognized for many years and it was used in the past as an argument in favour of preventing those with mental retardation from reproducing. It was over 50 years before an explanation for this observation emerged.

The DNA triplet repeat sequences are known to be unstable and typically expand in successive meioses. The size of the expansion correlates broadly with the severity of the clinical features of the disorder, so explaining the progressively increasing severity and earlier age of onset from one generation to the next.

The inheritance pattern of many trinucleotide repeat disorders is autosomal dominant, but there are also X-linked and autosomal recessive conditions (see table). The exact sequence that is repeated is also variable (see table) but the commonest is a CAG repeat resulting in an expanded tract of glutamine residues in the protein.

Infertility is not a typical feature of any of the disorders and, in most cases, males and females are equally affected. The exceptions to this are the X-linked disorders spinobulbar muscular atrophy (Kennedy's disease) and Fragile X. Spinobulbar muscular atrophy may be confused with motor neurone disease but can usually be distinguished by its more prolonged course. Female carriers may occasionally develop some mild clinical features but subclinical abnormalities on neurophysiological testing are probably more frequent.

Fragile X is a frequent cause of mental retardation affecting about 1 in 5000 males. Clinical features include accelerated growth, characteristic facies and macro-orchidism in post-pubertal males, and there may be a visible fragile site near the end of the long arm of the X chromosome. While both males and females can be symptomatic, as a general rule the mental retardation is more profound in males.

In some of the disorders there can be a difference in severity depending on whether it has been inherited from the mother or the father. The classic example is myotonic dystrophy where affected women, even those mildly affected themselves, have a high risk that an affected child will have the severe childhood or congenital form of the condition. This risk is especially high if the woman already has one such affected child but relatively low if she has no evidence of neuromuscular disease. There is a low risk that this form of the condition will affect offspring of affected males. The explanation for this seems to lie in the fact that the severity of the mother's symptoms correlates with the size of her expansion. The severe, congenital form is usually due to a large expansion and expansions greater than a certain size cannot be transmitted by sperm. In contrast, the juvenile form of Huntington's disease is almost always paternally transmitted.

Trinucleotide repeat disorder	Inheritance pattern	Triplet repeat sequence
Myotonic dystrophy	AD	CTG
Huntington's disease	AD	CAG
Fragile X	X-Linked	CGG
Friedreich's ataxia	AR	
Spinobulbar muscular atrophy	X-Linked	CAG
Spinocerebellar ataxias	AD	CAG

170
Question on p.57.

Answer D
40 hours

Warfarin has a half-life of 40 hours. The clinical relevance of this is that changes made to the warfarin dosage will not affect the INR for 2 days. This must be borne in mind when deciding the correct dosage to prescribe for a patient when serial INRs and previous dosages are considered.

171
Question on p.57.

Answer C
Albendazole

This boy has a symptomatic liver cyst. The differential diagnosis of a liver cyst includes a simple cyst, pyogenic or amoebic abscess, hydatid cyst or a necrotic tumour. The story that would fit best here is a hydatid cyst. ➤

Hydatid disease occurs when there is ingestion of *Echinococcus* eggs normally transmitted from dog faeces. The disease tends to be more prevalent in areas of sheep farming, i.e. Australia and Argentina. However, it is becoming more apparent in countries such as Russia and China. Typically eggs migrate from the gut through the wall of the gut and into the portal system where they are then carried to the liver. Here they form single thick-walled cysts that often contain smaller 'daughter' cysts. Cysts tend to occur in the liver but can be seen in any organ, e.g. brain, lung.

Diagnosis is aided by hydatid complement fixation test. Surgery to remove the cyst can be used, firstly injecting the cyst with formalin or alcohol to sterilize it. **Albendazole**, which penetrates the cyst, is the medical treatment of choice.

Praziquantel is used in helminthic infections such as Schistosomiasis and Cestodes (*Taenia*).

Metronidazole is an azole antibiotic used in the treatment of anaerobic and protozoal infections such as *Bacteroides*, *Giardia* and amoebiasis. Side effects include a disulphiram-like effect and peripheral neuropathy with long-term treatment.

Pentamidine is a drug used in the treatment of African trypanosomiasis and *Pneumocystis carinii* pneumonia occurring in the immunocompromised. Side effects include nephrotoxicity and pancreatic damage causing sudden hypoglycaemia by means of insulin release.

Doxycycline is a tetracycline antibiotic, it has a wide spectrum of activity against nearly all Gram-positive and Gram-negative bacteria. It is the drug of choice for infection with chlamydia, mycoplasma, rickettsiae, *Vibrio cholera* and borrelia. Side effects include dental enamel hypoplasia (contraindicated in pregnancy) and a rise in blood urea by means of inhibiting protein synthesis.

---

172 Question on p.57.

Answer B
Isoniazid

Hydralazine was the first drug that was found to cause an SLE-like syndrome with a positive ANA. The patients usually have a mild form of SLE characterized by arthritis, rash and fever. The disease usually disappears on stopping the drug. A number of other drugs have since been found to produce a similar picture and these include the following

Drugs causing an SLE-like picture
- Procainamide
- **Isoniazid**
- Chlorpromazine
- D-Penicillamine
- Sulphasalazine
- Sulphonamide
- Quinidine
- Methyldopa

The main side effects of the other drugs in the question are as follows:

- **Penicillin** – allergic/anaphylactic reaction in 1 in 50 000
- **Methotrexate**
  - liver fibrosis/cirrhosis after a cumulative dose of 5 g
  - bone marrow suppression
  - pulmonary fibrosis
- **Doxazosin** – well tolerated
- **Flecainide** – nausea, blurred vision, abnormal taste

---

173 Question on p.58.

Answer B
Pigmented retinopathy

Kearns–Sayre syndrome is one of the mitochondrial inherited diseases, which is covered in more detail in another question. Clinical features include small stature, retinitis pigmentosa (RP), ophthalmoplegia, bilateral ptosis, ataxia, diabetes, hearing loss and cardiac defects.

Conditions associated with **retinitis pigmentosa** include:

- congenital RP
- (Laurence–Moon) Bardet–Biedl syndrome
- Usher's syndrome
- abetalipoproteinaemia
- Refsum's disease
- Kearns–Sayre
- Friedreich's ataxia.

Causes of **blue sclerae** include:

- osteogenesis imperfecta
- pseudoxanthoma elasticum
- Ehlers–Danlos syndrome
- hyperthyroidism
- Marfan's syndrome.

➤

Loss of red reflex on fundoscopy suggests cataracts. Causes of cataracts include:

- diabetes
- steroids
- hypoparathyroidism
- myotonia dystrophica
- Down's syndrome
- Di George's syndrome
- Cushing's disease
- Rubella
- Galactosaemia
- Hurler's syndrome
- Refsum's disease
- (Laurence–Moon) Bardet–Biedl
- congenital hypothyroidism.

Angioid streaks are due to elastic fragmentation of Bruch's membrane and appear as dark lines radiating from the optic disc. These retinal streaks vary in colour from dark red or maroon to black. Causes are:

- pseudoxanthoma elasticum
- Ehlers–Danlos syndrome
- Paget's disease
- acromegaly
- sickle cell anaemia
- diabetic retinopathy
- neurofibromatosis
- hypercalcaemia
- lead poisoning
- tuberous sclerosis.

Causes of **optic atrophy** are:

- Hereditary
  - Friedreich's ataxia
  - Diabetes insipidus, diabetes mellitus, optic atrophy and deafness (DIDMOAD)
  - Leber's congenital amaurosis
- Acquired
  - glaucoma
  - retinal artery occlusion
  - multiple sclerosis
  - pituitary tumour
  - diabetes
  - tobacco/alcohol amblyopia
  - chronic papilloedema.

Answer C
Autoimmune chronic active hepatitis

This patient has abnormal liver biochemistry and a very raised IgG, which is characteristic of **autoimmune hepatitis**.

In patients with **primary biliary cirrhosis**, the IgM is elevated and in patients with alcoholic liver disease the IgA is often raised.

In **primary sclerosing cholangitis**, the alkaline phosphatase is disproportionately elevated and the immunoglobulins are usually normal.

In **non-alcoholic steatohepatitis**, there is usually an isolated rise in the ALT and the immunoglobulins are also normal.

Autoimmune hepatitis is more common in women and is characterized by hyperglobulinaemia, circulating autoantibodies and histological evidence of hepatitis with piecemeal necrosis.

Classification of autoimmune hepatitis

Autoimmune hepatitis is classified according to the circulating antibodies present.

	Antibodies
Type 1	Antinuclear antibody > 1:320
	Smooth muscle antibody > 1:320
Type 2	Anti-liver/kidney microsomal antibody (Anti LKM-1)
Seronegative	Nil

Patients usually present with non-specific symptoms of malaise. Occasionally, there is a more fulminant presentation with jaundice, a very high ALT and abnormal synthetic function (raised INR and reduced albumin). The diagnosis is based on a combination of the liver histology and the typical antibody profile. There are a group of patients who are seronegative. In these patients, the diagnosis is based on a high index of clinical suspicion, suggestive histology and exclusion of other possible diagnoses, such as chronic hepatitis C, acute viral hepatitis (A, B, C, E and EBV), primary biliary cirrhosis, primary sclerosing cholangitis and drug-induced hepatitis.

Autoimmune hepatitis is steroid sensitive. Patients are started on 30 mg of prednisolone for 1 month and then azathioprine is introduced as a steroid-sparing agent. The dose of steroids is gradually reduced over the next few months with close monitoring of the liver function tests to ensure that the disease remains in remission whilst this is being done.

Patients are treated with the lowest dose of prednisolone that keeps their LFTs normal plus azathioprine for 12–18 months. At the end of this time, a further biopsy is performed. If the patient has no inflammation, the prednisolone is withdrawn but the azathioprine continued. Recent data ➤

suggest that it may be safe to withdraw the azathioprine in patients with no liver inflammation after 4 years. However, most patients are treated with lifelong immunosuppression. Patients with type 2 disease are more likely to fail to respond to the above therapy and generally have more aggressive disease.

175
Question on p.58.

Answer D
Cerebral toxoplasmosis

New onset of fits in a known HIV-positive patient requires some form of imaging for a diagnosis. The diagnosis could either be cerebral **toxoplasmosis** or cerebral **lymphoma**, as they both cause multiple ring-enhancing lesions and present in a similar fashion. However, to differentiate the two would either involve performing a brain biopsy or treating and rescanning to monitor improvement. The latter of these is preferable, as biopsying the brain carries significant morbidity.

Forty-five per cent of AIDS patients who are positive for toxoplasmosis antibodies will develop cerebral disease (50% of the general population are antibody positive). Patients can present with headaches, confusion, focal signs or seizures. Treatment is with pyrimethamine and sulphadiazine. If there is no response to treatment, the alternative diagnosis of lymphoma is made.

Progressive multifocal leucoencephalopathy (PML) presents with focal signs, changes in personality and confusion. Seizures are uncommon. CT shows areas of abnormal signal in the white matter. There is no enhancement.

Patients with HIV are at higher risk of TB. **Tuberculomas** are ring-enhancing on CT and can often be multiple, but are much less common than toxoplasmosis.

Focal **cryptococcal** infection can present with seizures but this infection more frequently presents with meningitis in these patients.

176
Question on p.59.

Answer C
Ulnar nerve lesion

The main differential diagnosis in a patient who has wasting of the small muscles of the hand lies between a T1 root lesion and an ulnar nerve lesion. Sensory loss is sometimes helpful but is not always reliable. Assessment of motor function is usually the best way of distinguishing between the two.

	T1 Root lesion	Ulnar nerve lesion
Sensory loss	Medial aspect upper arm	Medial aspect of hand
Motor loss	All the small muscles of the hand especially abductor pollicis brevis	All the small muscles of the hand except **LOAF** **L** – lateral two lumbricals **O** – opponens pollicis **A** – abductor pollicis brevis **F** – flexor pollicis brevis

N.B. The muscles of **LOAF** are supplied by the median nerve.

The answer in this case is, therefore, an ulnar nerve lesion, as the patient does not have weakness in the LOAF muscles.

A **median nerve lesion** causes weakness in the LOAF muscles and sensory loss on the lateral aspect of the palmar surface of the hand.

A **C7 root lesion** causes weakness in shoulder adduction, elbow and wrist extension and wrist flexion. Typically the triceps reflex is absent. There may be sensory loss over the C7 dermatome (middle finger).

A lesion of the **lower trunk of the brachial plexus** (Klumpke paralysis) is usually caused by trauma, and results in a lesion in the C8 and T1 root distribution. There is loss of motor function of all the small muscles of the hand, and the long finger flexors and extensors.

177   Question on p.59.

Answer C
Low-molecular-weight heparin

The question states that this lady has had a significant pulmonary embolus and so she must receive some form of treatment to prevent further embolic events. The best therapy needs to be assessed on grounds of safety and efficacy.

Aspirin is of little benefit here. It will decrease platelet activity and adhesion, but will not impact on the coagulation system.

Warfarin is teratogenic and should not be given in the first trimester of pregnancy. In addition it crosses the placenta with risk of placental or fetal haemorrhage, especially during the last few weeks of pregnancy and at delivery. For this patient, in her second trimester, warfarin could be used for a short while, if there were no other alternatives. However as a general rule it is best to avoid warfarin in pregnancy if at all possible.

Heparins have been used safely in pregnancy, although osteoporosis has been reported with prolonged use. **Unfractionated heparin** needs to be given subcutaneously twice a day and is more of a burden than the once daily **low-molecular-weight heparin**. Low-molecular-weight heparin is commonly given during the pregnancies of females with known thrombophilias. ➤

Caval filters are umbrella-like devices that may be placed into the inferior vena cava under radiological guidance. The intention is to catch any thrombus that may travel from the venous system and prevent it reaching the lungs. This is not the best choice in this patient. It is an invasive procedure and does not completely abolish the risk of thromboembolism. In addition, some post-mortem studies have suggested that the relative stasis distal to the filter may cause thrombus formation on the other side of the filter, which could cause pulmonary emboli. Filters are often used temporarily and are difficult or impossible to remove after a few weeks due to intimal overgrowth.

178
Question on p.59.

Answer A
A 52-year-renal transplant recipient with a 1-day history of flu-like symptoms

Zanamivir is a drug used in the treatment of influenza. It reduces the replication of influenza A and B viruses by inhibiting viral neuraminidase. It is licensed for the treatment of influenza within 48 hours of first symptoms and the National Institute for Clinical Excellence (NICE) has recommended its use in at-risk individuals.

At-risk individuals are defined as those over 65 years or those who have one or more of the following conditions:

- chronic respiratory disease (including COPD and asthma)
- significant cardiovascular disease (excluding hypertension)
- chronic renal disease
- immunosuppression
- diabetes mellitus.

Zanamivir should be used with caution in asthma and COPD because there is a risk of bronchospasm. If necessary, short-acting bronchodilators should be available. In severe asthma, it should be avoided unless there can be close monitoring and appropriate facilities to treat bronchospasm.

179
Question on p.59.

Answer A
Ankylosing spondylitis

Most common disorders, unlike single-gene disorders, do not follow straightforward Mendelian patterns of inheritance (autosomal dominant, autosomal recessive, X-linked or mitochondrial). This is true for the more common birth defects, such as neural tube defects, as well as many chronic disorders of later life, such as diabetes mellitus. However, it has long been clear that, to some extent, they do show a familial tendency. Polygenic inheritance and multifactorial inheritance are both terms that have been used to describe the underlying genetic basis of these conditions but there are subtle differences in their true meanings.

Polygenic inheritance implies that there are many genes at different loci, each of which has a small but additive effect.

Multifactorial (also called complex) inheritance is the type of non-Mendelian inheritance shown by traits that are determined by a combination of multiple factors, both genetic and environmental. The relative role of each category can be widely variable for different conditions.

The best way to answer this question is to exclude any condition that you know is a single-gene disorder.

Friedreich's ataxia is autosomal recessive and **Huntington's disease, acute intermittent porphyria** and **achondroplasia** are autosomal dominant conditions.

This leaves **ankylosing spondylitis**, a chronic inflammatory disease of the spine and sacroiliac joints. There is a very strong association between the HLA allele B27 such that over 95% of AS patients are HLA B27-positive compared with less than 10% in the general population. This gives a relative risk of developing the condition of over 150 for people who carry the B27 allele compared with those who do not. However, less than 5% of all individuals who are HLA B27-positive will actually develop ankylosing spondylitis, although up to 20% of them may have very subtle, subclinical signs of the condition and remain asymptomatic.

Other conditions with a multifactorial inheritance include:

- cleft palate
- schizophrenia
- pyloric stenosis
- autism
- diabetes mellitus
- Crohn's disease
- multiple sclerosis
- coronary heart disease
- neural tube defects
- Hirschsprung's disease.

180 Question on p.60.

Answer A
19.2

$$\text{Number needed to treat (NNT)} = \frac{1}{\text{Absolute risk reduction (ARR)}}$$

$$ARR = \text{Control event rate} - \text{experimental event rate}$$
$$= 13.2\% - 8\%$$
$$= 5.2\%$$

Thus

$$NNT = \frac{1}{5.2\%}$$

$$\frac{1}{0.052}$$

$$NNT = 19.2$$

Answer C
Pathergy

Pathergy is when a sterile subcutaneous puncture, e.g. venepuncture, results in a sterile pustule after 24–48 hours. It is virtually pathopnemonic for Beçhet's disease, and is used as a diagnostic test in Middle Eastern countries and Japan.

Dermatomyositis is an inflammatory disease of the skin and striated muscle. It predominantly affects adults between the ages of 40 and 60, and is twice as common in females. It commonly presents with a rash on sun-exposed areas, general malaise and proximal muscle weakness. Rarely patients may have a diffuse arthralgia, Raynaud's phenomenon, dyspnoea and speech/swallowing difficulties.

The most common clinical signs are as follows:

- heliotrope rash
- Gottron's papules
- prominent nailfold capillaries
- proximal muscle weakness.

It is associated with underlying carcinoma or lymphoma.

Patients with malignancy are highly prothrombotic and anyone presenting with **venous thromboembolism** without obvious cause should be considered for underlying malignancy. The most highly thrombotic tumours include brain, pancreas, lung and kidney. Armand Trousseau first described the association between malignancy and thromboembolic disease, noting that the thrombosis was often superficial, migratory and often in unusual sites, e.g. upper arm.

Bullous pyoderma gangrenosum is a feature of leukaemia and myeloma.

Palmar keratoses are associated with carcinoma of the bladder or lung.

Dermatosis	Underlying tumour
Acanthosis nigricans	Lung, liver, gastrointestinal
Paget's disease of the nipple	Ductal breast carcinoma
Dermatomyositis	Lung, gastrointestinal, genitourinary
Erythema gyratum repens	Lung, breast
Tylosis	Oesophagus
Ichythyosis	Lymphoma
Necrolytic migratory erythema	Glucagonoma
Erythroderma	Lymphoma, leukaemia

182
Question on p.60.

Answer C
Upper GI endoscopy

This gentleman has polycythaemia, it may be primary, i.e. rubra vera, or secondary. The diagnosis is by demonstrating a raised haemoglobin and PCV/haematocrit. The WCC is often raised (70%) as are the platelets (30%).

This patient's haematocrit is elevated as are the white cell count and the platelets as one would expect in polycythaemia. However, the haemoglobin is much lower than one would anticipate in a patient with polycythaemia. Moreover, the MCV is low and causes of a low MCV include iron-deficiency anaemia. This gentleman actually has a relative anaemia given a previous diagnosis of polycythaemia, hence he needs investigation of his GI tract.

Patients with polycythaemia are more prone to develop peptic ulceration. It is, therefore, reasonable to perform an **upper GI endoscopy** as the first step. If this proves to be normal it would be important to then visualize the large bowel by either barium enema or colonoscopy.

Treatment consists of trying to maintain a normal haemoglobin and prevent thrombosis or haemorrhage. **Venesection** is normally successful, but is limited by iron deficiency. **Chemotherapy** with either hydoxyurea or busulphan is used successfully for those refractory to venesection or where it is contraindicated.

183
Question on p.61.

Answer A
Solitary parathyroid adenoma

Primary hyperparathyroidism and hypercalcaemia of malignancy are by far the most common cause of hypercalcaemia, accounting for about 90% of cases. In a case like this, the next step is to measure the PTH. If it is elevated, the diagnosis is likely to be primary hyperparathyroidism. If it is suppressed, it is likely to be malignancy. ➤

Causes of hypercalcaemia
- **Excess parathyroid hormone (PTH) secretion**
  - Primary hyperparathyroidism, e.g. adenoma, hyperplasia, carcinoma
  - Tertiary hyperparathyroidism
  - Ectopic PTH secretion
- **Malignancy**
  - Bony secondaries
  - PTH-related protein secretion
- **Excess action of Vitamin D**
  - Granulomatous disease, e.g. sarcoid
  - Lymphoma
- **Others**
  - Thyrotoxicosis
  - Familial hypocalciuric hypercalcaemia
  - Milk alkali syndrome
  - Vitamin D analogues
  - Thiazide diuretics

A calcium this high could be secondary to malignancy. This could either be due to secondary deposits in the bone, or more rarely due to ectopic PTH secretion. In the former, the PTH is normal and, in the latter, the PTH is elevated. True ectopic PTH secretion is, however, very rare and most cases are due to secretion of **PTH-related protein**.

Primary hyperparathyroidism can be caused by a **single solitary adenoma** (> 80%), **hyperplasia** (15–20%) or more rarely by **multiple adenomas**.

Parathyroid carcinoma accounts for less than 1% of all causes of hyperparathyroidism.

The correct answer is, therefore, single solitary parathyroid adenoma.

---

184 Question on p.61.

Answer B
Goodpasture's disease

The main differential diagnosis in a patient of this age with pulmonary and renal involvement is between Goodpasture's disease and Wegener's granulomatosis.

Patients with **Goodpasture's disease** usually have pulmonary symptoms for a month or so before the onset of glomerulonephritis. Presentation is usually with cough, haemoptysis and a systemic illness. The CXR typically shows transient blotchy shadowing owing to pulmonary haemorrhage. It occurs in adults at any age and is an autoimmune-mediated process. The circulating autoantibody is directed against the basement membrane (anti-GBM), which is present in both kidney and lung.

Wegener's granulomatosis can cause a very similar picture. However, the CXR changes in this case are more suggestive of Goodpasture's disease. In Wegener's granulomatosis the CXR characteristically shows single or multiple nodular masses, or infiltrates with cavitation. These CXR changes tend to come and go in a very transient manner.

Alveolar cell carcinoma accounts for 1% of malignant bronchial tumours. Patients often complain of huge volume sputum production and dyspnoea. The CXR shows single or multiple nodular shadows. It does not cause renal disease *per se*. However, in end-stage disease, renal dysfunction is more common. This is a very unlikely explanation to the question, as the patient has only been unwell for 1 month.

Systemic lupus erythematosus could also cause this picture. However, the patient is the wrong age and sex, and pulmonary involvement in SLE is usually either pleurisy or pleural effusions.

Post-streptococcal glomerulonephritis does not affect the lung.

---

185 Question on p.61.

Answer E
Amyloidosis

The term cardiomyopathy refers to a disease of the heart muscle itself. Infiltration of the cardiac muscle is seen in a few, relatively rare conditions. The diagnosis is suggested by the overall clinical picture, echocardiographic and angiographic findings. It is sometimes necessary to perform an endomyocardial biopsy to confirm the diagnosis. All the alternatives listed in the question are potential causes of an infiltrating cardiomyopathy but, of these, **amyloid** is the most common.

Amyloidosis affecting the heart is usually of AL origin, formally known as primary amyloidosis. The heart is stiff due to infiltration of amyloid protein between the myocardial cells. Patients normally present with congestive cardiac failure, but with a normally sized heart on CXR. Arrhythmias are common. The patients tolerate atrial fibrillation poorly. It is important to note that they are very sensitive to digoxin, which is best avoided in this situation. Other common arrhythmias include sinus arrest and AV block. The clinical picture can be difficult to differentiate from constrictive pericarditis. Echocardiography and cardiac catheterization can usually make this differentiation. Patients often have extracardiac features of AL amyloid. These symptoms include macroglossia and peripheral neuropathy. No treatment has been shown to slow the relentless progression of the disease.

Patients with AA amyloid have amyloid deposition secondary to a chronic inflammatory disease, such as rheumatoid arthritis or Crohn's disease. This often presents due to renal involvement, as a nephrotic syndrome. Cardiac involvement is much less common.

Small deposits of amyloid are found in the hearts of 80% of very elderly patients at post-mortem. This is not thought to have any clinical significance. ➤

Endomyocardial fibrosis and **Loeffler's eosinophilic endocarditis** are thought to be the same condition. There is infiltration of the myocardium by eosinophils, which causes fibrosis. The ventricular cavities become small in size and systemic emboli are common. This syndrome can be seen in equatorial Africa and is thought to be infective in origin. An identical picture is seen in eosinophilic leukaemia.

Five per cent of patients with **sarcoid** have cardiac involvement. The commonest cardiac problem is complete AV block. This occurs in up to 30% and is caused by granulomatous infiltration at the AV node.

In **scleroderma** focal fibrosis occurs in the myocardial cells, with associated microvascular involvement. This results in a restrictive or dilated cardiomyopathy. Conduction defects are common.

Causes of an infiltrating restrictive cardiomyopathy
- Amyloid
- Haemochromatosis
- Sarcoid
- Scleroderma
- Eosinophilic heart disease (Loeffler's)

---

186 Question on p.62.

Answer E
Contains heparin

Total parenteral nutrition (TPN) is reserved for patients who either do not have a functioning gut or where insufficient nutrition is absorbed through the gut, i.e. short bowel syndrome. Careful consideration must be given prior to commencing TPN since its administration has potential complications.

TPN comprises various nutritional elements as follows.

Energy
Glucose is the **main form of nutrition** with added calories coming from fat. Since soya fat is used it does not exclude its use in **vegans**.

Nitrogen
Synthetic L-amino acid solutions are used providing 9–17 g/L of nitrogen.

Electrolytes and trace elements
Electrolytes should initially be monitored daily, magnesium and calcium every other day. If long-term therapy is needed, a **trace element solution** can be added to the TPN.

> **Complications of TPN**
> - Catheter related
>   - Immediate (pneumothorax, air embolism)
>   - Chronic (sepsis)
> - Metabolic – hyperglycaemia (often requiring insulin)
> - Electrolyte disturbances
> - Hypocalcaemia
> - Liver dysfunction
> - Refeeding syndrome

187   Question on p.62.

Answer C
Had oesophageal pH and manometry studies

Gastro-oesophageal reflux disease (GORD) is a very common clinical problem. Typically the patient complains of positionally dependent retrosternal burning discomfort with or without an acid taste in the back of the mouth (water brash). In patients with GORD, typical features of reflux oesophagitis are seen at endoscopy in only 50% of patients. A normal upper gastrointestinal endoscopy does not, therefore, exclude the diagnosis of GORD.

The vast majority of patients will get good or complete symptomatic relief from full-dose proton pump inhibition, with or without the addition of promotility agents such as metoclopramide. However, when the proton pump inhibitor is withdrawn or the dose reduced, the symptoms promptly return. A common indication for considering a laparoscopic fundoplication is a patient in early adulthood with reflux symptoms fully responsive to proton pump inhibition who does not wish to stay on these drugs indefinitely.

All patients require **oesophageal manometry and pH studies**. There are a number of patients with reflux symptoms; particularly those who make only a partial response to proton pump inhibitors, who have a coexisting oesophageal motility problem. Performing a fundoplication on such patients produces disappointing results and may worsen the patient's original symptoms.

Following a fundoplication, in carefully selected patients, 95% of patients can discontinue proton pump inhibitors indefinitely. Complications include gas-bloat symptoms in 10% and dysphagia in approximately 2–3%. These symptoms are occasionally severe enough to warrant reoperation and taking down the fundal wrap. The incidence of these two common complications can be minimized by careful patient selection and meticulous attention to surgical technique by ensuring the wrap is not too tight.

188 Question on p.62.

Answer D
Ceftazidime

The treatment of cystic fibrosis (CF) has progressed such that now 90% of children survive into their teens and the median survival is now 40 years. The major hazard facing CF patients is infection with *Burkholderia cepacia*, previously known as *Pseudomonas cepacia*. Infection with this organism is associated with rapid acceleration of the disease and progression to death.

Transmission is from person to person and multiple drug resistance is common. It has been found that groups set up to support patients with CF can be a common place for transmission to occur and patients known to be colonized with the organism need to be excluded from these groups. Likewise colonized patients must be segregated during inpatient stays from other CF patients.

It is likely that this patient is now colonized and the choice of antibiotic needs to cover *Burkholderia cepacia* as well as normal infecting agents. The drug of choice is a third-generation cephalosporin such as **ceftazidime**.

Vancomycin has a narrow range of activity against Staphylococci and Streptococci and is often used in combination with other drugs.

Aztreonam is a β-lactam with good activity against Gram-negative aerobes including *Pseudomonas aeruginosa, Neisseria meningitides* and *Haemophilus influenzae*, but not *Burkholderia cepacia*. It should not be used 'blind', since it is not active against Gram-positive organisms.

Clarithromycin, a macrolide has no activity against *Pseudomonas* species.

Tobramycin is similar to gentamicin in action. It has good activity against Gram-negative aerobes including *Pseudomonas*, but this alone will not cover Gram-positive organisms.

189 Question on p.62.

Answer C
Eosinophilic inclusion bodies

This man has parkinsonism as demonstrated by his shuffling gait, increased tone and worsening of symptoms on haloperidol. He does, however, have other symptoms and signs and, therefore, he has one of the Parkinson's plus syndromes.

This is the name given to a group of disorders with parkinsonian symptoms but with additional features. In this case there are additional features of dementia, visual hallucinations and labile affect. This suggests the diagnosis of Lewy body dementia, which is characterized by **eosinophilic inclusion bodies**. Treatment is with conventional anti-

Parkinson's drugs, although this can worsen psychiatric symptoms. Avoidance of dopamine agonists is necessary. Atypical neuroleptics, such as risperidone and olanzapine, have been used with some success. Prognosis is poor, with patients often progressing to terminal disease rapidly.

Other Parkinson plus syndromes are listed in the table below.

1. Progressive supranuclear palsy	Parkinsonism + inability to move eyes vertically or laterally + axial rigidity + dementia
2. Multiple system atrophy	Parkinsonism + autonomic dysfunction
3. Corticobasal degeneration	Parkinsonism + dysarthria + dysphasia + myoclonus

Neurofibrillary tangles are a feature of Alzheimer's disease.

Multiple **grey matter infarcts** are seen in multi-infarct dementia.

Picks bodies (disorganized protein filaments) are seen in Pick's disease as well as shrinkage of the frontal and temporal lobe.

Neuritic plaques are found in a variety of diseases including Alzheimer's, Creutzfeld–Jacob, dialysis dementia and in middle age in Down's syndrome.

---

190 Question on p.63.

Answer A
History and clinical findings

The diagnosis of tetanus is a clinical one. To wait for wound cultures and other isolation techniques would be wasting valuable time when treatment could be instigated. There are few other diagnoses that imitate tetanus:

• meningitis – opisthotonus
• hypocalcaemia – tetany
• phenothiazine overdose, e.g. chlorpromazine – extreme rigidity.

---

191 Question on p.63.

Answer E
Methysergide 1–2 mg tds

• Migraine presents as an episodic pain with complete resolution between attacks.
• Attacks may last from a few hours up to several days.
• Pain is throbbing or constant.
• Temporal area unilateral or bilateral. ➤

- 90% experience nausea and 75% vomit.
- Aura may be experienced: transient hemianopia, fortification spectra, spreading scintillating scotomata.
- Unilateral paraesthesia, and face or hand weakness have been described.

All the drugs mentioned in the question have been used for migraine prophylaxis. **Methysergide** is less commonly used as, in the long-term, patients may develop retroperitoneal fibrosis.

In pregnancy paracetamol is the safest analgesic and prochlorperazine for nausea. Most migraines improve during pregnancy but, if prophylaxis is essential, **propranolol** is the safest.

Hormone replacement therapy (HRT) is not contraindicated and, since menopause can make migraine worse, HRT sometimes helps symptoms. Rarely, migraines get worse on HRT and then the patient should change formulation.

192

Question on p.63.

Answer E
Haemoglobin electrophoresis

Patients are very frequently referred for gastrointestinal investigations for 'iron-deficiency' anaemia on the basis of a low haemoglobin and a microcytosis. The problem with this is that, although iron deficiency is a very common cause of a microcytic anaemia, there are a number of other causes.

Causes of a microcytic anaemia
- Iron deficiency
- Anaemia of chronic disorders
- Thalassaemia trait
- Sideroblastic anaemia

Patients with a microcytic anaemia are often referred without any iron studies being performed. To make matters worse, the patient is often started on oral iron therapy. This therapy will not work if the patient has another cause for the microcytic anaemia. Furthermore, it will also cause diagnostic confusion as iron studies will be misleading if taken whilst the patient is on iron therapy or has been in the preceding 3–4 weeks.

The patient in the question has a profound microcytosis but normal iron studies. He is, therefore, not iron deficient and gastrointestinal investigations are entirely inappropriate. The patient, in fact, has β-thalassaemia trait and the correct answer is, therefore, E.

193 Question on p.64.

Answer D
Phenylalanine hydroxylase

Phenylketonuria is an inborn error of amino acid metabolism that comes from the deficiency of the enzyme **phenylalanine hydroxylase**. The incidence is 1 in 10 000–20 000 live births. If untreated, infants present at 6–12 months with spasms or developmental delay. Fortunately, most children are now detected using the Guthrie test when born. Treatment consists of dietary restriction of phenylalanine.

Alkaptonuria is also an inborn error of amino acid metabolism that is caused by a defect in the enzyme **homogentisic acid oxidase**. It is inherited as an autosomal recessive trait. The accumulation of homogentisic acid leads to increased pigmentation, e.g. in skin, cartilage, sclera and urine on standing. The main problem associated with alkaptonuria is premature arthritis, especially affecting knees, back and hips. Treatment is a low-protein diet.

Homocystinuria is caused by a defect in the enzyme **cystathionine synthetase**. This leads to cystathionine deficiency and an excess of homocystine. Homocystine is thought to affect cross-linking in collagen leading to the skeletal, ocular, neurological and vascular abnormalities found in this condition.

Glucocerebrosidase is a lysosomal acid glucosidase. Deficiency leads to the most common lysosomal storage disease – Gaucher's. It affects the liver, bone marrow and spleen by deposition of glucosylceramide.

A deficiency of **phosphofructokinase** leads to a muscle glycogen storage disease similar to McArdle's, i.e. cramps and myoglobinuria after exercise.

194 Question on p.64.

Answer C
Cyclosporin

Gingival hypertrophy may occur due to fibrous dysplasia, infiltration or as a result of inflammatory changes.

Causes of fibrous dysplasia include:

- hereditary gingival fibromatosis
- phenytoin
- cyclosporin
- nifedipine.

Inflammatory swellings may be due to:

- pregnancy
- gingivitis
- scurvy.

➤

Infiltrative causes include:

- acute promyelocytic leukaemia (AML-M3)
- Wegener's granulomatosis.

Since this patient has had a renal transplant, she will almost certainly be on immunosuppression. Tacrolimus and methotrexate do not cause gingival swelling. The most likely cause of the gingival swelling is cyclosprin. It occurs in up to 5% of transplant patients on the drug.

There is an increased risk of skin and lymphoproliferative malignancies amongst patients on any immunosuppressants, with an incidence of 1%. AML-M3 is not a common malignancy arising from long-term immunosuppression. Statistically the cause of hypertrophy in the question is five times more likely to be due to the cyclosporin itself rather than AML.

Since this patient has a history of chronic renal failure, it is possible that she may be on antihypertensives to control her blood pressure and nifedipine remains a possibility as the cause of her gum hypertrophy. Given the choice between cyclosporin, which she is almost certainly taking, or nifedipine, which she could possibly be taking, the best answer would be cyclosporin.

195

Question on p.64.

Answer C
Pulmonary fibrosis

Pneumocystis carinii **pneumonia** occurs in immunocompromised individuals. It is most commonly encountered in patients with HIV disease, where it is an AIDS-defining illness. It is extremely uncommon in patients with rheumatoid arthritis, even in those patients who are receiving high-dose immunosuppressive therapy.

Patients with rheumatoid arthritis are at slightly increased risk of developing thromboembolic disease. This is probably related to their general immobility rather than being an independent effect of the disease itself. A **pulmonary embolus** usually presents with acute dyspnoea, although occasionally the symptoms gradually worsen, as in this case.

Pulmonary nodules are a common finding on the CXR of a patient with rheumatoid arthritis. These are usually asymptomatic. In a patient with an associated pneumoconiosis, large cavitating nodules develop and the patient becomes breathless. This is termed Caplan's syndrome and is very rare.

Pulmonary oedema often presents as acute dyspnoea, but sometimes presents in a more indolent fashion as in this case. Patients with rheumatoid arthritis have an increased relative risk of between 2 and 3 of developing ischaemic heart disease and thus left ventricular dysfunction. This is a possible answer to this question.

However, the correct answer is **pulmonary fibrosis**. Patients with rheumatoid arthritis are at risk of developing fibrosing alveolitis (common) and obstructing bronchiolitis (rare). These usually present after 10 years and are more common in patients with seropositive disease. Furthermore, it is possible that this patient has also received methotrexate, which can also cause pulmonary fibrosis.

196   Question on p.65.

Answer E
He had his dog put down the day before the attempt

Of all people who kill themselves, 70% will be depressed, 15% are alcoholics and 6% will have other forms of mental illness, i.e. dementia, schizophrenia.

Increased risk factors for suicide include:

- male sex
- older age
- socially isolated
- previous suicide attempt
- presence of agitation or insomnia
- self-neglect
- impairment of memory
- pessimism
- poor physical health
- psychiatric illness
- unemployed.

The important features in assessing this man are those that identify his suicide intent. These include:

- timing of attempt
- attempts not to be discovered
- perceived dangerousness of the act
- anticipatory acts
- suicide attempt occurring in place of isolation
- presence of suicide note.

With regards to the male in question, the presence of **diabetes** and the fact that he **lives alone** are indicators of suicide risk but not as useful in assessing this particular attempt.

Using **alcohol to wash the tablets down** does not necessarily suggest a high intent. It is not possible to tell whether the attempt was a spontaneous decision whilst drunk or something he had planned for a long time.

The presence of a **suicide note** often indicates that the patient has made a serious attempt at suicide. Suicide notes are often written in parasuicides and also the absence of a note does not diminish the seriousness of the attempt. It merely suggests some planning. ➤

The fact that the man had his **dog put down** the day before the attempt demonstrates an anticipatory act which would have to be planned a day or so in advance. It suggests the man has planned the attempt and put his affairs in order. He has made sure his dog will not suffer (i.e. it will not starve with him gone or have to watch him kill himself) and the pre-planning of this act suggests a high intent to kill himself.

197

Question on p.65.

Answer C
A larger sample size will be required, if there is a precise outcome measure

For a clinical trial to be successful, it needs careful planning and design. It is essential to identify the necessary trial size that is required to stand a reasonable statistical chance of being able to answer the trial question. The power of a study is a measure of the likelihood of the study being able to do this.

Important definitions are covered below.

Type 1 error

The risk of a **false-positive** result, i.e. the chance of detecting a statistically significant difference when there is no real difference between treatments.

Type 2 error

The risk of a **false-negative** result, i.e. the chance of not detecting a significant difference when there really is a difference.

Power

The chance of not getting a false-negative result, i.e. the chance of spotting a difference as being statistically significant if there really is a difference. Higher power is better, aim for at least 90% power; 80% power is the minimum acceptable.

The sample size required will depend on several features. There will be a **bigger sample size** with:

- high power
- small difference to detect
- large standard deviation
- low chance of false positive.

There will be a **smaller sample size** with:

- low power
- large difference to detect
- precise outcome measure.

198 Question on p.65.

Answer B
Sotalol

The question is asking for the best drug to prevent paroxysmal atrial fibrillation.

Digoxin is a useful drug for rate control of patients already in atrial fibrillation and is particularly useful if there is accompanying congestive cardiac failure. It is of little use in preventing the arrhythmia.

Flecainide is indicated for paroxysmal atrial fibrillation in patients with disabling symptoms and should only be initiated in hospital. It is mainly used for the management of ventricular arrhythmias.

Disopyramide is indicated for ventricular arrhythmias, especially after myocardial infarction and supraventricular arrhythmias. It is not used for paroxysmal atrial fibrillation.

Amiodarone can be useful in the management of atrial fibrillation but its side-effect profile makes it a less appealing option for this patient.

Sotalol is licensed for the prophylaxis of paroxysmal atrial fibrillation and is the best choice for the question. Calcium channel blockers such as verapamil and diltiazem are also of benefit.

199 Question on p.65.

Answer D
Thiamine iv

This gentleman has the triad of signs associated with Wernicke's encephalopathy. It is a potentially reversible syndrome characterized by:

• ocular signs, e.g. nystagmus, ocular palsies, etc.
• ataxia
• confusion, varying levels of consciousness.

It is caused by ischaemic damage to the brainstem caused by a deficiency of **thiamine**. Treatment is parenteral replacement of thiamine. Doctors working with this type of patient should have a low threshold for giving thiamine, as failure to treat leads to the irreversible Korsakoff's syndrome. This causes a short-term memory problem, with often confabulation to 'make up' the lost memories.

Aspirin would be the treatment of choice for a cerebellar thrombotic event. These types of strokes can present with variable symptoms including nystagmus, ataxia, Horner's syndrome, loss of ipsilateral facial pain and temperature sensation, etc.

A **CT** of the head may well be the next investigation for this gentleman, if he fails to respond to initial treatment. A subdural haematoma may present with a decrease in the level of consciousness and focal neurological signs. They are particularly common in the elderly and ➤

alcoholics, and patients and relatives are often unable to remember the precipitating injury.

Fifty per cent dextrose is reserved for patients with hypoglycaemia. Symptoms are those of:

* adrenergic stimulation, e.g. sweating, palpitations, etc.
* neuroglycopenia, e.g. confusion, convulsions and coma.

In the elderly, hypoglycaemia can mimic symptoms of a CVA.

In this gentleman, giving dextrose would actually worsen his condition and may precipitate Korsakoff's syndrome. Thiamine must always be given before intravenous glucose/dextrose.

Hydroxycobalamin is given intramuscularly to treat vitamin B_{12} deficiency/pernicious anaemia.

200
Question on p.66.

Answer B
IgG and C3 along the dermoepidermal junction

There are two main types of immunofluorescence tests used.

* **Direct immunofluorescence** (DIF) – used to detect antibodies and complement deposited in the skin *in vivo*.
* **Indirect immunofluorescence** (IIF) – used to detect serum antibodies that react with normal skin *in vitro*. This is a less sensitive alternative than DIF in some diseases but, since it gives a measurement of antibody titre, it may be useful in monitoring disease progression.

The classic DIF finding in all forms of pemphigoid is IgG and C3 along the dermoepidermal junction (DEJ).

IgA and C3 in dermal papillae is found in dermatitis herpetiformis.
Intercellular IgG and C3 is found in pemphigus.
DIF may also be helpful in the investigation of the following diseases:

* systemic lupus erythematosus – IgG, IgM, IgA and C3 along the DEJ
* discoid lupus erythematosus – IgG, IgM, IgA and C3 along the DEJ
* lichen planus – fibrinogen along the DEJ.

201
Question on p.66.

Answer A
Anti-GBM antibody titres

Goodpasture's disease is a rare autoimmune disease characterized by the presence of anti-glomerular basement membrane (anti-GBM) antibodies causing glomerulonephritis and lung haemorrhage. A spectrum of disease can be seen and patients can present with either lung haemorrhage or glomerulonephritis alone. There is a bimodal incidence of distribution, the first peak occurring around the third decade and the second around the seventh. Haemorrhage is more commonly seen in young male patients.

A total of 60–70% of patients present with acute lung haemorrhage and are then also found to be in acute renal failure. In one-third of patients, presentation is with renal disease alone, symptoms being that of uraemia.

Chest X-rays are a relatively insensitive diagnostic tool in the presence of pulmonary haemorrhage; indeed, the patient may be anaemic but there may only be subtle radiographic changes. The most sensitive indicator of pulmonary haemorrhage is transfer factor. **Transfer factor** is of no use in assessing overall disease severity since lung haemorrhage is not seen in 30% of cases.

The **erythrocyte sedimentation rate** (ESR) is a marker of inflammation but is non-specific. Urinalysis normally shows a degree of haematuria, which can be considerable, red cell casts and mild proteinuria. Renal biopsy is essential both for diagnosis and prognosis. Appearances normally show a diffuse proliferative glomerulonephritis with variable crescents, necrosis and tubular loss. The presence of linear immunoglobulin deposition along the basement membrane is almost pathognomic.

Circulating **IgG anti-GBM antibodies** are invariably present, their titres at presentation correlating with disease severity. Treatment and relapses are mirrored by anti-GBM titres.

Treatment aims to reduce autoimmunity, and hence prednisolone and cyclophosphamide are used. Plasmaphoresis is also used in some centres.

202
Question on p.66.

Answer A
Chronic granulomatous disease

The nitroblue tetrazolium test is a simple screening test of reducing power of phagocytes. In patients with normal reducing ability, the dye turns from yellow to blue. In patients with impaired reducing ability, the dye remains yellow.

Chronic granulomatous disease (CGD) is a defect in the production of NADPH-oxidase. This enzyme is found in phagocytes and is important in the production of hydrogen peroxide and hydroxyl free radicals. These molecules have a bacteriocidal function. This means that patients with CGD have defective phagocytes that are able to engulf bacteria, but once engulfed they are unable to kill them. This leads to the formation of chronic granulomas and microabscesses. These can occur anywhere but are commonly found in the skin, live and bone.

Wiskott–Aldrich syndrome is a rare X-linked recessive immunodeficiency, with thrombocytopenia and eczema. It is ➤

characterized by recurrent infections and developmental delay and usually presents in infancy with bloody diarrhoea.

Di George's syndrome is a developmental abnormality of the 3rd and 4th branchial arches. It is caused by failure of neural crest cells. This leads to the following abnormalities:

- absence of parathyroid glands
- congenital heart disease
- thymic hypoplasia
- facial and ear abnormalities

X-linked agammaglobulinaemia is characterized by very low levels of circulating B cells and immunoglobulins. It presents in infancy with recurrent infections with *Streptococcus* and *Haemophilus* sp. Major sepsis is common, particularly meningitis and septic arthritis. Chronic infection with *Giardia lamblia* is frequently the cause of failure to thrive.

Hyperimmunoglobulinaemia E-recurrent infection syndrome is characterized by very high IgE levels. It is associated with atopic disease and recurrent Staphylococcal skin and chest infections. Eosinophilia on the blood film is nearly always present.

203

Question on p.67.

Answer B
Intramuscular human antitetanus immunoglobulin

This man has generalized tetanus. Tetanus is caused by *Clostridium tetani* found in soil and faeces of animals. They gain entry to the body by a wound. Here they multiply under anaerobic conditions and produce the potent neurotoxin tetanospasmin. The toxin travels in nerves to the spinal cord, where it interferes with the action of inhibitory neurones. There is also overactivity of the autonomic nervous system.

This man has lockjaw and spasm of the facial muscles. He is in danger of developing reflex spasms. These occur in response to a loud noise, a sudden movement or light. The time of onset of symptoms to the time of reflex spasms is called the *period time* and gives an indication as to the severity of disease. The shorter the time, the worse the prognosis.

Reflex spasms normally develop 24–72 hours after the onset of initial symptoms and progress to involve oesophageal, urethral and laryngeal muscles if not treated. Death is from aspiration, respiratory failure or cardiac arrest.

Treatment is **iv penicillin** and **im anti-tetanus immunoglobulin** in multiple sites. The immunoglobulin binds to any circulating toxin. It has no effect on that toxin that is already bound. Diazepam is used to treat spasms. Cleaning and debridement of the wound will remove any fixed neurotoxin. If severe, patients are intubated and ventilated.

Answer B
Stevens Johnson syndrome

Stevens Johnson syndrome is a form of erythema multiforme involving the limbs, especially the hands and feet. The main feature, which points to this diagnosis, is severe necrotic ulcers in the buccal mucosa. Conjunctivitis and ulcers of the genitalia are also found.

Bullous pemphigus is a potentially fatal blistering condition, which usually presents in middle age. Mucosal involvement is common and oral ulceration may be the presenting feature in 50% of cases. This is usually followed by flaccid blisters, predominantly involving the trunk.

Kaposi's varicelliform eruption is name given to a distinct cutaneous eruption caused by *Herpes simplex* virus. It is most commonly caused by disseminated HSV infection in patients with atopic dermatitis. It starts in areas of pre-existing dermatitis as clusters of vesicopustules and may be associated with pyrexia, malaise and lymphadenopathy. Buccal involvement is not a characteristic feature.

Primary *Varicella zoster* infection or chicken pox is usually a disease of children. In adults not previously exposed to the virus, the primary infection is more severe and sometimes fatal. It usually presents with a macular erythematous rash, papules and vesicles at the same time. It tends to start on the face and scalp before progressing to the trunk and later to the limbs. Individual lesions progress from being papular to vesicles to pustules, which then crust over. Adults tend to be systemically unwell, with fever, myalgia, headache and malaise. The more severe complications include pneumonitis and encephalitis.

Staphylococcal toxic shock syndrome is seen most frequently in menstruating females using high-adsorbancy polyacrylate-containing tampons. It usually presents with a rapid onset of fever with a diffuse macular erythema. The patient frequently experiences diarrhoea, vomiting, myalgia and shock. It is caused by toxic shock syndrome toxin-1 (TSST-1) produced by staphylococci. Blood cultures are negative with a low concentration of anti-TSST-1 antibodies in the serum. Treatment is supportive. It is rare, but not unheard of in males.

Answer C
Acute rheumatic fever

The diagnosis of rheumatic fever is based on the revised Jones criteria listed in the table below.

Major criteria	Minor criteria
Carditis including:	**Fever**
New murmurs	**Previous rheumatic fever**
Cardiac failure	**Raised ESR/CRP**
Pericardial effusion	**Arthralgia**
ECG changes:	**Prolonged PR interval**
ST elevation	
Flattened T waves	
AV block	
Arthritis	
Migrating polyarthritis of large joints	
Sydenham's chorea	
Erythema marginatum	
Subcutaneous nodules	

For a diagnosis to be made, the following need to be present:

• evidence of preceding streptococcal infection, i.e. raised antistreptolysin O titres (ASOT), positive throat swab

  plus either of the following:

• two or more major criteria, *or*
• one major and two minor criteria.

This patient has two major criteria: polyarthritis and a rash that may be erythema marginatum (erythema marginatum occurs in 20% of all cases). She also has two minor criteria: fever and prolonged PR interval.

Still's disease is a possible answer because it includes fever, pink maculopapular rash and arthritis. However, the cardiac involvement tends to present as a pericarditis.

Lyme disease is a tickborne infection caused by *Borrelia burgdorferi*. It consists of three stages. The first stage begins with fever, myalgia, arthralgia and the characteristic skin lesion erythema chronicum migrans. These symptoms then resolve. The second stage occurs weeks to months later and consists of either neurological or cardiac manifestations (including a prolonged PR interval). The third stage of the disease involves arthritis, which may occur months to years after the initial infection.

The principal signs in the question occur simultaneously. Lyme disease is, therefore, less likely as the corresponding features occur in different stages across the natural history of the disease.

Henoch Schonlein purpura includes arthralgia, a purpuric rash, abdominal pain and glomerulonephritis. Cardiac involvement is not seen.

Answer E
Rofecoxib

Rofecoxib potentiates the action of warfarin. However, the effect is minor, as the INR is rarely elevated by more than 10%.

All the others are non-steroidal anti-inflammatory drugs which significantly interact with warfarin. In addition, these drugs are all non-selective and have a much greater toxic effect on the upper gastrointestinal tract compared to rofecoxib, which is a COX-II inhibitor.

Answer A
Benign essential tremor

This is a condition that is often inherited in an autosomal dominant pattern. It tends not to be present at rest and gets worse with posture or stress. In over half there is associated titubation and a third have movements of trunk or legs. It is more common in the elderly and can be mistaken for parkinsonism; however, this is excluded by the lack of any other signs.

There is such a dramatic improvement with alcohol that frequently patients have overindulged to keep their tremor at bay. If treatment is needed, β-blockers or anticonvulsants may be tried. In these patients, it is best to try and avoid β-agonists such as salbutamol that can make the tremor worse.

It is highly unlikely to be **Parkinson's disease**, as there are no other signs of the disease, such as rigidity and bradykinesia. In addition, he is extremely young to present with this condition.

Huntington's disease is inherited in an autosomal dominant fashion and it is caused by a trinucleotide repeat on chromosome 4. Presentation is with dementia, psychiatric illnesses or chorea (fidgety, flitting, continual movements of limbs). Although presentation at 25 years of age is highly unlikely, it is theoretically possible.

Salbutamol therapy causes a fine hand tremor that is present consistently.

This is unlikely to be **delirium tremens**, a condition affecting alcoholics, whereby the body reacts to alcohol withdrawal. Symptoms do include a tremor; however, it would be usual to have other symptoms, such as confusion, hallucinations and agitation.

208 Question on p.68.

Answer B
Ankylosing spondylitis

No revision for the MRCP would be complete without learning the classic causes of upper and lower lung fibrosis.

Upper lobe fibrosis	Lower lobe fibrosis
'BREAST-X'	'CRABSS'
Bronchopulmonary aspergillosis	**C**ryptogenic fibrosing alveolitis
Radiotherapy	**R**heumatoid arthritis
Extrinsic allergic alveolitis	**A**sbestosis
Ankylosing spondylitis	**B**leomycin and other drugs
Sarcoid/silicosis	**S**ystemic lupus erythematosus
Tuberculosis	**S**cleroderma
Histiocytosis-**X**	

Causes of pulmonary fibrosis without loss of lung volume
• Histiocytosis-X
• Tuberous sclerosis
• Neurofibromatosis
• Lymphangiomyomatosis

209 Question on p.68.

Answer B
Proteus mirabilis

This woman has symptoms of a lower urinary tract infection, alkaline urine and a history suggestive of passing a renal calculus. This combination suggests an infection with *Proteus*, a Gram-negative rod.

Proteus mirabilis is an organism that promotes the formation of stones by means of alkalizing the urine and thus promoting stone formation. Proteus has the ability to hydrolyse urea, hence producing ammonium hydroxide, a strong base. The increase in the pH of the urine and the presence of ammonium ions encourage the formation of infective stones, mostly composed of magnesium ammonium phosphate and calcium.

The common causes of urinary tract infections (UTIs) are listed in the table below.

Organism	Frequency (%)
Escherichia coli	68
Proteus mirabilis	12
Staphylococcus	10
Enterococcus faecalis	6
Klebsiella	4

Pasturella is an uncommon Gram-negative rod that is a commensal of the nasopharynx and the gastrointestinal tracts of animals. The spectrum of diseases it causes includes cutaneous infection, sepsis, pneumonia, meningitis and renal abscesses

Candida is a commensal fungus. When infection occurs in the renal tract, it is normally in an immunocompromised individual and is common in diabetics. Treatment is with fluconazole.

210
Question on p.69.

Answer C
A 38-year-old man with glycosuria, plasma glucose of 6.8 mmol/L fasting and 10.8 mmol/L 2 hours after an oral load of 75 g glucose

Diagnosis of diabetes

1. Symptomatic + single random plasma sample ≥ 11 mmol/L (lab measured)
2. Asymptomatic + two fasting plasma samples > 7 mmol/L
3. Asymptomatic + two random plasma samples ≥ 11.1 mmol/L.

Symptomatic = evidence of end-organ damage due to microvascular or macrovascular disease, e.g. retinopathy, nephropathy, neuropathy, ischaemic heart disease.

Impaired glucose tolerance
Fasting plasma sample < 7.0 mmol/L and oral glucose tolerance test (OGTT) plasma sample ≥ 7.8 mmol/L at 2 hours.

Borderline cases
These should all go on to have an OGTT.

	Normal	Impaired glucose tolerance	Diabetes mellitus
Fasting	< 7 mmol/L	< 7 mmol/L	≥ 7.0 mmol/L
2 hours after 75 mg glucose	< 7.8 mmol/L	7.8–11.0 mmol/L	≥ 11.1 mmol/L

➤

Applying the above criteria to the cases in the question:

Case A = Symptomatic and a random plasma glucose ≥ 11 mmol/L

Diabetic

Case B = Fasting < 7 mmol/L but 2 hours after 75 mg glucose
     ≥ 11.1 mmol/L   **Diabetic**

Case C = Fasting < 7 mmol/L and 2 hours after 75 mg glucose
     7.8–11.0 mmol/L   **Impaired glucose tolerance**

Case D = Asymptomatic + two fasting plasma samples > 7 mmol/L

Diabetic

Case E = Symptomatic + single random plasma sample ≥ 11 mmol/L

Diabetic

211

Question on p.69.

Answer B
Intravenous broad-spectrum antibiotics

All the therapeutic options in the question have a place in the management of acute variceal haemorrhage. The mortality from acute variceal haemorrhage depends on the severity of the underlying liver disease. The severity of the liver diseases is assessed by the Child–Pugh classification:

Score	Ascites	Encephalopathy	Albumin	Bilirubin	INR
1	None	None	> 35	< 30	< 1.7
2	Moderate	Grade I–II	28–35	30–50	1.7–2.3
3	Severe	Grade III–IV	< 28	> 50	> 2.3

Scores < 6	Child-Pugh Grade A
Scores 7–9	Child-Pugh Grade B
Scores > 9	Child-Pugh Grade C

The more severe the disease, the worse the prognosis.

Banding, sclerotherapy and intravenous terlipressin have all been shown to reduce the incidence of rebleeding from oesophageal varices but they have not been shown to reduce mortality. **TIPS** is used to lower portal pressure and so achieve haemostasis in patients who have failed to respond to these three measures. It has not been shown to improve mortality.

Intravenous broad-spectrum antibiotics are a vital part of the management of bleeding oesophageal varices. Their use improves mortality by between 15% and 20%.

Answer B
Fever

Patients with classical Hodgkin's disease usually present with palpable non-tender lymphadenopathy. In most patients, lymph nodes are discovered in the cervical, supraclavicular and axillary regions. More than half the patients have **mediastinal lymphadenopathy** at diagnosis, and symptoms from a large mediastinal mass are often the initial presentation. **Superior vena caval** obstruction may be present but does not in itself carry prognostic implications.

The best long-term prognostic indicator for Hodgkin's disease is response to treatment. However, prognosis also depends upon the staging of the disease at presentation. The classic staging system is the Ann Arbor classification as detailed below.

- **Stage I** disease in single lymph node or lymph node region
- **Stage II** disease in two or more lymph node regions on the same side of the diaphragm
- **Stage III** disease in lymph node regions on both sides of the diaphragm are affected
- **Stage IV** disease is widespread, including multiple involvement at one or more extranodal sites (such as the bone marrow).

In addition, the staging will classify whether the patient has B symptoms, which include:

- fever
- weight loss of 10% body weight
- night sweats
- pain in the nodes on drinking alcohol.

The presence of B symptoms indicates more advanced disease and suggests a worse prognosis. **Pruritus** is a symptom experienced by patients but not strictly speaking a B symptom. It is not useful as a prognostic indicator.

Histological subtypes do not appear to have major independent prognostic significance. Patients with nodular sclerosing Hodgkin's disease have a better outcome than those with mixed-cellularity or lymphocyte-depleted Hodgkin's disease. However, adverse prognostic factors are more commonly found in patients with the latter histological subtypes and it is these rather than the subtype that has the implication. To put it another way, a patient with stage IV nodular sclerosing disease will have a worse prognosis than Stage I mixed cellularity.

One-third of patients with Hodgkin's disease present with **fever**, night sweats and/or weight loss. Fevers associated with Hodgkin's disease occasionally persist for days to weeks, followed by afebrile intervals and then reoccurrence of the fever. This pattern is known as Pel–Ebstein fever. ➤

From the choices in the question, fever is the only option that is a B symptom, suggesting more advanced disease. It is, therefore, the best answer.

213

Question on p.70.

Answer D
Inhibits osteoclast activity

Calcium haemostasis is mainly regulated by the effects of parathyroid hormone and $1,25\text{-}(OH)_2\text{-}D_3$ on intestinal absorption, renal tubular reabsorption and bone resorption. Changes in extracellaular calcium concentrations stimulate calcium-sensing receptors present in the parathyroids, kidneys and brain.

Parathyroid hormone has several actions, which serve to increase plasma calcium as outlined below:

- increases osteoclastic resorption of bone
- increases intestinal absorption of calcium
- increases synthesis of $1,25\text{-}(OH)_2\text{-}D_3$
- increases renal tubular absorption of calcium
- increases excretion of phosphate.

There is a homeostatic rise in **calcitonin** levels in the presence of increasing serum calcium. It tends to lower serum calcium via the following mechanisms:

- inhibiting osteoclastic bone resorption
- increasing renal excretion of calcium and phosphate.

1,25-Dihydroxycholecalciferol ($1,25\text{-}(OH)_2\text{-}D_3$) increases serum calcium by the following mechanisms:

- increases gut calcium absorption
- increases bone calcification
- increasess bone resorption.

Zoledronate is one of the newer **bisphosphonates** and is mainly used in patients with cancer. It is licensed for reduction of bone damage in advanced malignancies with bone involvement and is given with calcium and vitamin D supplementation. It is also used for treatment of hypercalcaemia of malignancy. Administered intravenously, it is adsorbed on to hydroxyapatite crystals in bone **inhibiting osteoclast activity**, slowing the rate of bone growth and dissolution. This results in a decreased rate of bone turnover.

214

Question on p.70.

Answer D
Add naproxen 500 mg bd and decrease morphine to 100 mg bd

Bone pain due to metastases is not always fully responsive to opioids. From the history the patient is either alert and in pain or pain free and drowsy. Cancer pains often require more than one analgesic to adequately control pain.

Non-steroidal anti-inflammatory drugs are useful in bony pain and the addition of **naproxen** would be sensible. It must be remembered that she is drowsy on the present dose of modified release morphine and it would be sensible to decrease this. There is little point in **retitrating** with immediate release morphine, as this will not alter the total morphine used to control her pain.

Converting to **transdermal fentanyl** is not a good idea for the following reasons:

- it is not particularly good for bony pain
- it should not be routinely used for unstable pain, as it is harder to titrate the dose
- the transdermal preparation takes at least 14 hours to reach a steady plasma level. If she becomes narcosed on fentanyl, it will take hours for the effects to wear off.

215

Question on p.70.

Answer C
Lown–Ganong–Levine

The history of someone with symptomatic tachyarrhythmia and the resting ECG as described suggests an accessory pathway syndrome of some sort.

The most common accessory pathway syndrome is **Wolf–Parkinson–White (WPW)**, which occurs as a result of an atrioventricular accessory pathway, separate from the atrioventricular node. This pathway is known as the Bundle of Kent and results in a shortened PR interval and a delta wave. The position of the accessory pathway will determine the morphology of the ECG and results in there being two types of WPW – Type A and Type B.

Type	Site of accessory pathway	ECG appearances
Type A	Posterior left atrial wall to left ventricle	Positive delta wave in leads V1–V6 Negative delta-wave in lead I
Type B	Lateral right atrial wall to right ventricle	Biphasic or negative delta wave in leads V1–V3 Positive delta wave in lead I

➤

Lown–Ganong–Levine Syndrome is due to the accessory pathway known as the bundle of James, which lies along atrionodal tracts. Since the pathway is so close to the atrioventricular node, there is no delta wave on the ECG. It does, however, have a shortened PR interval and is the correct answer in this question.

Romano–Ward and **Jervell–Lange–Nielson** are both syndromes associated with long QT intervals, which may precipitate ventricular arrythmias (most commonly torsades de pointes). More than 90% of cases have a positive family history of syncope or sudden death with a chromosome defect localized to chromosome 11.

216

Question on p.71.

Answer B
They are inherited from the mother

Mitochondrial diseases are a group of disorders caused by mutations in the mitochondrial DNA. The mitochondrial genome is small and circular, and replicates independently of the mechanisms that control chromosomal or nuclear DNA. The protein products are a series of oxidative enzymes that are involved in mitochondrial functions, although other enzymes involved in these functions are also produced by nuclear genes. Mitochondrial DNA is effectively exclusively **maternal in origin**, i.e. inherited from the egg and not the sperm.

In mitochondrial diseases, no children or other descendants of males, whether affected or unaffected, are at risk of developing the condition or being carriers of it. **Both sexes can be affected**, although the ratio of affected males and females may vary between different conditions and may be determined by other genetic and environmental factors.

In Leber's optic atrophy (Leber's hereditary optic neuropathy), one of the best-known mitochondrial diseases, males are more commonly affected than females. Females may be asymptomatic carriers but like affected females, all their children are at risk of developing the condition and all their daughters are at risk of transmitting it. The exact proportion of sons and daughters who will become affected is variable and not determined by any fixed rule. In Leber's optic atrophy, about 50% of sons and 30% of daughters will develop the condition.

Some examples of disorders with mitochondrial inheritance are:

- Leber's optic atrophy
- MELAS (mitochondrial encephalopathy with lactic acidosis and stroke-like episodes)
- MERFF (myoclonic epilepsy with ragged red fibres)
- Kearns–Sayre syndrome
- Pearson syndrome (lactic acidosis, pancreatic insufficiency, pancytopenia)

- deafness (antibiotic induced and some forms of progressive nerve deafness)
- various poorly classified central nervous system degenerations
- diabetes mellitus (some familial types).

Anticipation is the term used to describe the progressively earlier onset and increased severity of certain diseases in successive generations of a family. It is caused by expansion of the number of triplet repeats within or associated with the gene responsible for the disease.

Imprinted genes are those where the maternally inherited and paternally inherited alleles are differentially expressed. This phenomenon of imprinting is caused by an incompletely understood alteration in the chromatin that affects the expression of a gene but not its DNA sequence. Thus, it is a reversible form of gene inactivation but it is not a mutation. Several genetic conditions that apparently follow autosomal dominant inheritance are only fully manifested when they are transmitted by one particular parent. Examples of the role of genomic imprinting in human disease include Prader–Willi syndrome, Angelman syndrome, Beckwith–Wiedemann syndrome and Albright's hereditary osteodystrophy.

| **217** | Question on p.71. |

Answer D
Acquired hypogammaglobulinaemia

The key features in this question are:

- recurrent chest infections
- intermittent diarrhoea
- normal full blood count and electrolytes
- reduced IgG, IgA and IgM
- clinical examination is normal.

Kartagener's syndrome is a condition characterized by dysfunctional cilia resulting in poor mucociliary clearance and bronchiectasis with situs inversus. Immunoglobulins are not reduced and cardiorespiratory examination will be abnormal.

Yellow nail syndrome is a rare disorder of lymphatic drainage. Presenting with thickened slow-growing yellow nails, it is associated with pleural effusions and lymphoedema of the legs. The immunoglobulins are not altered in this condition and altered bowel habit infrequent. In addition, the examination will not be normal as described in the question.

Acquired hypogammaglobulinaemia frequently presents with recurrent infections due to an impaired immune response. Specific immune response is based on two major components: (1) humoral immunity supported by B-lymphocytes or B cells; and (2) cellular immunity ➤

supported by T lymphocytes or T cells. Immunoglobulins (Igs) produced by B cells play a central role in humoral immunity, and deficiency may result in dramatic consequences for the body's defence against infections. Disorders of the immune system that can result in hypogammaglobulinaemia can involve B cells, T cells or both.

Acquired hypogammaglobulinaemia commonly presents with infection. Knowing the type of microorganisms involved is helpful. Antibody deficiency and complement deficiency are associated with recurrent infections with encapsulated bacteria. *Giardia lamblia* infection is observed most often in patients with IgA deficiency. Opportunistic infections with viral and fungal pathogens suggest T-cell deficiency.

In this particular patient, the chronic diarrhoea is likely to be due to giardiasis. This occurs due to impairment of intestinal IgA production. Although all the Ig levels are below normal, the IgA appears particularly low.

Hypogammaglobulinemia also can result from lack of or decreased production caused by acquired lymphoproliferative disorders. Igs also may be lost in the urine or stools, or as a result of hypercatabolic states.

Causes of hypogammaglobulinaemia
- Catabolic disorders
  - Myotonic dystrophy
  - Nephrotic syndrome
  - Protein-losing enteropathy
  - Severe ovarian hyperstimulation syndrome
  - Thyrotoxicosis
- Decreased synthesis
  - Uraemia
  - Viral infections
  - Immunosuppressive therapy
- Severe malnutrition
- Lymphoproliferative malignancies
  - Multiple myeloma
  - Chronic lymphocytic leukaemia
  - Lymphomas, especially non-Hodgkin's lymphomas
- Prematurity in infants
- Drug-related: chlorpromazine, phenytoin, carbamazepine, valproate, D-penicillamine, sulphasalazine and hydroxychloroquine have been implicated in IgA deficiency

---

Although **Hodgkin's lymphoma** and **non-Hodgkin's lymphoma** could cause hypogammaglobulinaemia, it is unlikely that the patient would still have a normal full blood count, electrolytes and examination. Therefore, the best answer is D.

Question on p.71.

Answer E
Autoantibodies against gated-voltage calcium channels

Lambert–Eaton is a rare autoimmune condition of the neuromuscular junction causing weakness that characteristically improves with successive muscle contractions. It is seen as non-metastatic complication of small cell carcinoma of the bronchus. Antibodies to *pre*-**synaptic voltage-gated calcium channels** are found, unlike myasthenia gravis where the target is the *post*-**synaptic acetylcholine receptor**.

Post-synaptic acetylcholine receptors are present in 90% of patients with myasthenia.

Ten per cent of patients with myasthenia will have a **thymic tumour**. These patients are less likely to experience improvement following thymectomy than those without a thymoma. The reason for this is uncertain.

There is an association between myasthenia and **HLA B8**.

The main treatment of myasthenia is with anticholinesterases. Patients that show incomplete response to these may improve with **steroids**.

 Question on p.72.

Answer B
No treatment

The painful rash on the shins is erythema nodosum.

Causes of erythema nodosum
- Streptococcal infection
- Drugs, e.g. sulphonamides, oral contraceptive
- Sarcoidosis
- Idiopathic
- *Yersinnia* infection
- Fungal infections, e.g. histoplasmosis, blastomycosis
- Tuberculosis
- Leprosy
- Inflammatory bowel disease
- *Chlamydia* infection

---

220 Question on p.72.

Answer D
Pacemaker syndrome

Pacemaker syndrome is defined as symptoms related to the use of a pacemaker. It is usually seen in patients with single-chamber ventricular pacemakers, where ventricular pacing leads to retrograde conduction to the atria. The atria contract against closed atrioventricular valves, causing pulmonary and systemic venous distension.

Clinical examination may reveal signs of pulmonary oedema and a raised JVP. Cannon a waves may be seen as the right atrium contracts against a closed tricuspid valve. The ECG shows a normal ventricular paced rhythm. Retrograde P waves may be seen, but these are sometimes difficult to spot as they may be buried in the T wave.

Treatment is to change the pacemaker to a dual-chamber system.

221 Question on p.72.

Answer D
Streptococcal sepsis

This lady is shocked and clinically septic. Given her history of splenectomy, the most likely organism responsible is an encapsulated organism, i.e. streptococcus. **Streptococcal sepsis** can occur rapidly in asplenic patients. Patients being prepared for elective splenectomy are routinely vaccinated against *Pneumococcus* and *Haemophilus* at least 2 weeks prior to the operation. This woman should also have received immunizations at the time of operation and be given long-term prophylaxis with penicillin. It is not clear from the history whether this actually happened.

She is unlikely to have a **subphrenic abscess,** as this would have presented earlier than 6 weeks post-operation.

Malaria and **yellow fever** are not endemic to South Africa, and are very unlikely in this patient.

The transmission of **HIV** via blood products in South Africa is not common. Blood undergoes the same screening as blood in the UK, but the screening is not as rigorous. This patient has signs suggestive of septicaemia with a high fever and hypotension. This would be very uncommon in HIV seroconversion illness.

222 Question on p.73.

Answer E
Colonoscopy every 5 years

Acromegaly is a rare disorder caused by an increase in the level of circulating growth hormone and its mediator, IGF-1. Principally, mortality is secondary to the cardiovascular risk factors of the associated hypertension and diabetes. However, with better control of these factors and the improvement in neurosurgical intervention, it has become apparent that there is an increase in the risk of colorectal cancer in these patients. Studies suggest that in patients with acromegaly the increased risk of colorectal cancer is up to fourfold, and that the increased mortality is 2.5-fold.

With these figures in mind, the British Society of Gastroenterology have recommended some guidelines for the surveillance of people with acromegaly.

1. All those with acromegaly over the age of 40 should be offered regular colonoscopic screening.
2. The frequency of screening depends on the original findings and the severity of the underlying acromegaly.
3. Screening at intervals of 5 years should be offered to those with either:
   • a negative initial colonoscopy or
   • a hyperplastic polyp at initial colonoscopy.
4. Screening at intervals of 3 years should be offered to those with either:
   • raised IGF levels or
   • adenoma on initial colonoscopy.

Colonoscopy is required rather than **sigmoidoscopy**, as up to 50% of carcinomas have been found in the ascending or transverse colon.

---

223   Question on p.73.

Answer D
Distal (type 1) renal tubular acidosis

Lower back pain is a common complaint that faces GPs every day. The trick is to try and pick up on points that are uncharacteristic of mechanical backache. This woman is young, and her blood and urine tests are abnormal. She has a low plasma bicarbonate with a raised urine pH. This suggests that she is not acidifying urine correctly.

A diagnosis of **renal tubular acidosis** is made on the basis of the plasma bicarbonate being less than 21 mmol/L and a urine pH > 5.3. Type I renal tubular acidosis is associated with renal calcium stone formation, which would also explain her back pain and dipstick haematuria. Another clue lies with the normal anion gap metabolic acidosis, of which renal tubular acidosis is a cause.

Idiopathic hypercalciuria is more common in men and is diagnosed by the presence of > 7.5 mmol calcium in a 24-hour urine collection. They are more prone to stone formation. The basis of the disease is thought to be increased absorption of calcium from the gut despite normal levels of circulating calcium. Their acid–base status is normal. ➤

Bartter's syndrome is a rare defect of renal sodium and chloride absorption. This produces hypokalaemia, alkalosis, hypercalciuria, normal blood pressure and high plasma renin levels. Diagnosis is based on a high urinary potassium and chloride despite low plasma levels and high plasma renin levels. Treatment is with amiloride. This lady has not got Bartter's because she is acidotic not alkalotic.

Glomerulonephritis is unlikely in the presence of normal renal function.

Osteoporosis is a decrease in the density of bone. It is a disease of increasing age. Bone mass increases up until the age of about 40 and then drops off after this. Risk is greater in women suffering early menopause or prolonged periods of amenorrhoea. It does not cause any biochemical alterations. This lady should have no reason to have osteoporosis at the age of 33.

224

Question on p.73.

Answer C
Vertical transmission is rare

Hepatitis D is caused by the hepatitis Delta virus. It requires helper functions from the hepatitis B virus and thus only patients who have hepatitis B infection can develop hepatitis D. The hepatitis D virion is a particle of 36 nm coated by the hepatitis B surface antigen, inside which are found the **RNA** genome and the hepatitis D antigen.

Hepatitis D and hepatitis B can infect an individual at the same time. This is termed **coinfection**. Progressive liver disease with coinfection is rare (< 2%), although the acute coinfection may produce a very severe acute hepatitis.

Hepatitis D can infect individuals who have chronic hepatitis B. This is termed superinfection. This commonly affects asymptomatic patients who are hepatitis B surface antigen positive. Chronic progressive liver disease occurs in up to 70% of these patients. In patients with a superinfection with hepatitis D, 10% will become temporarily negative for hepatitis B surface antigen immediately after the onset of the hepatitis D infection. This is due to suppression of the hepatitis B surface antigen by the hepatitis D infection.

Transmission is by the same methods of transmission as hepatitis B, i.e. **parenteral** or close bodily contact. It is very rare after blood transfusion as most blood products are screened for hepatitis B. It does occur in outbreaks in intravenous drug users and prisoners, especially in the developed world. In some parts of the world, e.g. Central Africa, South America and the Mediterranean Basin it is endemic. Worldwide up to 5% of patients with hepatitis B carry hepatitis D. **Perinatal transmission** of hepatitis D is rare as the majority of mothers have inactive hepatitis B infection (anti-Hbe positive) and, therefore, do not transmit hepatitis B virus, which is a prerequisite for developing hepatitis D.

Immunization of individuals at risk of hepatitis B with recombinant hepatitis B vaccine offers complete protection against hepatitis D.

Treatment of chronic hepatitis D is difficult and shows a poor response to a range of antiviral chemotherapy. Hepatitis D usually recurs in the transplanted liver and patients who are hepatitis D positive are very carefully assessed prior to transplantation.

225   Question on p.74.

Answer D
Hypophosphataemia

This patient has the classical features of 'refeeding syndrome'. This occurs in any malnourished individual, from any cause when they are refed. When such patients are fed, there is a sudden shift from fat to carbohydrate metabolism with increased insulin secretion. This causes increased uptake of phosphate into the cells and can provoke quite marked hypophosphataemia. For this reason, patients who are being enterally or parenterally fed should have regular serum phosphate estimations. If the serum phosphate falls, below 0.5 mmol/L, they should be treated with intravenous replacement therapy.

Hypocalcaemia and **hypomagnesaemia** also commonly occur in this situation. This patient's calcium and magnesium are both low. The corrected value for her serum calcium and magnesium (allowing for the low serum albumin) are normal, and certainly not low enough to cause a grand mal seizure. It is very unlikely that these values have changed significantly in 24 hours to be the cause of this patient's problem.

Patients who are being artificially fed commonly develop **hypokalaemia**. The common symptoms attributed to this are weakness, malaise and cardiac rhythm abnormalities.

Craniopharyngioma can sometimes present as an anorexia-type syndrome, but usually presents in children or teenagers.

226   Question on p.74.

Answer E
Omeprazole

This question is about drug interactions with warfarin.

Warfarin is a racaemic mixture containing R and L isomers. **Omeprazole** interferes with the cytochrome P450 system in the liver. It does this by inhibiting the enzymes responsible for the degradation of the R isomer. Omeprazole lengthens the $t_{1/2}$ of the R isomer from 35 hours to 50 hours. In practice, omeprazole has a variable effect on the INR in patients taking warfarin, but on occasion there can be a very significant and potentially dangerous rise in the INR.

Patients who have a very high INR due to poor warfarin control can bleed from pre-existing upper GI pathology, e.g. peptic ulcer disease. However, as in this case, upper GI endoscopy frequently fails to establish ➤

a cause, the presumption being that they have bled from gastrointestinal telangectasia in the small bowel.

Lanzoprazole does not interact with warfarin.

Rofecoxib potentiates the action of warfarin. However, the effect is minor as the INR is rarely elevated by more than 10%. **Celecoxib** does not interact with warfarin.

Cocodamol is a combination of codeine and paracetamol. It does not interact with warfarin. This must not be confused with coproxamol, which is a combination of dextropropoxyphene and paracetamol. This does interact with warfarin. The mechanism of this interaction is not fully understood but seems more common in the elderly. In this situation, the interaction is often dramatic, producing very high INRs, which are potentially fatal.

Drugs which interact with warfarin via the P450 system

Enzyme inducers	Enzyme inhibitors
Mnemonic: PCBRAGS	Mnemonic: ODEVICES
• Phenytoin	• Omeprazole
• Carbamazepine	• Disulfiram
• Barbiturates	• Ethanol (acute)
• Rifampicin	• Valproate
• Alcohol (chronic use)	• Cimetidine, ciprofloxacin
• Griseofulvin	• Erythromycin
• Sulphonylureas	• Sulphonamides

227

Question on p.74.

Answer A
Haemophilia A

This patient has an increased APPT but a normal PT and bleeding time. The most likely diagnosis in a patient of this age is **haemophilia A**. Haemophilia B presents in the same way with identical results but is less common than haemophilia B.

Clotting results in various conditions

	PT	APPT	Bleeding time
Haemophilia A	Normal	Raised	Normal
Haemophilia B	Normal	Raised	Normal
Von Willebrand's disease	Normal	Raised	Raised
Chronic liver disease	Raised	Raised	Normal
Bernard–Soulier syndrome	Normal	Normal	Raised

Bernard–Soulier syndrome is a rare inherited defect in platelet function. It presents with easy bruising and spontaneous bleeding.

Answer B
Oral amoxycillin and erythromycin

When approaching this question, remember common things are common. Candidates that answer D may have done so on the assumption that this postal worker has been contaminated with anthrax spores via a 'bioterrorism letter'. Full marks for knowing that the treatment for anthrax is with a **quinolone** (or doxycycline) but unfortunately it is not the correct answer.

We assume that this young man is previously fit but now clearly has a community acquired pneumonia. The white cell count does not give much of a clue to the causative organism. A count above 15×10^9/L is seen in more than 50% of pneumococcal pneumonias but only 10% of *Legionella* or *Mycoplasma* cases.

A large percentage of organisms causing pneumonia, i.e. *Mycoplasma pneumoniae*, *Haemophilus influenzae* and *Legionella pneumophilia*, do not respond to **benzyl penicillin** or ampicillin/amoxycillin. Furthermore, it may be some time before the causative organism is identified. In this situation, the British Thoracic Society recommend that therapy is initiated with amoxycillin and a macrolide antibiotic. They also recommend that the oral route is preferred in most patients unless they are very sick or unable to take oral medication.

The best answer is treatment is with oral amoxycillin and erythromycin.

Recommended antibiotic regimens for pneumonias

Community-acquired pneumonia (uncomplicated)	Amoxycillin and macrolide Oral in most cases iv if the patient is toxic
Community-acquired pneumonia (severe) unknown aetiology	Cefuroxime or Co-amoxiclav and macrolide iv Add Flucloxacillin iv if staphylococci suspected
Pneumonia caused by atypical pathogens	Erythromycin Add Rifampicin for severe *Legionella* infections Tetracycline for Mycoplasma or Chlamydial infections
Hospital acquired pneumonia	Broad-spectrum cephalosporin Add aminoglycoside in severe illness

➤

Severe community-acquired pneumonia can be diagnosed by assessing which of the following prognostic features apply:

Adverse prognostic features in community-acquired pneumonia

Core
(Mnemonic: CURB)
  Confusion
  Urea > 7 mmol/L
  RR >30/minute
  BP systolic <90 mmHg and/or diastolic > 60 mmHg
Pre-existing
  Age > 50 years
  Presence of pre-existing disease
Additional
  Hypoxia – PO_2 < 8 kPa or saturations < 92%
  Bilateral or multilobe involvement on CXR

Patients with two or more core adverse prognostic features have severe disease. Patients with one core feature may be classified as severe or mild depending on the clinicians judgement. Patients with no core adverse features should be considered for early discharge or managed in the community.

The case in question has no adverse prognostic features.

229
Question on p.75.

Answer D
Parvovirus B19

Polyarteritis nodosa (PAN), rubella, SLE and **parvovirus B19** can all present as arthralgia and a rash on the face. **PAN** is very rare and more commonly affects men.

Rubella is unlikely to be the diagnosis as it is very likely that a patient of this age has been immunized.

SLE is a possibility, as it often presents in this kind of way. The onset of symptoms of SLE seems to be more common in the post-natal period. SLE is, however, an uncommon condition.

Parvovirus B19 causes a condition called erythema infectiosum. This is a disease of children and typically the child presents with a fever, arthralgia and a characteristic rash on the cheeks (slapped cheeks appearance). This condition can also affect adolescents and adults. The rash is less common in adults. Patients may give a history of other family members being affected at the same time.

Parvovirus B19 is far more common than SLE and, although this patient is in late adolescence and, therefore, rather less likely to get a rash, this is the most likely diagnosis in general practice.

Answer B
Tumour obstructing CSF flow

The lumbar puncture reveals xanthochromia, high protein and high opening pressure.

The presence of xanthochromia indicates an old bleed into the CSF owing to the presence of oxyhaemaglobin and bilirubin. An **acute subarachnoid bleed** would not show xanthochromia until at least 12 hours after the event. Likewise, xanthochromia is unusual in bacterial meningitis. Very rarely, subarachnoid bleeding may occur at the acute onset of bacterial meningitis. However, the protein level, although raised, is usually much lower than 4.6 g/L making **partially treated bacterial meningitis** unlikely.

Tuberculous meningitis may have a high CSF protein, but it tends to be turbid and is less likely to be the answer here.

The raised protein and opening pressure in non-turbid CSF is caused by only a few conditions, which are listed below:

- Guillain–Barré Syndrome
- acoustic neuroma
- Froin's syndrome
- subacute sclerosing panencephalitis
- lead poisoning.

Froin's syndrome is an alteration in the CSF, which is yellowish and coagulates spontaneously in a few seconds after withdrawal. This is due to its greatly increased protein level in the spinal fluid below the level of a partial or complete block of the spinal canal. The blockage is usually due to a **spinal cord tumour**.

An acute subarachnoid haemorrhage may be complicated by blood clots forming in the subarachnoid space, leading to obstruction of blood flow and **hydrocephalus**. It should be considered as a cause of deterioration of conscious level a few days after a subarachnoid haemorrhage. However, the history of quickly coagulating CSF makes the correct answer more likely to be B.

Answer A
Paired *t*-test

This trial is a crossover randomized controlled trial. Since the data is Gaussian, i.e. normally distributed, it cannot be evaluated by the **Wilcoxon** or **Mann–Whitney *U*-test**, which are used for non-Gaussian data.

Since the same patients are evaluated under both test conditions, they are considered paired and so a **paired *t*-test** would be the best statistical test. ➤

The table below may help in deciding which test should be used in different situations.

	Measurement from Gaussian population	Rank, score or measurement (from non-Gaussian population)	Binomial (two possible outcomes)
Describe one group	Mean, SD	Median Interquartile range	Proportion
Compare one group to a hypothetical value	One sample t-test	Wilcoxon test	Chi-square or binomial test
Compare two unpaired groups	Unpaired t-test	Mann–Whitney U-test	Fisher's test (chi-square for large samples)
Compare two paired groups	Paired t-test	Wilcoxon test	McNemar's test

232 Question on p.76.

Answer B
Review in 3 months

Diabetics should have a fundoscopy on an annual basis at the very least. In some patients fundoscopy should be performed on a 3-monthly basis:

- new/worsening lesions on fundoscopy
- **scattered exudates > 1 disc diameter from fovea**
- patient is at high risk of progression, e.g. hypertensive.

Urgent referral to an ophthalmologist is indicated under the following circumstances:

- unexplained drop in visual acuity
- macular oedema
- unexplained retinal findings
- pre-proliferative retinopathy
- new vessel formation
- pre-retinal haemorrhage
- vitreous haemorrhage
- rubeosis iridis

Immediate ophthalmic referral is indicated in patients with:

- sudden loss of vision
- retinal detachment

233   Question on p.77.

Answer B
0.6

The **standard error of the mean** = standard deviation ÷ square route of the sample size

$$= 1.8 \div \sqrt{9}$$
$$= 1.8 \div 3$$
$$= 0.6$$

The standard error of the mean is necessary to work out confidence intervals. This is calculated by adding or subtracting (1.96 × standard error).

Therefore, the **95% confidence interval** is:

$$= 80 +/- (1.96 \times 0.6)$$
$$= 80 +/- 1.176$$
$$= \textbf{78.824 to 81.176}$$

234   Question on p.77.

Answer E
None of the above

Barrett's oesophagus is diagnosed at endoscopy when the lower oesophageal stratified epithelium is replaced by gastric-type columnar epithelium. The endoscopist identifies this macroscopically because the columnar epithelium has a pink appearance, whereas the normal oesophageal mucosa has a white appearance. Biopsies are taken to confirm the diagnosis and to check for any signs of dysplasia.

Patients with Barrett's oesophagus have an increased risk of adenocarcinoma of the oesophagus. The lifetime risk has been estimated to be between 0.5% and 2%, and this probably varies with the length of the Barrett's change. Patient's with ultrashort segment Barrett's (<1 cm) may have little or no increased risk of developing oesophageal adenocarcinoma, whereas patients with a very long segment of Barrett's epithelium may have considerably greater risk.

No management strategy has been shown to improve mortality in patients with Barrett's oesophagus. Proton pump inhibition and antireflux surgery have not been shown to reduce the incidence of dysplastic change, or the incidence of adenocarcinoma. Many centres routinely screen patients with Barrett's oesophagus by regular endoscopy with multiple oesophageal biopsies. If high-grade dysplasia is found and the patient is fit, an oesophagectomy is offered. The optimum frequency of screening endoscopy is unknown and none of the studies performed to date have shown improved patient outcome. ➤

Adenocarcinoma of the oesophagus is rapidly becoming more common in the developed world. The reason for this is uncertain. It is probably as a result of the increased incidence of gastro-oesophageal reflux disease, which predisposes to Barrett's oesophagus, which in turn predisposes to oesophageal carcinoma.

Treatment options in a patient with high-grade dysplasia who is unfit for surgery are:

- photodynamic therapy
- laser ablation
- argon beam diathermy ablation.

235

Question on p.77.

Answer C
Idiopathic hypercalciuria

Stones	Causes
Calcium stones (80%)	Hypercalciuria
	Hyperoxaluria
	Hypocitraturia
Uric acid stones (10%)	Acid urine
	High purine intake
	High cell turnover
Infection stones (5%)	Chronic infection
Cysteine stones (2%)	Cystinuria
Other stones (3%)	Xanthine stones
	Renal chloride channel mutations

Up to 80% of stones are visible on plain radiology. Pure uric acid stones are radiolucent. Mixed infective stones are barely radio-opaque. Calcium and cysteine stones are radio-opaque.

236

Question on p.77.

Answer A
Maternity blues

It is important to be familiar with the various post-natal disorders that mothers may experience. The time of onset after the delivery will give a clue to the diagnosis. Be sure to identify the presence of psychotic symptoms.

	Maternity blues	Post-natal depression	Puerperal psychosis
Aetiology	First pregnancy History of PMT	Previous depression Marital conflict Young age Poor support	Past history of mood disorder Family history Hormonal factors Older age Primipara Caesarean section
Epidemiology	50–70% women 3–4 days post-delivery	10–15% women 2 weeks post-delivery	1 in 500 births 2 weeks post-delivery
Presentation	Labile mood Tearfulness Irritability	Non-psychotic depression	Similar to affective disorder 20% resemble schizophrenia
Treatment	Supportive Reassurance	Psychosocial support Antidepressants Counselling/group work	Specialist care required Conventional drugs
Prognosis	Good	If untreated can last up to 2 years	Good for recovery but 30–50% will recur in subsequent deliveries

Pseudocyesis is a rare condition in which the patient believes she is pregnant. She has amenorrhoea and abdominal distension, and is so convinced of her pregnancy that she prepares for her delivery, buying clothes, etc. Many patients claim to feel fetal movements and get morning sickness.

The patient does not give a clinical picture fitting **acute mania**.

237 Question on p.78.

Answer B
Serum electrolytes

Given this lady's history of treatment for bipolar affective disorder, it is likely that she is taking lithium. She exhibits some features suggestive of lithium toxicity, which are listed below:

- ataxia
- dysarthria
- coarse tremor
- nausea and vomiting
- drowsiness
- apathy
- increased muscular tone.

It is possible that she has overdosed on her lithium but the history suggests another possibility. Lithium has a narrow therapeutic window and toxicity may occur accidentally. The most common reasons are:

1. impairment of lithium elimination by the kidney
2. electrolyte imbalances especially hyponatraemia.

An episode of diarrhoea is quite likely to lead to hyponatraemia and deterioration in renal function, and may explain her present condition.

The most useful investigation needs to be one that will not only aid diagnosis but also guide management. **Urgent psychiatric referral** is not indicated at the moment, as organic causes of her current state have not been ruled out.

Serum lithium concentrations correlate poorly with the severity of acute lithium toxicity but high levels will give some indication of prognosis (levels in excess of 2 mmol/L can be fatal and levels above 5 mmol/L should be dialysed). The most useful investigation will be **serum electrolytes**, since it will demonstrate any reversible electrolyte abnormalities and identify how biochemically dry she is. In practice, the team should stop the lithium whilst awaiting levels, and check electrolytes urgently whilst giving intravenous fluids.

Thyroid function tests are unlikely to help in the acute stage, although hypothyroidism may present in a similar way. A **CT brain** would help rule out significant intracerebral pathology and should be considered if other pathologies have been ruled out.

238 Question on p.78.

Answer B
Nevirapine

There is no cure for HIV; however, there are drugs that can slow its progression to AIDS. People experienced in this field should undertake initiation of treatment, as these are potent and expensive medicines with a significant side effect profile. The aim of treatment is to reduce viral load and to try and keep the immune system functioning for as long as possible. Combinations of drugs are best as they offer synergism without increasing the potential for side effects. Commonly used combinations include two nucleoside reverse transcriptase inhibitors. These are given with either two protease inhibitors, or a non-nucleoside reverse transcriptase inhibitor and a protease inhibitor.

Drugs	Side effects
Nucleoside reverse transcriptase inhibitors e.g. zidovudine, didanosine, lamivudine	Pancreatitis, lactic acidosis, peripheral neuropathy, hepatitis
Non-nucleoside reverse transcriptase inhibitors e.g. efavirenz, nevirapine	Hepatitis, Stevens–Johnson syndrome, elevated cholesterol
Protease inhibitors e.g. ritonavir, indinavir, lopinavir	Pancreatitis, lipodystrophy, rhabdomyolysis, neutropenia

239 Question on p.78.

Answer B
Surreptitious sulphonylurea self-administration

This patient's symptoms are due to hypoglycaemia.

Causes of hypoglycaemia
- Reactive
  - Dumping syndrome
  - Maturity onset diabetes in the young
  - Thyrotoxicosis
  - Hormonal deficiency – Addison's, hypothyroidism, hypopituitarism
  - Alcohol
  - Drugs, e.g. lithium
  - Idiopathic
- Other
  - Overdose of insulin or oral hypoglycaemic agent
  - Surreptitious use of insulin or oral hypoglycaemic agent
  - Insulinoma
  - Fructose 1,6-diphosphatase deficiency

➤

Although a **phaeochromocytoma** can present with dizzy spells, this is not the diagnosis in this case. Typically patients with a phaeochromocytoma will run a high/normal blood sugar and 30% have glycosuria.

This is not **maturity onset diabetes in the young (MODY)** because this condition occurs in overweight teenagers. Patients with MODY can get reactive hypoglycaemia but would not have fasting glucose at the levels shown on 3 consecutive days.

The differential diagnosis, therefore, lies between surreptitious sulphonylurea, and insulin self-administration and insulinoma. Differentiating these three entities can be difficult, particularly in a health professional that has easy access to drugs. The investigations listed in the following table will give the correct diagnosis.

Test	Insulinoma	Surreptitious insulin	Surreptitious sulphonylurea
Insulin levels taken when hypoglycaemic	Raised	Raised	Raised
Insulin/glucose ratio	Raised	Raised	Raised
C-peptide	Raised	Low/normal	Raised
Pro-insulin	Raised	Low/normal	Low/normal
Insulin antibodies	Negative	Positive	Negative

This patient has a raised C-peptide and a normal pro-insulin, which makes the diagnosis that of surreptitious sulphonylurea self-administration. This diagnosis can be confirmed with a urinary drug screen for oral hypoglycaemic agents.

240
Question on p.79.

Answer D
Bioavailability following intravenous administration

The **bioavailability of a drug** is a term used to describe the proportion of administered drug that reaches the site of action. When an intravenous dose of the drug is given, it all enters the systemic circulation, producing 100% bioavailability. By definition, this will be unaltered by renal impairment.

Renal metabolism
Many drugs and their metabolites are excreted via the kidney by glomerular filtration, tubular secretion or, in some cases, both. Renal impairment thus has a significant effect on the clearance of these drugs, with important clinical consequences. Drugs such as digoxin and opioids will accumulate with an increased likelihood of developing toxicity.

Gastrointestinal absorption of drug
Ammonia production in the stomach occurs in chronic renal failure, concomitant with urea accumulation and hydrolysis. Ammonia buffers hydrochloric acid, causing an increase in gastric pH. Consequently, there may be reduced absorption of drugs, such as ferrous sulphate, chlorpropramide, folic acid, pindolol and cloxacillin whose absorption is greater at acid pH.

Volume of distribution
Protein binding is affected by renal impairment, which is accompanied by increased concentrations in plasma of a number of acidic compounds that compete for binding sites on albumin and other plasma proteins. As a consequence, the proportion of free to bound drug is increased, and there are greater fluctuations in the free drug concentration following the administration of each dose.

Hepatic metabolism
Pre-systemic ('first-pass') metabolism by the liver of some drugs such as propranolol and cimetidine, may be reduced in renal impairment causing increases in plasma concentrations.

---

241 Question on p.79.

Answer B
Oesophageal carcinoma

Hereditary tylosis is a rare autosomal dominant condition causing hyperkeratosis of the palms and soles which take on a characteristic yellow/green colour. It is associated with 95% lifetime risk of oesophageal squamous cell carcinoma.

Nasopharyngeal carcinoma has an increased incidence in carpenters.
Coeliac disease is a pre-malignant condition, the incidence of all intestinal malignancies, including **duodenal,** are increased. T-cell lymphoma and adenocarcinoma of the small bowel are more common in coeliac disease.

Pancreatic adenocarcinoma is more common in smokers and patients with chronic pancreatitis.

Anal carcinoma is more common in homosexuals, being seen more frequently in those with anal warts. Those patients with anal warts tend to have a degree of intraepithelial neoplasia. This is a pre-malignant state. Fifty per cent of tumours contain viral DNA.

---

242 Question on p.80.

Answer B
Upgaze paresis

Creutzfeldt–Jacob disease (CJD) is one of the prion diseases. It has become more topical over the past 10 years following the increase of evidence supporting the link between bovine spongiform encephalopathy (BSE) and variant Creuzfeldt–Jacob disease (vCJD).

Genetic analysis suggests that BSE is only transmitted to humans with the prion protein gene (PRNP) codon 129 methionine homozygous genotype.

The definitive method of diagnosing CJD is by post-mortem neuropathological examination. However, there are several clinical features that may suggest a diagnosis of vCJD or sporadic CJD as outlined below.

	Variant CJD	Sporadic CJD
Mean presenting age	29 years	60 years
Mean disease duration	14 months	5 months
Presenting features	Cerebellar signs	Altered sensations
	Upgaze paresis	Occipital blindness
	Pyramidal signs	Personality/behavioural
	Grasp and pout	changes
	reflexes	Dementia
	Myoclonus	Myoclonus
EEG findings	Slow waves	Periodic spike and wave
		complexes

243

Question on p.80.

Answer C
Serum C2 levels are reduced

Hereditary angioedema is caused by a deficiency of C1 esterase enzyme. It is inherited in an **autosomal dominant** fashion and there is sometimes a family history of sudden unexplained death. The disease is manifest by reduced levels/reduced function of C1. **Serum C2** and C4 levels are also low but serum C3 is usually normal. Occasionally patients with lymphoma can develop an acquired form of the disease.

Typically, patients present with attacks of angioedema which last up to 3 days. **Urticaria** is not a feature. Patients may also have abdominal pain caused by intestinal oedema. Life-threatening laryngeal oedema may occur.

An acute attack is treated with fresh-frozen plasma or C1 esterase inhibitor concentrates. **Adrenaline and hydrocortisone** are ineffective in this setting but are often coprescribed when laryngeal involvement is also present.

Anabolic steroids, such as **danazole**, can be used as maintenance treatment. They work by inducing hepatic enzymes and hence the synthesis of C1 estrase inhibitor.

244   Question on p.80.

Answer E
Lower incidence of post-infarction angina

This lady has suffered a non-Q-wave myocardial infarction, in that she had coronary symptoms an elevated troponin I and an ischaemic ECG without developing Q waves.

The incidence of non-Q-wave myocardial infarction is rising, and currently accounts for up to 50% of all acute myocardial infarctions. Non-Q-wave infarction tends to involve a smaller area of myocardial necrosis but a larger potential area at risk of ischaemic injury. Thus, patients are less likely to have significant LV dysfunction and a lower in-hospital mortality rate. However, studies have shown a higher incidence of re-infarction, post-infarction angina and mortality at 1 year.

245   Question on p.80.

Answer C
***Klebsiella* pneumonia**

This is really a question about pneumonia with abscess formation. The clue is the 'bulging fissure' on the chest radiograph. This radiological sign is usually seen when there is an underlying abscess. The abscess may not be otherwise immediately apparent as a cavity on the chest X-ray.

Causes of cavitation on the chest X-ray

Abscess	*Staphylococcus aureus*
	Klebsiella
	Anaerobes, e.g. *Bacteroides* sp.,
	Peptostreptococcus sp., *Prevotella* sp.
Carcinoma	Usually small cell
Tuberculosis	
Wegener's granulomatosis	Rare
Infarction	
Hydatid cysts	Rare
Fungal infection	Rare

***Klebsiella* pneumonia** is caused by a Gram-negative rod and shows a predilection for the elderly with a history of heart or lung disease, alcoholics and the immunocompromised. It accounts for 1–2% of all community acquired infections and is frequently fatal.

Classically, the patient has a high fever, myalgia and rapidly progressive dyspnoea. There is production of red current jelly sputum. There are variable signs in the chest. *Klebsiella* pneumonia often produces lung abscesses. These may not be immediately apparent on the chest ➤

radiograph but the bulging fissure sign is highly suggestive of underlying cavitation.

The treatment of choice is determined by *in vitro* sensitivity tests but an intravenous cephalosporin is usually required pending these results.

246

Question on p.81.

Answer E
Multiple cerebrovascular events

This is a question about pseudobulbar palsy. It is a term that describes bilateral upper motor neurone lesions affecting the lower cranial nuclei. Symptoms include dysarthria and difficulty swallowing. Signs are of a spastic tongue, preserved gag and exaggerated jaw jerk.

This is in contrast to bulbar palsy, where there is principally a lower motor neurone type weakness, i.e. wasted, fasiculating tongue.

Causes of a pseudobulbar palsy include **bilateral cerebrovascular events**. Such patients also exhibit emotional lability and bilateral pyramidal signs, both of which are evident in this case.

Motor neurone disease can produce signs of pseudobulbar palsy; however, there is often a LMN component as well, e.g. wasted fibrillating tongue.

Multiple sclerosis can give a pseudobulbar palsy when there is brainstem involvement. However, this tends to occur late on in the disease. Brainstem involvement more frequently takes the pattern of either an internuclear ophthalmoplegia or an isolated cranial nerve palsy.

A **pontine glioma** is a rare brainstem tumour presenting most frequently in children or those suffering from neurofibromatosis. It produces symptoms of a cerebello-pontine angle lesion.

247

Question on p.81.

Answer C
Presence of anti-IgA antibodies in recipient

It is very unlikely that the cause of the major transfusion reaction is **ABO or rhesus incompatibility**. This patient is receiving cross-matched blood. Under these circumstances, the only way in which the patient can have a major transfusion reaction due to ABO or rhesus incompatibility is if he is given the wrong blood. This occasionally does happen in clinical practice, but its incidence has been minimized by rigorous checking procedures in the laboratory and on the ward.

Given this patient's background history of asthma and recurrent infections, it is likely that he has an underlying primary IgA deficiency. This is the most common cause of primary immunodeficiency in the UK and the prevalence may be as high as 1 in 700. Primary IgA deficiency presents with asthma/hay fever and recurrent infections of the ear, sinuses, and upper respiratory and gastrointestinal tracts. The diagnosis is confirmed by serum immunoglobulins, which shows a low serum IgA. The other immunoglobulins are normal.

Patients with IgA deficiency frequently have **IgA antibodies**. These can cause an often fatal transfusion reaction when even appropriately ABO or rhesus crossed-matched whole blood is given. Patients with IgA deficiency requiring transfusion should ideally have an autologous transfusion. This is clearly not possible in this clinical situation. An alternative is for patients to receive ABO or rhesus crossed-matched blood from a donor who is also IgA deficient.

---

248   Question on p.81.

Answer A
Avascular necrosis of the femoral head

In a patient with pain in a single joint, it is always necessary to exclude a **septic arthritis**. This is very important in immunosuppressed rheumatoid patients who are particularly susceptible.

The diagnosis and treatment of suspected septic arthritis is an orthopaedic emergency. An early diagnosis is essential to avoid joint destruction. The best way to exclude a diagnosis of septic arthritis is joint aspiration. The aspirate is analysed by microscopy and culture, and microscopy can be achieved very rapidly. A negative result makes the diagnosis of septic arthritis extremely unlikely in this patient. Patients who are found to have a septic arthritis on microscopy should have an emergency joint washout plus appropriate intravenous antibiotics.

Posterior subluxation of the femoral head is more common in patients who have had hip replacements and trauma. It could present in the way described in the question. It can often be missed on a plain anterior/posterior X-rays, and lateral films should always be taken if this diagnosis is suspected.

Osteomyelitis presents with pain and swelling over the infected area of bone. This is commonly the highly vascular areas of bone, i.e. distal femur and proximal tibia.

It is unlikely that this patient has a **flare of her arthritis**, as she is currently receiving treatment with prednisolone and methotrexate. If this were a flare, it would be unusual to have only one joint involved.

The most likely diagnosis is **avascular necrosis of the femoral head**. This condition is more common in patients on high-dose corticosteroids. Avascular necrosis presents as acute onset of severe pain in the affected joint, commonly the hip. The exact aetiology of this condition is not fully understood but it is thought to be a microangiopathic process. X-ray changes occur 1–2 weeks after the onset of the hip pain. Immediate diagnosis in this patient should be by bone scan or MRI. ➤

> **Risk factors for avascular necrosis of the femoral head**
> - Corticosteroids therapy
> - Alcoholism
> - Sickle cell disease
> - Divers
> - Heparin therapy

249

Question on p.81.

Answer E
Intravenous glucagon

The blockade of β-receptors results in decreased production of intracellular cyclic adenosine monophosphate (cAMP) with a resultant blunting of multiple metabolic and cardiovascular effects of circulating catecholamines. β1-receptors increase the force and rate of myocardial contraction and atrioventricular (AV) node conduction velocity.

β-Blockers, therefore, reduce heart rate, blood pressure, myocardial contractility and myocardial oxygen consumption. β2-receptor blockade inhibits relaxation of smooth muscle in blood vessels, bronchi, and the gastrointestinal and genitourinary tract. In addition, β2-blockade inhibits glycogenolysis and gluconeogenesis.

Other than the direct effects of the β-adrenoreceptor blockade, toxicity may result from other mechanisms including sodium and calcium channel blockade, a centrally mediated cardiac depression, and alteration of cardiac myocyte energy metabolism.

The most appropriate drug is **intravenous glucagon**. It stimulates production of cAMP through non-adrenergic pathways, resulting in enhanced contractility, heart rate and AV conduction.

250

Question on p.82.

Answer E
SCL-70

There is no one test that is diagnostic of systemic sclerosis. However, the diagnosis is made more likely by the presence of certain autoantibodies. The results of the autoantibody tests must always be interpreted in the light of the clinical findings.

Patients with systemic sclerosis may present with the following.

- Hand symptoms/signs:
  - Raynaud's
  - nailfold infarction
  - sclerodactyly
  - pulp calcinosis.

- Oesophageal symptoms:
  - dysphagia (strictures and motility abnormalities)
  - reflux symptoms.
- Hypertension
- Renal failure
- Lung fibrosis
- Cardiac arrythmias

Autoantibodies and disease associations

Autoantibodies	Disease association
Anti-Ro	SLE, Sjögren's
Anti-La	Sjögren's
Anti-Ds-DNA	SLE
Anti-Sm	SLE
Anti-histone	Drug induced SLE
Anti–Jo-1	Polymyositis
Anti-centromere	Limited cutaneous scleroderma (CREST)
Anti-SCL-70	Systemic sclerosis

---

251 Question on p.82.

Answer A
Course of antibiotics

Mucosa-associated lymphoid tissue (MALT) forms part of the lymphatic system and is present in mucosal surfaces in the gut, the respiratory system and the eyes.

A MALToma is an unusual form of B-cell lymphoma. It is normally low grade and represents about 5% of all cases of lymphoma. It presents from the teenage years through till old age but tends to be more common in those over 50 years. The most common site for occurrence is the stomach, representing two-thirds of all MALTomas. Mostly they are due to infection with *H. pylori*. Symptoms are vague and tend to be that of loss of weight and appetite, indigestion and occasionally GI bleeding.

Treatment depends on the stage however, spread is much less common than with other lymphomas. Initial treatment should be a course of **triple therapy** to eradicate the *H. pylori*; this leads to remission in most cases. For the few that spread, treatment then consists of **surgery, chemotherapy and radiotherapy**.

---

252 Question on p.82.

Answer C
Hypothermia

The ECG may give a clue to metabolic or biochemical abnormalities. The following ECG changes may be observed: ➤

- **Hypokalaemia**:
  - Flattened T wave, which may become inverted
  - Prominent U wave
  - Shortened ST segment
  - Prolonged PR interval
  - Rarely, complete SA block occurs and there is an increased risk of torsades de points.
- **Hypothermia**:
  - Bradycardia
  - J waves (also known as Osborn waves)
  - Prolongation of QT interval.
- **Hypomagnesaemia** (usually goes hand in hand with hypokalaemia):
  - Flattened T waves
  - Prolonged QT interval
  - Shortened ST segment.
- **Hypocalcaemia**:
  - Prolonged QT interval.

Hypothyroidism is a well-recognized cause of hypothermia. ECG changes may include bradycardia and, if hypothermic, J waves. From the question, it is unlikely that a 23-year-old female with hypothyroidism severe enough to cause ECG changes would be well enough to go out clubbing for the night. The more likely scenario is that she came home drunk, passed out and slipped into ketoacidosis. Her night clubbing clothes will have been too flimsy to keep her warm and she will have become progressively colder.

253
Question on p.82.

Answer C
Fundoscopy

Cytomegalovirus (CMV) retinitis is the commonest cause of eye disease and blindness in patients with AIDS, and occurs in 25–30% of cases. It is usually unilateral to start with but commonly progresses to involve both eyes. Symptoms depend on the part of the retina involved and include floaters, loss of acuity, scotomata and orbital pain.

The diagnosis is clinical and made on the basis of the characteristic fundoscopic appearances with haemorrhages and exudates along the line of the vessels in the retina. Patients who are not treated go blind. The treatment consists of iv gangcyclovir.

Causes of visual disturbances in patients with AIDS
- CMV retinitis
- *Toxoplasma* retinitis
- Progressive multifocal leucoencephalopathy
- Lymphoma
- Syphilis
- *Pneumocystis*

Question on p.83.

Answer A
Phenytoin

First-order kinetics is a term describing the metabolism of a drug in which the rate is proportional to the drug concentration.

In the metabolism and excretion of a drug by **zero-order kinetics**, a constant amount of drug is eliminated per unit time. This means that the rate of metabolism is saturable and small changes in dose can give dramatic changes in concentration.

Drugs metabolized by zero-order kinetics
- Alcohol
- Phenytoin
- Hydralazine
- Disulfaram

 Question on p.83.

Answer A
Hypomagnesaemia

This gentleman has symptomatic hypocalcaemia with a normal phosphate, albumin and alkaline phosphatase. The clue here is the parathormone level. This helps to differentiate the causes.

Patients with **hypomagnesaemia** are very frequently hypocalcaemic. The reason for this is that magnesium is a cofactor in the production of parathormone. Patients who have significant hypomagnesaemia, therefore, have a low PTH and low calcium as in this case (see box).

Di George syndrome is a developmental abnormality whereby the branchial arches fail to develop. Hence the parathyroid glands are absent. When children are born with this condition, they have seizures shortly after birth because of the severe hypocalcaemia. It also means that there is an absent thymus and they present later in life with recurrent infections, in particular, *Pneumocystis carinii* pneumonia and candidiasis. ➤

> **Causes of hypocalcaemia include:**
> - Hypoparathyroidism
>   - Idiopathic
>   - Post-neck surgery
>   - Magnesium deficiency
> - Vitamin D deficiency
>   - Rickets/osteomalacia
>   - Secondary to lack of sunlight, dietary, malabsorption
>   - PTH levels high
>   - Associated low phosphate, raised alkaline phosphatase
> - Renal disease
>   - Kidneys fail to synthesize 1,25 DHCC
>   - Subsequent overproduction of PTH can lead to bone destruction
>   - Associated raised phosphate
> - Pseudohypoparathyroidism
>   - Failure of end organ receptors to respond to PTH
>   - PTH levels high
> - Miscellaneous
>   - Acute pancreatitis (saponification in retroperitonium)
>   - Acute rhabdomyolysis
>   - Malignancy

256

Question on p.84.

Answer B
DR2

The possession of the HLA DR2 antigen carries a relative risk of 130 of developing narcolepsy. Important HLA antigen associations are listed below.

Disease	HLA antigen	Relative risk
Narcolepsy	DR2	130
Goodpasture's syndrome	DR2	16
Haemochromatosis	A3, B14	90
Ankylosing spondylitis	B27	70
Reiter's syndrome	B27	40
Psoriatic arthritis	B27	10
Coeliac disease	DR3	10
Dermatitis herpetiformis	DR3	17
Pemphigus	DR4	15
Type I diabetes mellitus	DR4	5
Addison's disease	Dw3	10

257 Question on p.84.

Answer A
1/150

In order to answer this question it is necessary to know:

- the inheritance of CF (autosomal recessive, see box)
- the risk that the patient is a CF carrier
- the risk that her partner is a CF carrier
- the risk that two parents who are carriers of a recessive condition will have an affected child.

For any autosomal recessive condition, if both parents are carriers, there is a 1/4 chance that they will have an affected child. The family tree below shows two carrier parents (Rr) and the four possible outcomes of any pregnancy they may have. Only if the child inherits the mutated gene (r) from both parents will it be homozygous (rr) and develop the condition.

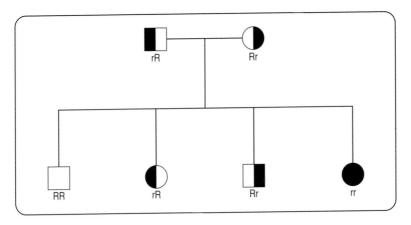

The chance that this patient is a CF carrier is 2/3, not 2/4 as is commonly thought, because the homozygous affected category has been excluded (the question tells us she is healthy). She must, therefore, be RR, rR or Rr (two of these three possibilities would mean she is a carrier).

Since we have not been told otherwise, we must assume that her partner does not have a family history of CF. (Of course, in actual clinical practice, it is essential to confirm this by taking a detailed family history from both sides). Therefore, he is at population risk, which we have been told is 1/25.

The calculation is then a straightforward multiplication of these three risk figures:

$$2/3 \times 1/25 \times 1/4 = 2/300 = 1/150$$

Most errors in this sort of calculation occur because the carrier risk of the patient (in this case the mother) is mistakenly believed to be 2/4 or ➤

possibly 1, leading to a final risk of 1/200 or 1/100, respectively. Alternatively, the 1/4 risk of having an affected child is forgotten, leading to a final risk of 2/75. A combination of these errors would be necessary to produce a risk of 1/50.

Autosomal dominant conditions
- Huntington's disease
- Myotonic dystrophy
- Adult polycystic kidney disease
- Acute intermittent porphyria
- Familial adenomatous polyposis
- Marfan's syndrome
- Tuberous sclerosis
- Neurofibromatosis Type 1
- Achondroplasia
- Peutz–Jeghers' syndrome
- Von Hippel–Lindau's syndrome

Autosomal recessive conditions
- Cystic fibrosis
- Phenylketonuria
- Wilson's disease
- Haemochromatosis
- Ataxia telangiectasia
- Alpha-1 antitrypsin deficiency
- Hurler's syndrome
- Tay Sachs' disease
- Galactosaemia
- Pseudoxanthoma elasticum
- Xeroderma Pigmentosum

X-linked recessive conditions
- Duchenne's muscular dystrophy
- Haemophilia A
- Fragile X mental retardation
- Hunter's syndrome
- Becker's muscular dystrophy
- Kennedy's disease
- G6PD deficiency
- Lesch–Nyhan's syndrome
- Chronic granulomatous disease
- Adrenoleucodystrophy
- Fabry's disease

Answer C
CEA

Tumour markers are substances that can be related to the presence or progress of a tumour. They include enzymes, other proteins and smaller peptides, which are secreted into body fluids by tumours, and antigens expressed on cell surfaces.

Carcinoembryonic antigen (CEA) is present in elevated concentrations in the plasma of 60% of patients with colorectal cancer. In patients with advanced disease it may be raised in 80–100%. CEA is neither specific nor sensitive enough to be used in screening for colorectal carcinoma but following surgical resection of a tumour, plasma CEA concentration can be expected to fall. However, while a subsequent rise suggests a recurrence, recurrence is not always heralded by such a rise. In addition other conditions may cause a raised CEA. Nevertheless, it is the best answer from the choices given and used routinely in oncology clinics.

Causes of a raised CEA include:
- Colorectal carcinoma
- Liver disease
- Pancreatitis
- Inflammatory bowel disease
- Heavy smokers

CA 19-9 is used for the monitoring of patients to treatment for adenocarcinoma of pancreas. Plasma CA 19-9 concentrations are elevated in more than 80% of patients with carcinoma of the exocrine pancreas but only occasionally in benign disease. However, its potential value as a marker is diminished by the fact that pancreatic cancer tends to present late, when no effective treatment is available. It may also have a role in the monitoring of colorectal and gastric carcinoma.

CA-125 is a specific tumour marker for ovarian cancer. Its level at diagnosis is of little prognostic significance but serial measurements at follow-up are valuable in monitoring patients following resection of a tumour.

Prostate specific antigen (PSA) is used to monitor disease progression in prostatic cancer. It is detectable in all men with concentrations increasing with age and in benign prostatic hypertrophy. The finding of an elevated level of PSA in a patient with prostatism is not diagnostic of prostatic cancer but should prompt the patient's admission for biopsy and histological diagnosis.

Other tumour markers, which are of potential value in monitoring the response of patients to treatment, include CA 50 for colorectal carcinoma and CA 15-3 for carcinoma of breast. In carcinoma of the breast, both CA 15-3 and mucin-like carcinoma-associated antigen (MCA) may help to identify patients who have metastases at the time of diagnosis.

Question on p.84.

Answer C
iv magnesium sulphate

The British Thoracic Society has recently revised its guidelines on the management of acute asthma.

Features of acute–severe asthma
- Unable to complete sentences
- Peak flow 33–50% of best
- Pulse > 110/minute
- Respiratory rate > 25/minute

Features of life-threatening asthma
- Peak flow < 33%
- Oxygen saturation < 92%
- Cyanosis, silent chest, feeble respiratory effort
- Bradycardia, dysrhythmia or hypotension
- Exhaustion, confusion or coma

This man has life-threatening asthma as judged by his peak flow of less than 33% of normal and oxygen saturations of 90%. The intensive care team need to be alerted along with a senior clinician.

The next step would be to commence **intravenous magnesium sulphate.**

The guidelines state that the senior clinician should consider the use of intravenous β_2-**agonists** or **aminophylline**.

A **chest X-ray** is not indicated unless a pneumothorax or consolidation is suspected.

 Question on p.85.

Answer D
Mamillary body atrophy

Wernicke–Korsakoff's syndrome is an amnesic syndrome resulting from thiamine deficiency in association with chronic alcoholism. It is sometimes associated with malnutrition or malabsorption.

The Wernicke phase of this disorder is characterized by confusion, nystagmus, abducent and conjugate gaze palsies (ophthalmoplegia), and ataxia. These features are commonly accompanied by peripheral neuropathy. Prompt treatment with thiamine replacement is vital in order to avert a chronic and disabling amnesic disorder (the Korsakoff syndrome).

The neuropathology of amnesic disorders usually involves lesions within the limbic system, including the thalamus and posterior hypothalamus, medial temporal lobes, and mamillary bodies. There may be many changes seen in these patients but the question asks for the 'characteristic pathological changes'. The characteristic changes in Korsakoff's syndrome involve neuronal loss, gliosis and microhaemorrhages that produce disruption of mamillary bodies. Pathology elsewhere in the grey matter, including the **frontal lobes,** and in white matter pathways traversing the diencephalons, are common accompanying features.

Chronic, heavy alcohol consumption causes structural changes in the brain, particularly in the **cerebellum**, limbic system, diencephalon and cerebral cortex. **Cerebral atrophy** may result in enlargement of the ventricles, and widening of the fissures and sulci.

Central pontine myelinolysis, also known as osmotic demyelination syndrome, occurs in patients with severe hyponatraemia. It is not certain whether this is caused by the hyponatraemia itself or by overzealous treatment of that hyponatraemia. Cerebral demyelination is thought to result from large shifts of intracellular water, resulting in quadriplegia and pseudobulbar palsy. Neurological signs usually develop 2–4 days after rapid correction of hyponatraemia.

---

261 Question on p.85.

Answer B
Minimal change nephropathy

This man has presented with nephrotic syndrome. The causes of nephrotic syndrome are listed below.

- All glomerulonephritides and minimal change lesion
- Systemic vasculitides, most commonly SLE
- Diabetic glomerulosclerosis
- Amyloidosis
- Drugs, e.g. penicillamine
- Allergies.

Minimal change accounts for about 20% of cases of nephrotic syndrome in adults. However, in children, that figure is nearer 90%. Minimal change is included in the GN classification even though there is no evidence for inflammation on biopsy. The change seen on light microscopy is a fusion of the podocytes; however, this can be seen occasionally as a non-specific finding. Despite this, it is thought to have an immunological basis because:

1. it responds to immunosuppressive therapy
2. there is an association between Hodgkin's disease and subsequent remission with successful treatment
3. there is a higher incidence in people with asthma/eczema and remission with desensitization. ➤

Membranous nephropathy is the most common cause of nephrotic syndrome in adults. Associations include SLE, colorectal carcinoma, hepatitis B and infection with *Plasmodium malariae*.

AA amyloid is associated with chronic inflammatory conditions such as rheumatoid arthritis and inflammatory bowel disease. However, it is AL amyloid (immunoglobulin light chains) that is associated with haematological malignancies.

IgA nephropathy is the most common cause of asymptomatic microscopic haematuria. It can cause nephrotic syndrome but this occurs in less than 5% of cases.

Kimmelsteil–Wilson nodules are the pathognomic lesions seen in glomerulosclerosis in diabetic patients. Their presence is normally associated with a significant degree of proteinuria that manifests a number of years after the diagnosis of diabetes.

262

Question on p.86.

Answer C
Left parietal lobe

This man has a right inferior homonymous quadrantinopia.

A basic knowledge of neuroanatomy is required when performing a neurological examination, subsequently trying to localize the signs and coming to the appropriate diagnosis.

Fibres from the retina of each eye join together to form the right and left optic nerve. These fibres join at the optic chiasm where the fibres are split. The optic chiasm sits in the sella turcica and can be compressed by lesions affecting the pituitary. This causes a bitemporal hemianopia that spreads down from the upper to lower field.

The lateral fibres conveying the nasal fields continue along the optic tract on the same side, whereas the medial fibres conveying the temporal fields decussate. From here the newly formed right and left optic tracts synapse at the lateral geniculate bodies. Lesions at this point, therefore, would cause a homonymous hemianopia.

From here fibres pass in the optic radiation through the parietal and temporal lobe. Those fibres travelling through the **parietal lobe** carry information from the lower visual field. A lesion here would cause a lower quadrantic hemianopia, which is how this man has presented.

Fibres travelling through the **temporal lobe** carry information from the upper visual field. A lesion here would cause an upper quadrantic hemianopia.

The fibres then pass into the **occipital lobe** where they terminate. Lesions here are frequently caused by posterior cerebral artery infarction and produce a homonymous hemianopia. However, there is macular sparing as the macular region has a separate blood supply from the middle cerebral artery.

Question on p.86.

Answer E
Isoniazid, rifampicin, pyrazinamide, streptomycin plus pyridoxine

	Pyogenic	Viral	Tuberculous	Cryptococcal
Cell count/mm^3	> 1000	< 500	< 500	< 150
Predominant cell type	Polymorphs	Lymphocytes	Lymphocytes	Lymphocytes
Protein concentration (g/L)	> 1.5	0.5–1.0	1.0–5.0	0.5–1.0
CSF: blood glucose	< 50%	> 50%	< 50%	< 50%

The history of iv drug use raises the question of immunocompromise and tuberculous, or cryptococcal infection. Both these conditions show a predominance of lymphocytes in the CSF, and a glucose ratio of <50%. In cryptococcal infection the cell count would be lower than in this case. The protein count is markedly raised and highly suggestive of tuberculous meningitis.

The other 'spanner in the works' is the fact that the GP has already given 2 g of cefotaxime and it is important to be aware that partially treated bacterial meningitis will have a different CSF result than that in the table with:

• fall in cell count
• increase in lymphocytes
• fall in protein level
• persisting low glucose.

These results look very similar to those of the patient in the question, but the raised protein makes tuberculous meningitis the most likely diagnosis. Treatment is with **antituberculous chemotherapy** as outlined in Answer E.

Answer D would be the treatment for **cryptococcal meningitis**.

Answer C is the treatment for **bacterial meningitis** in a previously healthy adult over 50 or someone who is immunocompromised.

Answer B would be appropriate treatment for *Herpes simplex* **encephalitis**.

Answer A would not adequately cover pneumococcal meningitis on its own. If Gram stain suggests pneumococcal infection, **vancomycin** needs to be added. If pneumococcal infection is not suggested by Gram stain, then **ceftriaxone alone** will be appropriate.

264   Question on p.86.

Answer D
Long-term diuretic therapy

The results of the blood tests demonstrate the following:

- hyponatraemia
- hyperkalaemia
- alkalosis
- mild dehydration (as suggested by a disproportionately raised urea to creatinine).

We do not know the cause of his dyspnoea, but the five potential answers direct us to diagnoses we should be considering.

1. Chronic obstructive pulmonary disease

COPD is likely to have been treated with steroids over time and Addison's disease may develop owing to long-term adrenal suppression. It can result in hyponatraemia, hyperkalaemia, alkalosis and raised urea. The glucose is often low and hypercalcaemia is sometimes seen.

2. Restrictive lung disease of some sort

A restrictive lung disease may lead to a compensated respiratory acidosis owing to hypoventilation. Chronic respiratory acidosis leads to a compensatory increase in urinary hydrogen ion secretion, resulting in a rise in plasma bicarbonate concentration. The raised bicarbonate could be a function of this.

3. Congestive cardiac failure (CCF)

CCF is a possibility because it is a common cause of dyspnoea and is treated with diuretics. Usually a loop diuretic would be prescribed with a potassium sparing diuretic to prevent hypokalaemia. This would explain the low sodium and high potassium. Long-term use of these diuretics would also result in an alkalosis owing to increased renal loss of hydrogen ions. ACE inhibitor therapy may be used in CCF but is less likely to cause an alkalosis as seen with this patient. Hyperkalaemia and mild hyponatraemia are recognized.

4. Chronic pulmonary emboli

This possible diagnosis is given in the answers but is less likely to be true as an isolated answer. Chronic hypoxia *per se* would not cause this biochemical picture. The only possible explanation would be that the patient had gone on to develop cor pulmonale. This would lead to congestive cardiac failure, which may be treated with diuretics. Although this would explain the blood tests, it is a rather tenuous explanation and less likely.

Several of these answers are plausible and so we need to choose the most likely. Consider which answer is clinically most common and which answer most completely explains the findings. The two answers that best fit the biochemical picture are diuretic use and Addison's disease. In practice, diuretic use tends to be long term and ongoing, whilst steroids are often given intermittently at varying doses. Not all patients on steroids will develop biochemically apparent Addison's whilst hyponatraemic. Hyperkalaemic alkalosis is a common finding with long-term diuretics. In addition, if the Addison's were the correct answer, the glucose would be lower to remove all doubt.

---

265   Question on p.87.

Answer B
Cervical rib

This patient has signs and symptoms suggestive of a T1 root lesion, caused by either a **cervical rib** or a **Pancoast's tumour**. Both typically cause pain and numbness in the axilla, which radiates down the medial part of the arm and down into the hand. The patient may have reduced sensation to pinprick in the T1 dermatome on the medial aspect of the upper arm. The T1 root supplies motor innervation to all the small muscles of the hand. However, the abductor pollicis brevis appears particularly susceptible to injury from a T1 root lesion and weakness in this muscle may be the only physical sign. This patient is much more likely to have a cervical rib than a Pancoast's tumour because of his age and the length of the history.

Carpal tunnel syndrome often presents as pain in the hand at night. Typically the pain wakes the patient at night and occurs in the lateral part of the palmar aspect of the hand. It is very common. The usual physical signs are weakness in the lateral two lumbricals, the opponens pollicis, flexor pollicis and abductor pollicis brevis. However, frequently weakness can only be demonstrated in the abductor pollicis brevis. Objective sensory signs may be absent.

Radial nerve compression causes weakness of the triceps, wrist and finger extensors and brachioradialis. Sensory signs are usually absent due to overlapping sensory fibres from the median and ulnar nerves.

A **C6 radiculopathy** usually occurs in patients with cervical spondylosis and it would be uncommon in a patient of the age of 40. The C6 root is the most commonly affected and T1 lesions are very rare. Patients complain of pain in the C6 root territory (lateral aspect of forearm and hand), which is worse on neck movement. In a C6 radiculopathy there is loss of the biceps and supinator reflexes (C5 and C6), and loss of power in the biceps and supinator muscles.

266

Question on p.87.

Answer C
Long synthacten test

This patient is likely to have hypoadrenalism secondary to long-term corticosteroid use. **Withdrawal of corticosteroids**, even very cautiously, can precipitate an adrenal crisis. For this reason, it is essential to be certain what functional reserve the pituitary–adrenal axis has. This is best established by a long synthacten test.

A **long synthacten test** involves administering 1 mg of intramuscular ACTH. Blood is assayed for cortisol levels hourly for 4 hours, and at 8 and 24 hours following. A rise of cortisol of 550 nmol/L, or an absolute level of over 1000 nmol/L excludes adrenal suppression. In this situation it is safe to withdraw corticosteroids, although this should still be done very cautiously as outlined in option A. Patients who have been on steroids for this length of time often get severe muscular aches and pains on withdrawal. This must not be confused with a recrudescence of the symptoms of polymyalgia. This distinction can be difficult to make clinically, but in steroid withdrawl-induced myalgia the ESR will be normal.

The **short synthacten test** is used in the diagnosis of Addison's disease. Cortisol is measured at 0 and 30 minutes after ACTH injection. A rise in cortisol of over 330 mmol/L excludes the diagnosis.

267

Question on p.87.

Answer C
Bronchial carcinoma

For this question you have to know your lists of causes of cerebellar symptoms and gynaecomastia. If there is a cause that links the two lists, that's the answer.

Gynaecomastia	Cerebellar syndrome
Physiological – puberty, old age	Phenytoin overdose
Hyperthyroidism	Hypothyroidism
Starvation/refeeding	Alcohol abuse
Liver disease	CO poisoning
Carcinoma of the breast	Strokes – infarct/haemorrhage
Oestrogen-producing tumours, e.g. testis, adrenal	HIV
	MS
hCG-producing tumours, **e.g. lung**	Non-metastatic malignancy **e.g. lung**
Digoxin	Inherited, e.g. Friedreich's ataxia
Oestrogens	Compression by tumour, e.g. acoustic neuroma
Antiandrogens, e.g. spironolactone, cyproterone	Tumour – primary or secondary
Kleinfelter's syndrome	

On review of the lists, it can be seen that lung cancer is the only condition that accounts for both gynaecomastia and cerebellar signs. Therefore, the answer is C.

Answer A
Loa loa and *Chrysops silicea*

Loaiasis is confined to Africa and adult worms are transmitted by *Chrysops* flies. They migrate through subcutaneous tissues and may cross the front of the eye.

Malaria is of course transmitted by the *Anopheles* mosquito, whilst *Aedes* species are the vectors of Dengue fever and yellow fever.

Onchocerciasis is a tissue-dwelling nematode that may localize to the eye causing river blindness. It is transmitted by the female blackfly, *Simulium domnosum*, and not *Glossina morsitas* (a tsetse fly), which is the main insect vector for Rhodesian sleeping sickness.

Tick-borne **relapsing fever** is transmitted by soft ticks (e.g. *Ornithoderus moubata*).

Ixodid ticks carry Lyme disease (*Borrelia burgdorfei*).

Rats are a reservoir host for **Leptospirosis** but not classified as a vector.

Answer C
Ipsilateral loss of proprioception and vibration sense belowT1

To answer this question, you need to know the wiring diagram of the spinal cord.

Temperature sensation is carried to the brain via the spinothalamic tract. The sensory fibres enter the ipsilateral spinal cord and immediately cross over to the contralateral spinal cord. They then pass up the contralateral spinal cord until they reach the thalamus. Thus, a hemicord lesion atT1 will cause contralateral loss of pain and temperature sensation. Occasionally patients will also lose pain and temperature sensation in the ipsilateral distribution of theT1 root and sometimes this is associated with hyperaesthesia above this region.

Proprioception is carried to the brain via the dorsal columns. The sensory fibres enter the ipsilateral cord and pass straight up the ipsilateral dorsal nuclei in the brainstem. At this level they cross over to the contralateral cerebellum and its connections. Thus a hemicord lesion atT1 will cause an ipsilateral loss of joint position, vibration and light touch sensation.

Motor fibres are carried from the brain to the brainstem, where the main pyramidal tracts cross over (the area of decussation in the medulla). They then pass down the contralateral spinal cord in the corticospinal tracts to innervate the contralateral motor peripheral nervous system via the spinal nerve roots. Thus, a hemicord lesion atT1 will cause ➤

ipsilateral upper motor neurone (UMN) signs (brisk reflexes and upgoing plantars) below the level of the lesion.

Motor fibres leave the spinal cord starting at the anterior horn cells via the motor roots to supply the ipsilateral musculature innervated by that root. **Lower motor neurone** signs can only be produced by damage to this final nerve fibre anywhere along its length, from the anterior horn cell to the motor end plate. Thus a hemicord lesion at T1 will cause ipsilateral lower motor neurone (LMN) signs in the T1 root distribution.

Abdominal reflexes are primitive cutaneous reflexes elicited by stroking the skin over the abdominal wall and watching the muscles contract. These reflexes are absent if there is a UMN lesion above the level of T9. Thus abdominal reflexes would be absent in this case.

270
Question on p.88.

Answer B
Staphylococcus

Staphylococcus aureus is responsible for over 90% of cases of osteomyelitis. Treatment is with flucloxacillin. Fusidic acid is often preferred, as it penetrates bone better than flucloxacillin. Prolonged treatment for 6 weeks or more is usually necessary. In addition, surgical debridement is occasionally required.

Streptococcus spp. rarely, if ever, cause osteomyelitis. They are a common cause of cellulitis.

Patients with sickle cell disease are prone to infarction of the bone during a crisis. Occasionally an infracted area becomes infected. A common infecting organism in this situation is *Salmonella*.

Haemophilus is a very rare cause of osteomyelitis and accounts for less than 2% of cases.

Mycobacterium tuberculosis can affect bone causing an osteomyelitis. It usually does this by haematogenous spread (Pott's disease). Tuberculous osteomyelitis is very rare in the UK.

271
Question on p.88.

Answer D
Sensitivity 80%, specificity 94%

Blood test	Diagnosis		Totals
	DVT	No DVT	
Positive	12	5	17
Negative	3	80	83
Total	15	85	100

Sensitivity = Proportion of patients with DVT correctly diagnosed by blood
test
=12/15
= 80%

Specificity = proportion of patients without DVT correctly diagnosed by
negative blood test
= 80/85
= 94%

---

272   Question on p.89.

Answer A
Translocation (9, 22)

This patient has got chronic myelocytic leukaemia. More than 95% of
patients with this condition have the Philadelphia chromosome, which is a
translocation between chromosome 9 and 22. The small minority without
this translocation have a much worse prognosis.

A **translocation of 15/17** is associated with acute promyelocytic
leukaemia. This type of leukaemia is of particular importance owing to its
relationship to disseminated intravascular coagulation (DIC).

A **translocation of 8/14** is associated with Burkitt's lymphoma and was
one of the first tumours in which cytogenetic change was noted.

A **deletion of chromosome 7** is associated with myelodysplasia.

A **duplication of chromosome 17** forms the genetic basis of
Charcot–Marie–Tooth syndrome or HSMN type II.

---

273   Question on p.89.

Answer A
Stimulates antithrombin III

Heparin works mainly by **stimulating antithrombin III**, (see figure) which
is a naturally occurring inhibitor of thrombin and activated Factor Xa. This
is involved in both the intrinsic and extrinsic pathways.

Urokinase works by **activating plasminogen**, which, in turn, is converted
to plasmin, and it is this that dissolves fibrin.

Production of **faulty Factor VIIIc** is the pathological basis of haemophilia
A. A decrease or **absence of protein C** is seen in prothrombotic conditions.
Testing for the absence/low levels of this protein make up part of the
thrombophilia screen. There is no drug that increases levels of this
protein.

An increase in the production of **faulty vitamin K-dependent factors** is
the basis of treatment with warfarin (II, VII, IX and X). ➤

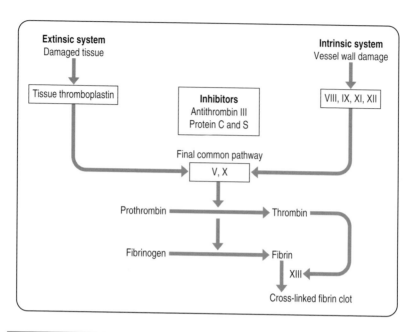

Extrinsic system
Damaged tissue

Intrinsic system
Vessel wall damage

Tissue thromboplastin

Inhibitors
Antithrombin III
Protein C and S

VIII, IX, XI, XII

Final common pathway
V, X

Prothrombin → Thrombin

Fibrinogen → Fibrin

XIII

Cross-linked fibrin clot

---

274 Question on p.89.

Answer B
Erythema nodosum

Panniculitis relates to an array of conditions that involves inflammation of the dermis and subcutaneous tissue. The causes are diverse but all tend to give the same clinical appearance. The skin feels thick and 'woody', pigmentation is brown or dark red. It is tender to touch and the area affected tends to be raised.

Treatment is of the underlying cause, rest and elevation, simple analgesics and occasionally compression hosiery. In severe cases, oral steroids, dapsone and colchicine have been used to good effect.

Typically, if panniculitis is seen on biopsy, the most likely diagnosis is erythema nodosum. Other rarer causes include polyarteritis nodosa (PAN), necrobiosis lipoidica and rheumatoid nodules.

Causes of erythema nodosum (EN)
- Streptococcal infections
- Sarcoidosis: CXR is essential in those presenting with EN. Bilateral hilar lymphadenopathy is the most common finding
- Drugs, e.g. sulphonamides, salicylates, gold
- Pregnancy and the oral contraceptive pill. It can occur in the first pregnancy, clears on delivery and then reoccurs in subsequent pregnancies

- Tuberculosis
- Inflammatory bowel disease
- Yersinia
- Fungal infections, e.g. histoplasmosis
- Idiopathic

275   Question on p.90.

Answer D
Pregnancy

In **pregnancy** there is an increase in thyroid binding globulin (TBG) levels, which lead to an elevated total T3 and T4. Free T4, if measured, is normal, as is TSH. The results above show an increased T3, T4 and TBG with a normal TSH and, therefore, pregnancy is the correct answer.

Hyperthyroidism is diagnosed by the presence of an elevated T4, less commonly T3 together with a low/undetectable TSH.

Sick euthyroid syndrome describes a disturbance in the normal regulation of hormone secretion that occurs in systemic illness. Increased amounts T4 are converted to the biologically inactive reverse T3 rather than to T3. However, this does not lead to an increase in the level of TSH. In fact, TSH is also suppressed, thus further lowering the levels of T3 and T4. Binding proteins are also decreased, this being classical of the metabolic response to illness.

Papillary carcinoma of the thyroid is the most common thyroid malignancy. It commonly presents with a nodule in the gland or cervical lymphadenopathy, but generally there is no change in the thyroid function tests.

Exogenous thyroxine ingestion would produce a similar picture to that seen in autoimmune hyperthyroidism. Thyroxine tablets contain T4, thus T4 would be elevated, as would T3 with a low TSH due to the feedback mechanism.

Causes of abnormal thyroid binding globulin

Increase	Decrease
• Genetic	• Genetic
• Pregnancy	• Protein-losing states, e.g. nephrotic syndrome
• Newborn	• Malnutrition
• Oestrogens, including the oral contraceptive pill	• Malabsorption
• Acute viral hepatitis	• Acromegaly
• Phenothiazines	• Corticosteroids (high doses)
• Hypothyroidism	• Cushing's syndrome
	• Severe illness
	• Androgen excess
	• Chronic liver disease
	• Thyrotoxicosis

276   Question on p.90.

Answer D
Ramipril

The patient has already made a significant step in secondary prevention
by stopping smoking. Weight loss in overweight patients reduces
comorbidity but has not been shown to improve survival.

It is likely that the patient will need to be on all the medications listed in
the question. Each of these drugs has been evaluated in large clinical
trials and the number of patients needed to treat to prevent one death
(NNT) calculated. These are summarized in the table below.

Drug	NNT	Study
Aspirin	42	ISIS 2
β-Blocker	143	ISIS 1
ACE inhibitor	22	SOLVD
Statin	33	CARE

From this it can be seen that ACE inhibitor use will prevent one death for
every 22 patients treated and is the best answer to this question.

277   Question on p.90.

Answer D
Nitrofurantoin

Routine urine culture is now part and parcel of obstetric screening.
Asymptomatic bacteriuria is found in 2–6% of pregnant women. Unlike
non-pregnant females, where bacteriuria tends not to lead to
pyelonephritis and is often not treated if asymptomatic, treatment must
always be commenced in pregnant women. During pregnancy,
asymptomatic bacteriuria has a much higher chance of going on to cause
acute pyelonephritis and premature labour.

Once this decision to treat has been established, this is really a question
about what antibiotics are safe during pregnancy. The table facing shows
some antibiotics to avoid in pregnancy and why.

Group	Action	Use	But
Tetracyclines, e.g. doxycycline	Interfere with protein synthesis by binding to bacterial ribosomes. Bacteriostatic	*Chlamydiae* *Mycoplasma* *Vibrio* *Rickettsiae*	Taken up by growing teeth – enamel hypoplasia
Trimethoprim	Inhibits dihydrofolic acid (DHF) reductase, hence limits production of bacterial DNA. Bacteriostatic	Gram-positive Gram-negative anerobes Not active against *Pseudomonas*	Teratogenic (by its inhibition of DHF reductase)
Quinolones, e.g. ciprofloxacin	Inhibition of bacterial DNA gyrase. Bactericidal	Gram-negative, e.g. UTIs, GI tract *Chlamidiae* Less active against *Strep. pneumoniae*	Arthropathy documented in immature animals – best avoided

Answer E
Amyloid cardiomyopathy

Amyloid deposits in the myocardium give the muscle a 'rubbery rigidity'. Infiltration between myocardial cells results in a small stiff heart with high right and left ventricular end-diastolic pressures. Systolic function remains normal. Tachyarrhythmias such as atrial fibrillation are common, as is bradycardia with 2:1 or complete heart block.

Digoxin is more likely to precipitate heart block in **amyloid cardiomyopathy** and there is an increased risk of digoxin toxicity. Isolated amyloid fibrils have been shown to bind digoxin. This may explain why such patients are particularly sensitive to the drug.

Digoxin increases the risk of ventricular tachyarrhythmias in patients with impaired left ventricular function. It should be used with caution in patients with **hypertrophic obstructive cardiomyopathy** and only prescribed in established irreversible atrial fibrillation.

Answer A
Valproate

All the drugs in the question are known to cause weight gain.

Phenytoin causes hirsuitism rather than alopecia.

Valproate, **carbamazepine**, **gabapentin** and **vigabatrin** are all reported to cause alopecia and so the problem is deciding which one is the most likely answer. The examiners are looking for the drug that most commonly causes these side effects and this would be valproate.

Furthermore, looking at this question practically, this patient has only recently been diagnosed and started on epilepsy medication. Gabapentin and vigabatrin are highly unlikely to be prescribed as first-line medicines. Gabapentin is usually prescribed as an adjunct to other medicines and vigabatrin is used for partial seizures when other medications have failed.

This leaves valproate and carbamazepine. Alopecia is a rare side effect of carbamazepine, making valproate the more likely answer.

Drugs causing alopecia
• Cytotoxics
• Methotrexate
• Warfarin
• Heparin
• Valproate
• Atenolol
• Sulphasalazine
• Vitamin A

Question on p.91.

Answer C
Human immunodeficiency virus

HIV is not a notifiable disease in the UK. A notifiable disease is one where the attending medical practitioner must notify a local authority officer as to its presence. In practice, this is normally the consultant for communicable disease control.

A list of notifiable diseases in the UK is given below.

Anthrax
Cholera
Diphtheria
Dysentery
Encephalitis
Food poisoning
Viral haemorrhagic fever (including
   Marburg's disease)
Viral hepatitis
Leprosy
Leptospirosis
Malaria
Measles
Meningitis
Meningococcal septicaemia
   (without meningitis)

Mumps
Ophthalmia neonatorum
Paratyphoid fever
Plague
Poliomyelitis, acute
Rabies
Relapsing fever
Rubella
Scarlet fever
Smallpox
Tetanus
Tuberculosis
Typhoid fever
Typhus
Whooping cough
Yellow fever

Question on p.91.

Answer B
Thrombolysis

The most likely diagnosis in this lady is a left ventricular (LV) aneurysm but the differential diagnosis includes:

• acute myocardial infarction (MI)
• angina, which is refractory to GTN
• dissection of thoracic aorta
• oesophageal spasm.

An LV aneurysm is the most likely diagnosis. The history and ECG suggest this lady has had not only a previous MI but also a TIA. Being on amiodarone suggests she has also had a ventricular or atrial arrhythmia. The clinical picture is in keeping with the presence of a ventricular aneurysm. Thrombolysis would be highly inappropriate because it would expose the patient to unnecessary risks of thrombolysis. Also, a ➤

dyskinetic ventricle is likely to be thrombogenic (as evidenced by previous TIA) and thrombolysis may disperse multiple thrombi.

This patient could be having a myocardial infarction, although this is less likely as there are no reciprocal changes on the ECG. However, **thrombolysis** should not be used in this patient as patients with LV aneurysms are at significant risk of ventricular rupture when given this treatment.

Thoracic aortic dissections can have ECG changes suggestive of an acute MI, if the dissection extends down to the coronary vessels. The patient usually describes the pain as tearing in nature. Regardless, thrombolysis for acute aortic dissection would be disastrous and likely to kill the patient.

Left ventricular aneurysm
- Late complication post-MI
- Presents with heart failure, arrhythmias or emboli
- Ventricular asynergy with double impulse
- Fourth heart sound
- Persistent ST elevation on ECG
- CXR may show ventricular bulge and or calcification
- Diagnosis with 2-D echocardiography
- Drug therapy for heart failure and arrhythmias
- Anticoagulation to prevent emboli
- Some patients require surgery (aneurysmectomy)

Low-molecular-weight heparin would treat her refractory angina, **CT** would rule out a dissection and confirm the presence of an aneurysm, and her **old notes** would show the residual ST elevation when she was initially admitted and on subsequent attendances.

Oesophageal spasm can mimic angina pain and may resolve with GTN. However, it is clear that thrombolysis in this and the other situations would not only be inappropriate but potentially dangerous.

---

282 Question on p.92.

Answer A
Carcinoma of the head of the pancreas

There are a limited number of conditions that cause dilatation of both the common bile duct and pancreatic duct:

- carcinoma of the head of the pancreas
- carcinoma of the ampulla of Vater
- Sphincter of Oddi dysfunction (type 1).

Gallstones rarely, if ever, cause dilatation of both duct systems. Moreover, when a stone gets impacted at the ampulla of Vater, the patient has very considerable pain, which is absent in this patient.

The correct answer is, therefore, **carcinoma of the head of the pancreas**. This condition is uncommon in patients below the age of 50 years but it does occur. Over 90% are inoperable at the time of diagnosis. The 5-year survival rate is 5%. Most patients are dead within 4–6 months from diagnosis but a small cohort of patients survives 18 months. The reason for a longer survival in this group is uncertain but probably represent biological heterogeneity of the tumour.

In **primary biliary cirrhosis** the common bile duct is normal at ERCP, the pathology being confined to the intrahepatic biliary cannaliculi.

In patients with **cholangiocarcinoma**, ERCP shows dilation of the biliary system proximal to the tumour. The bile duct downstream of the tumour is normal, as is the pancreatic duct. Similar findings are seen in patients with metastatic carcinoma involving the lymph **nodes at the portahepatis**.

---

283 Question on p.92.

Answer E
97%

	Pregnant	Not pregnant
Positive test	66	2
Negative test	4	28

The positive predictive value is the proportion of those who test positive who actually have the disease.

$$\text{Positive predictive value} = 66 \div (66 + 2)$$
$$= 97\%$$

The negative predictive value is the proportion of those who test negative who do not have the disease.

$$\text{Negative predictive value} = 28 \div (28 + 4)$$
$$= 87.5\%$$

---

284 Question on p.92.

Answer D
She has a normal bone mineral density for her age

The best method of detecting osteoporosis is by dual-energy X-ray absorptiometry (DEXA) scanning. Standard bone X-rays are virtually useless. ➤

DEXA scans are reported as a Z and T score.

The Z score is a comparison of the patient's bone mass to age-matched controls. This is expressed as the number of standard deviations above or below the mean of the control population. A Z score of 0 means that the patients bone density is equal to the mean of a population of aged-matched controls.

The T score is a comparison of the patient's bone age to young normal subjects. This is expressed as the number of standard deviations above or below the mean of the control population:

T > −1	Normal
T − 1 to −2.5	Osteopenia
T < −2.5	Osteoporosis

The correct answer is, therefore, D.

285
Question on p.92.

Answer C
FEV$_1$ < 1.2 L

The tumour appears technically respectable and so the two main issues that will prevent surgery are:

- if the patient's general health is too poor to withstand surgery
- if there is evidence of metastatic spread of disease or local spread not apparent on the CT scan.

Hypercalcaemia in lung cancer may suggest metastatic spread, but both small cell and non-small cell tumours can produce ectopic hormones leading to hypercalcaemia.

Hyponatraemia likewise may be from ectopic hormone production. A **pleural effusion** does not indicate malignant spread. It is not known whether this is a transudate or exudate, let alone whether it has malignant cells present. Further investigation would be required. Even if the effusion is an exudate, surgery is not contraindicated unless malignant cells are demonstrated.

Bone pain is not a contraindication as hypertrophic osteoarthropathy occurs in 3% of all lung tumours. This is characteristically a severe pain in the ankles and wrists, but can produce global stiffness. If bone metastases are suspected, a bone scan should be carried out prior to consideration of surgery.

Owing to the close association between smoking and lung cancer, many patients have concurrent lung disease, e.g. COPD or emphysema or cardiac disease, e.g. angina, arrhythmias. These features alone may prevent a patient having surgery because they are unfit for the anaesthetic. In addition, some of the patient's lung will be removed and so it is important that their remaining lung has the capacity to compensate.

An **FEV$_1$ < 1.5 L** is a contraindication to such surgery.

Question on p.93.

Answer D
Right jugular foramen, outside the skull

This patient has a right Horner's syndrome together with ipsilateral lesions of cranial nerves IX and X (dysphagia, nasal regurgitation and hoarse voice), XI (wasting of trapezius) and XII (deviation of the tongue towards the side of the lesion). This places the lesion at the jugular foramen outside the skull where the sympathetic nerve fibres on the right carotid artery lie adjacent to cranial nerves IX, X, XI and XII. This is known as Villaret's syndrome.

Causes of Villaret's syndrome

Secondary deposits (e.g. from bronchus)	Glomus/carotid body tumours
Meningiomas	Diabetes
Epidermoid tumours	Syphilis

Horner's syndrome

This consists of unilateral miosis (small pupil), ptosis, enophthalmos (sunken eye), impaired sweating over the ipsilateral forehead and conjunctival suffusion. It is unusual for a patient to have a 'full house' of these signs, and the latter three are often absent and certainly difficult signs to illicit.

The sympathetic pathway starts in the hypothalamus, and travels to the posterolateral brainstem and down to the lateral grey matter of the spinal cord. It then exits the spinal cord via the T1 root and back up the cervical sympathetic chain towards the skull. In the neck the sympathetic chain becomes intimately related to the carotid artery, and the sympathetic fibres follow this vessel through the carotid syphon and into the cavernous sinus. Here it leaves the carotid artery and splits into several branches that innervate the levator muscles of the eye, the pupil and the blood vessels of the eye. A lesion anywhere along this tortuous pathway can cause a Horner's syndrome. The anatomy of Horner's syndrome is a common examination question. The learning points below should help you determine the site of the lesion.

Horner's syndrome: key facts
- The lesion causing the Horner's is *always* ipsilateral.
- In the brainstem, the sympathetic pathway lies adjacent to the spinothalamic tract. Horner's at this level is associated with contralateral loss of pain and temperature sensation, e.g. lateral medullary syndrome.
- In the cervical cord, the pathway is vulnerable to central cord lesions, e.g. syringomyelia. This will produce bilateral lower motor neurone signs, and bilateral loss of pain and temperature sensation in the arms, and sometimes a *bilateral* Horner's syndrome.
- At the T1 root level, problems at the root of the neck (cervical rib) or apex of the lung (Pancoast tumour) can damage the pathway. Lesions here ➤

cause an ipsilateral T1 root lesion (wasting of the small muscles of the hand).
- A jugular foramen lesion (IX, X, XI and XII) with a Horner's is due to a lesion outside the skull.
- Lesions above the cervical sympathetic ganglion may not alter sweating at all, as the main outflow tract to the facial vessels is below this level.
- Lesions in the cavernous sinus and orbit may affect the parasympathetic pathway as well. In such patients, the pupil is semidilated and fixed to light. There are associated ipsilateral extraocular nerve palsies.
- In congenital Horner's syndrome, the iris fails to become pigmented and remains a blue colour.

Causes of Horner's syndrome

Site of lesion	Causes	Associated findings
Brain stem	Lateral medullary syndrome Multiple sclerosis Pontine glioma Brainstem encephalitis	Contralateral pain and temperature loss in cranial nerve V
Cervical cord	Syringomyelia Glioma (ependymoma)	Bilateral pain and temperature loss in both arms, with reduced reflexes
T1 root	T1 disc Cervical myelopathy Pancoast tumour Secondary deposits Cervical rib Avulsion of lower brachial plexus	Ipsilateral T1 root lesion
Neck	Secondary deposits Post-surgical (thyroid or laryngeal surgery)	

Note: A massive intracerebral bleed can produce an ipsilateral Horner's, owing to the removal of cortical control of the ipsilateral hypothalamus.

---

287 Question on p.93.

Answer D
Sri Lanka

When considering fever in a returning traveller, a knowledge of malarial endemicity is useful.

The last documented case of malaria endemically transmitted in the UK was in Stockwell in London circa 1955. One hundred years earlier it was a considerable cause of mortality throughout the Fenlands and even in the

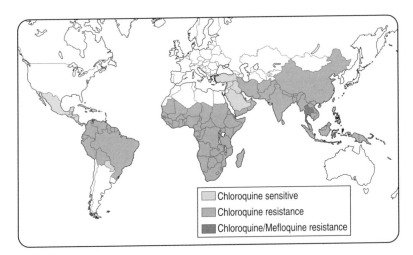

World map of malaria

lowlands of Scotland. Sporadic airport malaria continues to occur from mosquitoes hitch-hiking in the cabins of airliners and has been reported around Gatwick Airport from time to time.

Malaria has been eradicated from certain parts of Sri Lanka, particularly around Colombo and the southwest of the island. It is, however, very common in most of the island.

288 Question on p.93.

Answer D
Plasma aldosterone and renin levels

This young woman has hypertension in association with hypokalaemia.

Essential hypertension (primary) is the cause of elevated blood pressure in 95% of cases. However, in 5% of cases there is a primary endocrine or renal cause. These causes of secondary hypertension should be considered if there is resistance to control, associated electrolyte abnormalities or clinical suspicion, particularly in the younger patient.

Hypertension in association with hypokalaemia raises the possibility of primary hyperaldosteronism (Conn's syndrome) or Cushing's syndrome.

Cushing's syndrome is caused by an excess of glucocorticoid. The causes of Cushing's syndrome include:

- pituitary tumour (Cushing's disease)
- ectopic ACTH production
- adrenal adenoma
- adrenal carcinoma
- iatrogenic.

➤

341

Clinical suspicion from the body habitus of the patient, together with either hypertension or diabetes, is enough to justify investigation. Initial tests are performed to establish that the patient has an excess of circulating glucocorticoid and include 24-hour urinary free cortisol and a dexamethasone suppression test. Once the diagnosis of Cushing's syndrome is confirmed by these tests, further investigations are performed to try to elucidate the cause. These will include a **pituitary MRI**, CXR and abdominal CT.

Primary hyperaldosteronism causes sodium retention and potassium loss. A useful test in the diagnosis of this condition is a 24-hour urinary potassium level. This is characteristically elevated in Conn's syndrome. The diagnosis is confirmed by a combination of urinary potassium loss, hypokalaemia, elevated plasma **aldosterone levels** and suppressed **renin levels**. Once the diagnosis is confirmed, it is then appropriate to perform an **adrenal CT/MRI** and **adrenal scintillation scans**. Adrenal adenomata account for 60% of cases, commonly occurring in young females. Bilateral hyperplasia is much more common in males over the age of 40.

ACTH stimulation testing, also known as the short synacthen test, is used in the diagnosis of Addison's disease (primary hypoadrenalism).

In practice, this patient should initially have her 24-hour urinary free cortisol and potassium, and her serum aldosterone and renin levels checked. The results of these tests will guide subsequent cross-sectional and functional imaging. The best answer is, therefore, D.

---

289 Question on p.94.

Answer D
Chronic renal failure

Burr cells are irregularly shaped cells seen on the blood film in patients with uraemia. They get their name from 'burrs', which are the sticky bits of plants that adhere to your jumper when you go for a walk in the English countryside.

---

290 Question on p.94.

Answer C
Ulcerative colitis

The incidence of ulcerative colitis in patients who smoke or who have smoked is considerably reduced compared to patients who have never smoked. The reasons for this are unclear. Patients who have recently give up smoking seem particularly prone to develop the disease in the months following cessation.

Nicotine replacement therapy is sometimes helpful clinically, in patients with ulcerative colitis who are unresponsive to conventional treatment. Nicotine patches are usually used in this situation. However, in patients who have never smoked the side-effect profile is high and a significant number of patients have to stop nicotine replacement therapy for this reason.

There are very few illnesses that have a reduced incidence in smokers. These include Parkinson's disease and Alzheimer's disease, but the evidence in these two disorders for this effect is not as compelling as for the effect seen in ulcerative colitis. Part of the reason for this is that smokers are at increased risk of diffuse cerebrovascular disease, and this effect 'muddies the waters' somewhat from an epidemiological point of view.

 Question on p.94.

Answer C
Renal artery stenosis

This patient has type 1 Von Recklinghausen's disease, which is an autosomal dominant condition occurring in 1 in 3000 births. It is the most common type of the disease and is due to an abnormality on chromosome 17. The diagnosis is based on having two or more of the following criteria:

- six or more café au lait macules: > 5 mm pre-puberty, > 15 mm post-puberty
- two or more neurofibroma of any type *or* one or more plexiform neurofibroma
- freckling in the axillary or inguinal region
- optic glioma
- two or more Lisch nodules (iris hamartomas)
- neurofibromas in the bone
- one first-degree relative diagnosed by the above criteria.

The patient in question fulfils the first two criteria and, therefore, has Von Recklinghausen's disease.

Hypertension occurs in 6% of patients with Von Recklinghausen's disease. There are several causes of hypertension including:

Essential	4%
Renal artery stenosis	1.5%
Phaeochromocytoma	< 1%
Coarctation of the aorta	< 0.5%

Type 2 Von Recklinghausen's disease occurs in 1 in 35 000 births and is due to an abnormality on chromosome 22. It is also autosomal dominant. The diagnostic criteria include one of the following:

- bilateral vestibular schwannomas
- a first-degree relative with type 2 Von Recklinghausen's disease and either:
  – unilateral vestibular schwannoma ➤

or one of the following:
- – neurofibroma
- – schwannoma
- – glioma
- – juvenile cataract.

292 Question on p.94.

Answer C
G6PD levels

Glucose 6-phosphate dehydrogenase (G6PD) deficiency may precipitate haemolytic anaemia following treatment with Fansidar (sulfadoxine and pyrimethamine). A haemolytic screen for bilirubin, haptoglobins and reticulocytes would also be indicated as well as assessing the patient for G6PD deficiency.

There are various tests available that screen for antigens in *falciparum* infection with low-level parasitaemia, which is often difficult to detect on blood films. The **parasite F test** uses a monoclonal antibody specific to the histidine-rich protein of *P. falciparum* and is used in specialist centres.

293 Question on p.95.

Answer B
This patient's GCS is 9:

Eye opening	**2/4**
Spontaneous	4
To speech	3
To pain	2
No response	1
Motor response	**4/6**
Obeys verbal commands	6
Localizes to pain	5
Withdraws to pain*	4
Flexion response to pain*	3
Extension response to pain*	2
No response	1

*Withdrawal to pain is a coordinated movement using a balance of muscle groups to move the limb away from the source of the pain. This is in contrast to a flexion response, where the limb is slowly flexed and adducted. A flexion response implies significant impairment of cortical function. An extension response results in extension, adduction and internal rotation, and implies global cerebral impairment (decerebrate response).

Verbal response	3/5
Orientated	5
Disorientated	4
Inappropriate words	3
Incomprehensible words	2
No response	1

Answer A
Disability living allowance

To answer this question, one needs a basic understanding of a few of the benefits available to patients in the UK. What follows is a very basic explanation that should be enough to get you through the exam. In practice, it is much more complicated and any social worker reading this would be horrified by the oversimplification.

In assessing someone for benefits, there are several things that must be known:

- patient's age (whether they are younger or older than 65)
- the prognosis of their condition (i.e. whether their prognosis is less than 6 months)
- whether they were working before they became ill and paid national insurance contributions.

Attendance allowance is paid to individuals over the age of 65 who need help looking after themselves. So it pays for carers to 'attend' on the patient.

The **disability living allowance** is paid to people under the age of 65 who need help looking after themselves.

Incapacity benefit is for people who have worked and previously made National Insurance contributions. They usually claim it once **statutory sick pay** (SSP) has ended or if they do not qualify for SSP.

Those who have not paid enough National Insurance and do not qualify for incapacity benefit are entitled to claim **income support**.

The **carers allowance** is not claimable by the patient. Someone who is providing care for the patient can claim it and in this situation the 22-year old daughter would be entitled.

The **DS-1500** is a way of claiming benefits for patients under 'special rules'. This is usually when the patient has a terminal condition with a prognosis of less than 6 months.

The patient in question cannot claim carers allowance, although her daughter can. She is too young to claim attendance allowance and has not paid National Insurance so does not qualify for incapacity benefit. Her local slow-growing spinal cord meningioma is unlikely to kill her in the immediate future, although she will clearly be significantly disabled by it. Nevertheless, she may be unable to claim under special rules with a DS-1500. ➤

She is entitled to the disability living allowance, which is the correct answer. It is important to note she is also entitled to income support, although this was not one of the possible answers.

295

Question on p.95.

Answer C
Herpes simplex encephalitis

Herpes simplex encephalitis is clinically characterized by headaches and fever in its early stages. Seizures are also common. The virus tends to localize initially in the temporal lobe of the brain resulting in hallucinations, behavioural abnormalities and personality changes in 90% of patients early on. Classically patients experience auditory or gustatory hallucinations, and musical hallucinations are not uncommon. Other clinical manifestations and their frequency are listed below:

- headache (81%)
- psychiatric symptoms (71%)
- seizures (67%)
- vomiting (46%)
- focal weakness (33%)
- memory loss (24%)
- other findings include the following:
  - altered mental status
  - photophobia
  - movement disorders.

There are no *specific* signs for *Herpes simplex* encephalitis, but it should be considered in all adults presenting with fever, bizarre behaviour and altered neurology.

Useful investigations include cerebrospinal fluid analysis, which shows lymphocytic pleocytosis and a raised protein level. CT of the brain may show temporal lobe changes, although MRI is more sensitive. The electroencephalogram classically shows spike and slow wave activity in the temporal lobes. Polymerase chain reaction for HSV-DNA is a useful tool to support the diagnosis but rarely practical in the acute stage of diagnosis. Historically, the condition was diagnosed by brain biopsy, which showed focal haemorrhagic necrotizing encephalitis, affecting the temporal lobes.

Treatment of suspected cases should be immediate with intravenous acyclovir. This is a potentially fatal condition, which even with antiviral treatment results in a large number of patients experiencing permanent neurological effects (i.e. seizures, memory loss and personality changes) more than 6 months after treatment.

The other options do not fit the clinical presentation so well. The onset of symptoms is too quick for **vCJD** and a **cocaine-induced cerebrovascular**

event is more likely to present as a focal stroke without pyrexia. There is a possibility that she may have a **malignant hyperpyrexia** from ecstasy ingestion, but this would not present with temporal signs. Also the patient would exhibit muscular rigidity.

She is not presenting with any specific psychotic symptoms. The hallucinations are not characteristic and the main angle that this question is addressing is that *Herpes simplex* encephalitis must be considered in this presentation. Writing this off as a **drug-induced psychosis** would have disastrous consequences and be indefensible in court.

---

296   Question on p.96.

Answer D
Cyclophosphamide

Cyclophosphamide has no place in the management of Crohn's disease.

Treatment	Use
Elemental diet	Induces remission in a flare of Crohn's with similar efficacy to oral corticosteroids.
Methotrexate	Can induce remission in patients with chronic active disease unresponsive to other therapies. It is usually given by intramuscular injection (oral absorption is unreliable) weekly for 12 weeks. Up to 60% of patients show a sustained response
6-Mercaptopurine (6 MP)	6MP and its pro-drug azathioprine are used in patients with chronic active disease and induce a sustained response in 70% of patients. Treatment is usually continued for up to 4 years in patients who respond
Anti-TNF antibodies	Induces remission in chronic active disease, unresponsive to other therapies

---

297   Question on p.96.

Answer A
She has a nearly normal life expectancy

Cigarette smoking is a major public health issue, as it is one of the greatest avoidable causes of death and disability. Helping a patient give up smoking is one of the most effective interventions in disease prevention. The risk of death from smoking-related diseases declines steadily for 15 years in patients who quit. In patients who quit before the age of 35 years, their life expectancy is virtually the same as lifelong non-smokers. ➤

Smoking–related diseases
- Vascular disease – ischaemic heart disease, peripheral vascular disease, aortic aneurysms
- Chronic obstructive pulmonary disease
- Pneumonia
- Cancers – lung, oesophageal, throat and mouth, bladder
- Stroke
- Osteoporosis
- Male infertility
- Impotence
- Cataracts
- Fetal abnormalities – increased perinatal death and reduced birthweight

---

The risk of **fatal coronary artery disease** declines rapidly after stopping smoking and within a year the risk is halved. Within 20 years, the absolute risk of fatal coronary artery disease is nearly identical to a lifelong non-smoker.

Quitting smoking before the age of 30 years reduces the lifetime risk of developing **lung cancer** by more than 90% compared to a lifelong non-smoker. The older the patient is when she quits, the greater is the risk of subsequently developing lung cancer.

The risk of developing **oesophageal cancer** is reduced by 50% within 5 years of stopping smoking.

Smokers have an accelerated age-related decline in lung function and, therefore, have an increased lifetime risk of developing **COPD** at whatever age they quit. When a patient gives up smoking, there is a small improvement in lung function. Furthermore, within a year their age-related decline in pulmonary function becomes the same as that of a non-smoker.

298
Question on p.96.

Answer A
Growth hormone level with oral glucose tolerance test

The gold standard for diagnosis of acromegaly is still measurement of **growth hormone during an oral glucose tolerance test (OGTT)**. Growth hormone should suppress to below 4 mU/L within 2 hours of a 50 g oral loading dose. In those with acromegaly there is a failure to suppress or indeed a paradoxical rise in growth hormone.

The **insulin tolerance test** is used to assess pituitary function in patients with suspected panhypopituitarism. It has no role in the assessment of patients with acromegaly.

A **serum growth hormone level**, taken at any time of the day, is of no benefit as growth hormone is secreted in an episodic manner and so levels may vary quite widely.

An **MRI of the pituitary** gives a three-dimensional picture of any tumour or space occupying lesion; however, there is no capacity for functional evaluation or dynamic testing in this setting. Pituitary adenomas are benign lesions that can be functional or non-functional, and can cause symptoms by mass effect or by secretion. Non-functioning tumours cause symptoms by mass effect alone. Pressure upon the optic chiasm causes an upper bitemporal quadrantinopia (as pressure is from below the chiasm) progressing to a bitemporal hemianopia. Production of hormones, such as prolactin, ACTH and GH, by pituitary tumours need dynamic functional assessment by means of suppression testing and hormone levels.

An MRI will be carried out as a pre-operative assessment to document the size and structure of any adenoma, if acromegaly is proved by means of an OGTT.

Insulin-like growth factor 1 (IGF-1) is used as a screening test for acromegaly and for monitoring post-treatment. Levels are much more stable than GH and are almost always elevated in active disease. Raised IGF-1 levels are not diagnostic for acromegaly, as they are also elevated in other conditions, e.g. pregnancy.

---

299 Question on p.96.

Answer E
Giant cell arteritis

This patient is exhibiting some of the classical features of **giant cell (temporal) arteritis**. This is a granulomatous arteritis affecting large vessels. It occurs mainly in the over 60s and does not occur in patients below the age of 50 years. Common presenting symptoms include general malaise, fever, tenderness of the scalp over the temporal area (worse on combing the hair) and jaw claudication.

Suspected temporal arteritis is a medical emergency. The reason for this is that the arteritis can affect the ophthalmic arteries. This results in sudden visual loss, which may be permanent. The diagnosis is based on the clinical features and a raised ESR (often over 80 mm/hour) and confirmed by temporal artery biopsy. Treatment with high-dose oral corticosteroids should be started in a patient with a suggestive history and a raised ESR. It is important not to delay treatment whilst awaiting a temporal artery biopsy, as whilst waiting the patient may suddenly go blind. Note that corticosteroids are unlikely to interfere with the biopsy result for 36–48 hours. A negative biopsy does not completely exclude a diagnosis of temporal arteritis, as sometimes the vasculitic change may be patchy. ➤

Polymyalgia rheumatica is a related condition and presents with pain and stiffness of the limb girdle muscles. It occurs in the over 50s only. The ESR is usually raised. Some patients with polymyalgia rheumatica go on to develop temporal arteritis at a later date.

300 Question on p.97.

Answer C
Zero

To work this out, you need to know the diagram of electrical vectors.

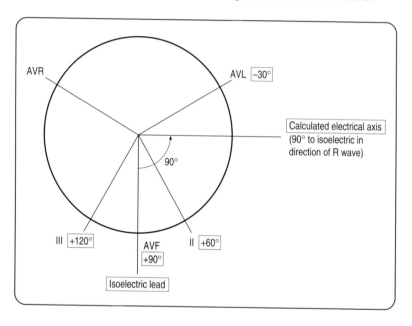

First find the isoelectric lead, i.e. the one in which the size of the R wave is closest to the size of the S wave. In this case, it is lead AVF. Check this against the diagram of electrical vectors. In this case the isoelectric lead is AVF, i.e. at +90 degrees. The electrical axis of the heart lies at 90 degrees to the isoelectric lead in the direction of the large R waves. The large R waves are found in lead I. Therefore, the electrical axis in this case is zero degrees. The normal cardiac axis ranges from +90 degrees to −30 degrees

Causes of left-axis deviation
- Left anterior hemiblock
- Q waves of inferior myocardial infarction
- Artificial cardiac pacing
- Emphysema
- Hyperkalaemia
- Wolff–Parkinson–White syndrome Type B – right-sided accessory pathway
- Tricuspid atresia
- Ostium primum ASD
- Injection of contrast into left coronary artery

Causes of right-axis deviation
- Normal finding in children and tall thin adults
- Right ventricular hypertrophy
- Chronic lung disease even without pulmonary hypertension
- Anterolateral myocardial infarction
- Left posterior hemiblock
- Pulmonary embolus
- Wolff–Parkinson–White syndrome – left-sided accessory pathway
- Ostium secundum ASD
- Ventricular septal defect

301　　　　　　　　　　　　　　Question on p.97.

Answer D
Gestodene/ethinylestradiol combination pill

Phenytoin and **amitriptyline** do not increase risk of venous thromboembolism (VTE). There have been reports suggesting that there is an increased risk of VTE with the oral contraceptive pill (OCP).

The incidence of VTE in healthy non-pregnant women on an oral contraceptive is about 5 cases per 100 000 women per year. Different pills are believed to have different risks of VTE and this is also related to length of use of the pill.

For combined OCPs containing second-generation progestogens, i.e. **levonorgestrel,** the incidence of VTE is 15 per 100 000 women per year of use.

For OCPs containing third-generation progestogens, i.e. **desogestrel** and **gestodene**, the incidence is 25 per 100 000 women per year of use.

302 Question on p.97.

Answer E
Atrioventricular septal defect

Trisomy 21 (Down's syndrome) is the most common trisomy, and occurs in 1:650 of live births. A total of 40% of patients with Down's syndrome have congenital heart disease.

Congenital heart disease in Down's syndrome

Type	Incidence
Atrioventricular septal defect	40%
Ventricular septal defect	30%
Atrioseptal defect[a]	10%
Tetralogy of Fallot	6%
Miscellaneous	14%

[a] Primum is more common than secundum ASD

303 Question on p.98.

Answer C
Adult polycystic kidney disease

This woman had hypertension, blood on dipstick and a family history of subarachnoid haemorrhage. The diagnosis that must be thought of first is **adult polycystic kidney disease** (APKD). This is a common disease being inherited as an autosomal dominant manner. It has a prevalence of 1 in 700 and accounts for up to 10% of patients requiring dialysis. The defect lies on chromosome 16 in most cases. Presentation occurs from the second decade onwards with a variety of symptoms:

- haematuria
- loin pain (haemorrhage into a cyst, infection or stone formation)
- recurrent/resistant urinary tract infections
- abdominal pain/discomfort (due to mass effect of enlarging kidneys)
- hypertension – or evidence of end-organ damage, e.g. stroke
- subarachnoid haemorrhage
- symptoms of chronic renal failure.

Increasingly, patients are being diagnosed at an asymptomatic stage as a result of family screening. Screening is performed by either ultrasound (which is best delayed until the third decade as there is a high rate of false-positive examinations in younger patients) or genetic testing.

Thirty per cent of patients have associated polycystic disease in the liver. This rarely causes any problems but just occasionally the liver becomes so large that a transplant is required.

Eight per cent of patients with AKPD have asymptomatic Berry aneurysms. In patients with AKPD with a family history of Berry aneurysms this risk is doubled.

All of the other possibilities could cause dipstick haematuria except **phaeochromocytoma**. This causes episodic hypertension associated with glycosuria.

Takayasu's arteritis is a very rare, large-vessel vasculitis first described in young women in Japan. It usually affects the aortic arch and its branches, causing a systemic illness, hypertension and absent pulses. This progresses to heart failure and cerebrovascular events.

Von Hippel–Lindau disease or retinocerebellar angiomatosis is a rare autosomal dominant condition that consists of retinal and cerebellar haemangioblastomas. Adrenal, pancreatic and renal tumours also occur, the latter causing microscopic haematuria.

Renovascular disease is the same pathological process that occurs to cause MIs in the heart except that the renal artery is 'furred' instead of the coronary arteries. It occurs in the setting of an arteriopathy and is more common with advancing age. It causes worsening renal function and blood can be present on dipstick. This lady has no other symptoms of vascular disease and normal renal function, therefore, this is unlikely. Furthermore, although renovascular disease can occur at this age, it is uncommon.

---

304   Question on p.98.

Answer B
No therapy

The blood results show an incidental finding of a 'lymphocytic picture' in an asymptomatic elderly gentleman.

This suggests the diagnosis of chronic lymphocytic leukaemia. This is the commonest leukaemia affecting adults and usually affects the elderly. In the early stages, there is a lymphocytosis in the blood and bone marrow. In these stages, it requires **no treatment** and many elderly patients are managed on supportive therapies. These include prompt treatment of infections with antibiotics **and polyvalent immunoglobulin**, if infections become frequent. Anaemia caused by marrow infiltration requires transfusion.

Indications for **chlorambucil** or **cyclophosphamide** are the appearance of symptoms related to the disease, e.g. lymphadenopathy, thrombocytopenia, anaemia.

Question on p.98.

Answer B
Intravenous sodium bicarbonate

The clinical situation suggests an overdose and the history suggests that she would have access to antidepressants.

The clinical picture is highly suggestive of a tricyclic overdose, i.e.

* reduced consciousness
* tachycardia
* ECG changes
* hypotension

Tricyclic antidepressants, such as amitryptyline, are still prescribed for depression and chronic neuropathic pain. Most of their common side effects are due to their anticholinergic actions, e.g. dry mouth, blurred vision, urinary retention, etc. The more serious side effects that occur in overdose are probably unrelated to this. They include:

* convulsions
* coma
* hypotension
* tachyarrhythmias with prolongation of the QRS complex
* cardiorespiratory collapse
* metabolic acidosis.

The patient requires airway protection, cardiac monitoring and admission to intensive care. The recommended treatment is intravenous bicarbonate, which is effective even if the patient is not acidotic. Bicarbonate should be considered if any of the following are present:

* systemic acidosis
* QRS > 160 milliseconds
* ventricular arrhythmia
* hypotension
* cardiac arrest.

Naloxone is the antidote for opioid overdose. The patient usually has pinpoint pupils and mild myoclonus. It is a useful diagnostic tool, fast acting but short lasting.

Flumazenil is used to counteract the effects of benzodiazepines. Although benzodiazepines and opioids can cause drowsiness, the broad complex tachycardia is not usual. It is important to note that flumazenil should be given with caution (especially in patients who have been treated for epilepsy), as it can precipitate symptoms of withdrawal including convulsions.

Calcium gluconate is used to stabilize the myocardium in the presence of hyperkalaemia and is covered in another question.

306   Question on p.99.

Answer C
Coeliac disease

Coeliac disease most commonly presents as iron-deficiency anaemia in adults and can present at any age. Patients are often diagnosed a having irritable bowel syndrome. Patients may give a history of delayed menarche, recurrent anaemia, mouth ulceration or rashes (dermatitis herpetiformis). Patients presenting with iron-deficiency anaemia should always have a duodenal biopsy as part of their gastrointestinal work-up.

Crohn's disease is less likely as the ESR is normal.

Carcinoma of the colon is a possibility but uncommon in patients under 45, especially in the absence of a family history.

If the patient's anaemia is due to **fibroids**, she is unlikely to be anaemic 6 months after the hysterectomy.

Bacterial overgrowth is a cause of iron-deficiency anaemia but this is uncommon in patients of this age with an anatomically normal gastrointestinal tract. It occurs in patients with previous GI surgery (blind loop syndrome) and jejunal diverticulosis. It is seen occasionally with structurally normal GI tracts, but these tend to be elderly or diabetic patients.

307   Question on p.99.

Answer D
Oral dapsone

Dermatitis herpetiformis is characterised by the presence of intensely itchy papules and vesicles over the extensor surfaces, i.e. elbows, knees, buttocks, etc, presenting in the teens to the thirties. The condition is named herpetiformis because the rash tends to occur in groups, similar to the lesions of *Herpes*.

It is thought of as 'coeliac disease of the skin', as it is associated with a gluten-sensitive enteropathy and the typical autoantibody profile is present. However, duodenal biopsies are rarely completely typical for the changes of coeliac disease.

Diagnosis can be difficult but skin biopsy shows subepidermal blisters and microabscesses in dermal papillae. Immunofluorescence demonstrates IgA in the dermal papillae and basement membrane.

Treatment should always consist of a gluten-free diet, as the need for **dapsone** in the long term may be minimal or even unnecessary. In the acute setting, dapsone relieves the feeling of itching and burning within hours. The dose is then adjusted for maintenance requirements.

An important side effect of dapsone is haemolytic anaemia owing to its oxidant effect on haemoglobin. Iron is oxidized to the ferric state, resulting in methaemoglobin. This leads to a decrease in NAPDH and hence a ➤

decrease in the stability of the red cell membrane. Methaemoglobin also has a high affinity for oxygen, leading to a left shift in the oxygen dissociation curve. In most cases, this is a dose-related effect, which is reversed when the drug is stopped. However, in patients with G6PD deficiency, there can be a catastrophic drop in haemoglobin.

308

Question on p.99.

Answer C
Iron overload in β-thalassaemia major

Venesection is the primary treatment for **genetic haemochromatosis**. Patients with this disorder undergo weekly venesection after diagnosis, until their iron stores are normalized (serum ferritin < 50 and iron saturation < 50%). Once the iron stores have been normalized, most patients require maintenance venesection every 3–4 months. Iron deposition can occur in many organ systems, and the clinical response to venesection varies as shown below:

Clinical consequence of iron overload	Response to venesection
Cirrhosis	No
Diabetes	Yes
Cardiomyopathy	Yes
Pyrophosphate arthropathy	No
Hypopituitarism	Yes

Cirrhosis of the liver is irreversible and is associated with a particularly high incidence of hepatocellular carcinoma in patients with haemochromatosis (25% over 20 years).

Patients with **polycythaemia** (either primary or secondary) are at risk of thromboembolic disease and stroke if their PCV is more than 55. Such patients are treated with venesection, sometimes on a regular basis, to keep the PCV below this figure.

Iron overload is often seen in **porphyria cutanea tarda**, and is usually associated with excessive alcohol intake. The main symptom of this disorder is a photosensitive blistering rash, particularly on the hands. It is treated by total sun block and alcohol withdrawal. In patients who have biochemical evidence of iron overload, the skin disease responds well to venesection. In patients with no evidence of iron overload, it responds to low dose chloroquine.

Iron overload is a common problem in β-**thalassaemia major**. It is an inevitable consequence of multiple transfusions that these patients require because of their abnormal haemoglobin production. Venesection would make them anaemic again, and the iron overload in these patients is treated with chelation therapy, e.g. with desferrioxamine.

Answer C
Anterior spinal artery occlusion

Anterior spinal artery thrombosis results in infarction of the anterior half of the spinal cord. Causes include the following.

- Surgical
  - sympathectomy
  - thoracic surgery
  - intercostal nerve blocks.
- Medical
  - aortic dissection
  - emboli, e.g. atrial fibrillation, infective endocarditis
  - diabetes
  - coagulopathy
  - decompression sickness
  - sickle cell disease
  - syphilis.

Typically, a patient with anterior spinal artery thrombosis has an acute onset of flaccid paraplegia with retention of urine. Loss of pain and temperature sensation occurs below the level of the lesion. These signs are due to damage to the pathways in the anterior half of the cord (corticospinal and spinothalamic tracts, respectively). There is complete preservation of light touch and joint position sense. These modalities are transmitted by the dorsal columns, which lie in the posterior part of the cord and are thus unaffected. Patients often also complain of back pain at the level of the lesion.

Spinal cord compression secondary to **malignant infiltration, prolapsed intervertebral disc and spinal meningioma** all cause extrinsic spinal cord compression and usually motor signs predominate. When sensory signs do develop, this implies irreversible spinal cord damage. Local pain is common in all three.

A **prolapsed intervertebral thoracic disc** is extremely uncommon. Over 90% of disc prolapses occur at L5–S1 and 5% at L2–4. Prolapsed intervertebral discs are more common in the cervical region than in the thoracic region.

The most common site of a **spinal meningioma** is between T3 and T6, but it is far more common in women (F:M 9:1).

Syringomyelia causes an intrinsic cord lesion as the cyst expands out. Typically pain and temperature sensation are affected first at the level of the lesion owing to damage to the spinothalamic tracts as they cross the cord. A Horner's syndrome may then develop followed by wasting of the small muscles of the hand (anterior horn cell damage). The lesion is slowly progressive and pyramidal signs in the legs may take years to develop. Dorsal column loss occurs late.

Question on p.100.

310

Answer A
Cryptogenic fibrosing alveolitis

The FEV_1 and FVC are both reduced, and the FEV_1/FVC is 84%, suggesting that it is a restrictive defect. All the possible answers have restrictive lung defects, but it is the transfer factor (TLCO) and the transfer coefficient (KCO) that help identify the correct answer.

Transfer factor is a measure of the transfer of gas across the alveolar capillary membrane and reflects the uptake of oxygen from the alveoli into the red cells. It is usually reduced in patients with severe degrees of emphysema or fibrosis. It is unchanged in patients with thoracic cage deformity/neuromuscular defects and pneumonectomy.

The transfer coefficient is a function of the transfer factor taking into account lung volume.

Spirometry	Obstructive defect	Restrictive defect
FEV_1 (L)	↓↓	↓
FVC (L)	↓	↓↓
FEV_1/FVC	< 70%	> 80% (normal is 70–80%)
TLC (L)	↑	↓
RV	↑	↓
TLCO (L)	↓	↓
KCO (mmol/minute per kPa)	↓	↓
e.g.	Emphysema	Interstitial lung disease
	Asthma	Pulmonary emboli
	Bronchiectasis	Neuromuscular disease
	Chronic bronchitis	Guillain–Barré
		Motor neurone disease
		Thoracic cage defects
		Pulmonary haemorrhage
		Goodpasture's
		Pulmonary oedema
		Lymphangitis

↓, reduced; ↓↓, greatly reduced; ↑, increased.

Causes of increased KCO
- Pulmonary haemorrhage
- Polycythaemia
- Left to right shunts
- Asthma
- Thoracic cage deformities

Causes of decreased KCO
- Interstitial lung disease
- Anaemia
- Multiple pulmonary emboli
- Lymphangitis
- Primary pulmonary hypertension
- Obstructive airways disease

Answer D
Regular outpatient review

The most common cause of aortic stenosis presenting in adults over 60 years of age is senile calcification of a normal valve. The three cusps of the aortic valve are immobilized by heavy calcification, although the commisures are rarely fused.

Symptoms due to aortic stenosis vary with severity and include:

- asymptomatic
- angina – even with normal coronary arteries
- dyspnoea
- syncope/dizziness
- systemic emboli
- sudden death
- endocarditis
- congestive cardiac failure.

Aortic stenosis is classed as severe if there is a peak systolic gradient of **> 100 mmHg** or valve area is < 0.5 cm^2. The average survival of medically treated patients who are symptomatic is poor (2–3 years with angina or syncope, 1–2 years with cardiac failure).

Aortic valve replacement is indicated once symptoms develop. In patients who are asymptomatic but have documented severe stenosis and a deteriorating ECG, valve replacement may be considered but, in practice, are usually kept under regular review. Since this patient is asymptomatic, urgent or routine surgery is not indicated.

Aortic valvuloplasty is indicated for elderly patients with severe aortic stenosis who are considered inoperable owing to poor lung, liver or kidney function, or severe coronary artery disease.

Patients are at risk of systemic emboli, usually cerebral or retinal. Amaurosis fugax may be the presenting symptom in calcified aortic stenosis. The embolus is usually calcific, not thrombotic and unlikely to be improved by **anticoagulation**.

Answer B
Paget's disease

This man has bone pain and a raised alkaline phosphatase with the remainder of his biochemistry normal. This is Paget's disease.

Paget's disease is a common disorder of bone metabolism. It is thought that 10% of people aged 90 have some form of the disease. There is extreme remodelling of bone leading to a rapid turnover but the new bone formation is faulty. This makes it prone to fractures. The majority ➤

of people are asymptomatic. However, it can cause bony pain, pathological fractures, deformities of the bone, secondary compression of nerves, high output cardiac failure and rarely (< 1%) osteosarcoma.

Typically affected sites include the pelvis, tibia, skull, femur and lumbosacral spine. Treatment is with simple analgesics initially and, if still symptomatic, with oral bisphosphonates, which limit the activity of osteoclasts.

This is not **polymyalgia rheumatica** because, even though you can get a *small* rise in alkaline phosphatase in one-third of patients, this patient has not got other symptomatology that is associated with this syndrome, such as fever, night sweats, loss of weight, malaise, proximal symmetrical muscle pain, etc.

Osteomalacia is the adult form of rickets. There is a lack of mineralization of the bone because of a lack of vitamin D. It is seen in those who cover up in sunlight and in vegans. The biochemical profile shows a raised alkaline phosphatase, low phosphate and low/normal calcium. Treatment is supplementation of the diet. This gentleman does not have osteomalacia.

Both **myeloma** and **metastatic prostatic carcinoma** can cause back pain by infiltration of the bones of the spine. In both these cases the calcium is often raised in conjunction with such a high alkaline phosphatase. In addition, patients with advanced malignancy develop an anorexia/cachexia syndrome owing to the hypercatabolic state and systemic release of tumour necrosis factor. This patient has a brief history with a normal albumin. Furthermore, the patient has a normal total protein implying his globulin is also normal making myeloma highly unlikely.

---

313 Question on p.101.

Answer E
Legionella urinary antigen

Legionella pneumonia is a serious condition that needs prompt treatment with the correct antibiotics. To establish a prompt diagnosis, one must have a high degree of suspicion from the history:

- males affected more than females
- high fever
- prodromal viral-like illness
- hyponatraemia
- lymphopenia
- associated diarrhoea.

A prompt and accurate diagnosis is needed. **Culture** can take up to 3 weeks on special medium. **Direct immunofluorescent** staining of bronchial washings, pleural fluid or sputum is available and highly reliable. However, to get washing, a bronchoscopy has to be performed, which is not always convenient when a patient is admitted. A quick method of obtaining a diagnosis is **urinary *Legionella* antigen**. It has a yield of 90% in the first week of illness.

Treatment is clarithromycin or ciprofloxacin. Rifampicin can be added in if patients are particularly unwell.

---

314 Question on p.101.

Answer D
Change morphine to diamorphine 40 mg via syringe driver in 24 hours.

In choosing the correct parenteral opioids for the patient, the following need to be taken into account:

- the opioid needs to be equianalgesic to the 60 mg bd of morphine sulphate so that the patient does not have any breakthrough pain
- the conversion needs to be quick
- the patient's pain may improve as the calcium comes down and so the morphine needs to have a relatively short half-life, in case the dose needs reducing.

Fentanyl is not appropriate in this case because it takes at least 14 hours for the drug to reach steady state in the body. Subcutaneous diamorphine is the best option. To convert oral morphine to subcutaneous diamorphine, the total oral morphine in 24 hours should be divided by three.

$$\text{Therefore, } 60 \text{ mg bd} = 120 \text{ mg in 24 hours}$$
$$120 \text{ mg} \div 3 = 40 \text{ mg diamorphine in 24 hours}$$

Hence, the correct answer is D.

---

315 Question on p.102.

Answer C
Isoniazid

Bactericidal drugs	Bacteriostatic drugs
• Penicillins	• Trimethoprim
• Cephalosporins	• Erythromycin
• Aminoglycosides	• Sulphonamides
• Isoniazid	• Tetracyclines
• Co-trimoxazole	• Linocomycin
	• Clindamycin
	• Chloramphenicol

316   Question on p.102.

Answer D
Hypertrophic obstructive cardiomyopathy

Indications for permanent pacing include:

- hypertrophic cardiomyopathy
- dilated cardiomyopathy
- long QT syndrome
- chronotropic incompetence
- post-AV nodal ablation for arrhythmias
- post-cardiac transplantation.

   Asymptomatic 2:1 block Mobitz Type I (Wenckebach phenomenon) does not require pacing, although Mobitz type II is a more sinister bradyarrhythmia, which does need pacing.
   Complete heart block is not uncommon following an **inferior myocardial infarction** because the right coronary artery supplies the AV node in 85% of patients. It almost always resolves and pacing support if required is usually via a temporary wire.
   Asymptomatic bifasicular block will not need pacing. Trifasicular block may need a permanent pacemaker, if the patient has symptoms. Pre-operatively, a temporary pacing wire is indicated for trifasicular block.
   Permanent pacing is not the treatment of choice for **Wolf–Parkinson–White**. The definitive treatment is radiofrequency ablation. Rarely complete heart block may occur after the procedure and then a permanent pacemaker is indicated.

317   Question on p.102.

Answer C
Corneal microdeposits

Amiodarone may be used in the treatment of arrhythmias including:

- paroxysmal nodal, ventricular and supraventricular tachycardias
- atrial fibrillation
- atrial flutter
- ventricular fibrillation.

   It has a very long half-life (several weeks) and may take months to achieve steady-state plasma concentration. It can be given orally or intravenously into a large vein. It is an excellent antiarrhythmic but has many side effects, and is best used after other drugs have been ineffective or are contraindicated. A helpful way to remember the main side effects is with the mnemonic **BITCH**:

- **b**radycardia
- **i**nterstitial pulmonary fibrosis
- **t**hyroid disorders
- **c**orneal microdeposits
- **h**ypersensitive skin/**h**epatitis.

Most patients taking amiodarone develop **corneal microdeposits**. These are reversible on stopping treatment and rarely interfere with vision. There is a possibility of **skin photosensitivity** and patients should be advised to shield the skin from sunlight and use a wide-spectrum sunscreen to protect against long ultraviolet and visible light. The classic skin discoloration is a slate-grey colour.

Amiodarone contains iodine and can cause disorders of thyroid function. Both **hypothyroidism** and **hyperthyroidism** can occur, and patients should have their thyroid function tests checked prior to treatment and every 6 months subsequently.

The most serious complication is pneumonitis leading to **interstitial pulmonary fibrosis**. It should always be suspected if patients develop new or progressive dyspnoea or cough.

Other side effects include peripheral **neuropathy**, **hepatitis** and **bradycardia**. It is important to be aware that amiodarone **prolongs the QT interval** and should be avoided in torsades de pointes.

318

Question on p.102.

Answer D
Lead

Toxins that can be removed by haemodialysis include:

- alcohols – ethanol, methanol and ethylene glycol
- salicylates – aspirin
- theophylline
- phenobarbitone
- lithium.

Lead poisoning is best treated by chelation therapy with calcium ethylene diamine tetracetic acid (EDTA), D-penicillamine and dimercaprol.

319

Question on p.103.

Answer A
Acute tubulointerstitial nephritis

This lady has classical **tubulointerstitial nephritis** secondary to the course of amoxicillin. Penicillins are a common cause of this florid hypersensitivity reaction that results in acute oliguric or non-oliguric renal failure. Clues to the diagnosis in this case are the initial course of ➤

antibiotics, which presumably treated the UTI, and then a space of 2 weeks. During this time there will be an increasing inflammatory response in the kidneys to the drug. This is manifest clinically as fever, arthralgia and a feeling of general malaise.

The blood tests help in the diagnosis in this case, as they show an eosinophilia and renal impairment. Raised eosinophil counts are seen as a consequence of parasitic infections, some vasculitides and hypersensitivity, as in this case.

A renal biopsy should be carried out in this case. This will not only clarify the diagnosis, by showing interstitial infiltrate, eosinophils and tubular necrosis, but also give an idea as to the severity of the disease process and ultimately the prognosis. Initial treatment is withdrawal of the offending drug and then a course of steroids. Some patients may need a short period of dialysis but most recover, leaving a degree of interstitial scarring.

Acute pyelonephritis is unlikely after treatment with amoxicillin. This is a good choice of antibiotics for treatment of UTIs because most common pathogens are sensitive. It would be unlikely to present in this way as a rapid deterioration would be expected if the initial course of antibiotics did not clear any infection.

Churg–Strauss is a rare systemic vasculitis characterized by eosinophilic infiltrates. Typically presentation is with symptoms of rhinitis and asthma. As the disease progresses, other organ systems are affected including the skin, kidneys and nervous system. It tends to affect young males. This diagnosis is highly unlikely in this case.

Post-streptococcal glomerulonephritis is an immune-mediated post-infectious inflammatory response resulting in a nephritic syndrome normally occurring in children. It occurs 2–3 weeks post-exposure to streptococcal tonsillitis, pharyngitis or cellulitis. UTIs are rarely caused by this organism and it would be extremely rare for this to progress to glomerulonephritis.

Renal abscesses are rarely seen nowadays. If caused by a bacterium, the patient is usually very sick. However, the presence of an abscess in a patient with no signs of sepsis must raise the possibility of a cold abscess caused by *Mycobacteria*.

---

320 Question on p.103.

Answer C
Magnetic resonance imaging and metaiodo-benzylguanidine metaiodo-scintiscan

Most phaeochromocytomas have a diameter greater than 3 cm and such tumours are usually easily detectable by cross-sectional imaging. High-quality **spiral CT** has a sensitivity of 98% and a specificity of 70%. High-quality **MRI** yields similar results.

MIBG scans rely on the fact that MIBG is actively taken up by adrenergic tissue and concentrated in phaeochromocytomas. This allows the detection of small lesions, including metastatic lesions, which are undetectable on CT or MRI.

Selective angiography with venous sampling was used fairly extensively in the past to localize tumours. It is now rarely used and has largely been superseded by high-quality cross-sectional imaging.

The correct answer to this question is MRI and MIBG scintiscan. This will detect nearly all those with phaeochromocytomas. MRI is preferred to CT as there is no radiation exposure and possibly has a slightly higher sensitivity.

Phaeochromocytomas have an incidence of 1/100 000.

Rule of ten for phaeochromocytomas
- 10% are extra-adrenal (bladder, aortic bifurcation, mediastinum, etc.)
- 10% are bilateral
- 10% are familial (MEN 2A or 2B, often bilateral)
- 10% are malignant

Intravenous pyelogram (IVP)	Positive in only 40%
Ultrasound	Positive in 85%
Angiography	Selective angiogram has risks of anaesthesia but localizes 90% – digital subtraction angiogram better
Selective renal venography	
CT scan	As good as the selective angiograms, but may miss the smaller phaeochromocytomas
Scintiscan	Metaiodobenzylguanidine 90% accuracy

---

321 Question on p.104.

Answer B
Loss of the corneal reflex on the left

The natural history of an acoustic nerve tumour can rage from 2 to 10 years plus. The first **symptom** that the patient usually notices is **tinnitus** in the affected ear. This is followed by slowly progressive and usually unrecognized **loss of hearing**.

The most consistent early physical sign is **depression of the corneal reflex**. The fifth nerve passes directly over the internal auditory canal and, when an acoustic neuroma expands, it lifts this nerve and stretches it. The afferent fibres for the corneal reflex are very sensitive to distortion. Subsequent numbness over the face nerve may occur though a complete fifth nerve lesion is rare. ➤

The tumour tends to extend medially and distorts the brainstem and cerebellum. This produces **ipsilateral ataxia** worse in the upper limbs. Some patients also develop vertigo and a mild spastic paraparesis with upgoing plantars. By this stage the patient is usually profoundly deaf in the affected ear.

In the final stages, the brainstem may be so distorted that the cerebral aqueduct becomes blocked producing hydrocephalus and papilloedema. There are numerous other cranial nerves in the vicinity of an acoustic neuroma, which include VI, IX, X and XI. These are all involved late in the natural history.

322

Question on p.104.

Answer A
Confusion

Hypercalcaemia causes shortening of the QT interval not lengthening. Likewise Trousseau's sign is a feature of hypocalcaemia.

One of the difficulties in diagnosing hypercalcaemia in advanced malignancy is that the symptoms are similar to the advanced disease itself. In addition, the patient is receiving chemotherapy, which will result in other symptoms.

Lethargy is the commonest symptom due to chemotherapy and is frequently reported in patients with advanced cancer. **Nausea** is commonly associated with chemotherapy, although the calcium should be routinely checked as part of assessment for cancer-related nausea.

Confusion is unlikely to be due to chemotherapy. Although there are several causes for confusion in advanced malignancy, i.e. drugs, cerebral metastases, infection, etc.

Hypercalcaemia should be considered first because it is treatable and may have prognostic implications.

Clinical features of hypercalcaemia	Clinical features of hypocalcaemia
• Weakness, lethargy	• Stupor
• Muscle weakness	• Numbness, paraesthesia
• Confusion	• Muscle cramps, spasm
• Drowsiness	• Laryngeal stridor
• Abdominal pain	• Convulsions
• Polyuria, dehydration, renal failure	• Chvostek's sign
• Short QT interval	• Trousseau's sign
• Cardiac arrhythmias	• Prolonged QT interval
• Bone pain	

Answer B
Papule

Dermatological terminology

Macule	Flat, circumscribed, non-palpable lesion
Papule	Small, circumscribed, palpable lesion (< 0.5 cm)
Vesicle	Small fluid-filled blister
Nodule	Large papule (> 0.5 cm)
Pustule	Pus-filled lesion

Answer E
Domperidone

To answer this question correctly you need to:

1. diagnose the mechanism of this man's vomiting
2. choose an antiemetic to counteract this mechanism
3. avoid any drug that may exacerbate his Parkinson's disease.

The most likely cause of his nausea is delayed gastric emptying. It is likely that this is a functional rather than a mechanical obstruction, as he has recently had an ERCP, implying patency of the upper GI tract at least as far as the ampulla of Vater. He has some of the symptoms suggestive of gastric outflow obstruction detailed below:

- gradual increase in nausea
- large-volume vomit
- relief after vomiting
- succussion splash
- belching.

The choice of drug should, therefore, be a prokinetic to increase gut motility and encourage gastric emptying. **Metoclopramide** and **domperidone** are such drugs. However, metoclopramide is also a partial dopamine antagonist and may worsen the patients Parkinson's symptoms.

Levomepromazine (also known as methotrimeprazine) is an antipsychotic with a broad spectrum of antiemetic activity, including antidopaminergic effects, and should be avoided in this case.

Prochlorperazine is most effective for labyrinthine-related nausea, such as travel sickness. It can cause extrapyramidal symptoms.

Cyclizine is an antimuscarinic and histamine-receptor antagonist. It acts centrally on the vomiting centre and is unlikely to cause any untoward side effects in a Parkinsonian patient. In fact, the antimuscarinic effects may help rigidity and tremor (but not bradykinesia). However, it is less appropriate as an antiemetic because it will not alter gastric outflow. ➤

The best choice would, therefore, be **domperidone**.

Sometimes, patients with inoperable carcinoma of the head of the pancreas develop complete obstruction of the second part of the duodenum. This presents with symptoms of gastric outflow obstruction as described above. The treatment of choice in this condition is radiological placement of an expandable metal mesh stent across the stricture.

325 Question on p.105.

Answer B
Left bundle branch block

Reversed splitting occurs when the aortic valve closes after the pulmonary valve. It is caused by a delay in left ventricular emptying.

Splitting of the second heart sound

Physiological

| | Expiration | ▌‖ | Children, young adults |
| | *Inspiration | ▌ ‖ | |

Wide splitting

| | Expiration | ▌ ‖ | RBBB |
| | Inspiration | ▌ ‖ | |

Fixed splitting

| | Expiration | ▌ ‖ | ASD |
| | Inspiration | ▌ ‖ | |

Reverse splitting

| | Expiration | ‖ ▌ | LBBB, Aortic stenosis, LVF |
| | Inspiration | ‖ ▌ | |

Note: ▌ = A_2 ‖ = P_2

*inspiration increases venous return to the right side of the heart and lengthens the time it takes the right ventricle to empty.

Answer E
Libman–Sacks endocarditis

The important results to identify from the question are:

- new left-sided murmur
- new renal impairment with haematuria
- raised ESR with normal CRP.

The **erythrocyte sedimentation rate** is a measure of the rate of fall of red blood cells in a calibrated tube. During an acute-phase response, there is an increase in plasma proteins, such as fibrinogen, immunoglobulins and α_2-macroglobulin, and these increase the ESR. However, the ESR can also be influenced by other changes in the blood. The presence of other plasma proteins, e.g. in myeloma, will cause a raised ESR. Also certain hyperglobulinaemic states such as Sjögren's syndrome and SLE will give a high result.

C-reactive protein is a protein synthesized in the liver in response to proinflammatory cytokines (IL-1, IL-6 and TNF) during the acute-phase response. It is not influenced by changes in plasma proteins.

In a 26-year-old female with new-onset renal impairment and haematuria, the diagnosis must be SLE. This particular condition is known as **Libman–Sacks endocarditis**. Some patients with SLE have a very high ESR owing to the high gammaglobulins but a relatively normal CRP. This is a classical membership question.

It is not **atrial myxoma** because patients tend to have right-sided murmurs and the CRP would also be raised.

It is not **rheumatic fever** because the patient does not fit the diagnostic criteria.

Marantic endocarditis usually occurs in patients with cancer (gastric and pancreatic) or some other debilitating illness. Fibrin is deposited on damaged valve leaflets of the heart, more commonly the left side. Her story and age make this unlikely to be the answer.

Answer A
JC virus

Progressive multifocal leucoencephalopathy is a progressive demyelinating disease occurring in the immunocompromised. Disease descriptions were first noted in the 1930s but it was not diagnosed as an entity until the 1950s, where characterization of the pathological basis was described. The **JC virus** is the underlying infection, seemingly causing demyelination and alteration of primary brain cells. ➤

Its incidence has grown exponentially with the burden of HIV disease. It commonly seems to affect men between the ages of 25 and 50 with a male to female ratio of 8:1. It is an AIDS-defining illness and is the first presentation of the infection in 1% of people. Presentation tends to be with rapidly progressive focal neurology, e.g. weakness or speech disturbances, associated with an alteration in mental state or dementia.

Diagnosis is by CT of the brain showing characteristic changes of hypodense lesions in the white matter with no mass effect. CSF examination shows few cells but often there is an elevated protein level. PCR of the CSF to detect JC virus is sensitive and specific. The prognosis is poor, median survival from diagnosis being 6 months.

HIV infection of the nervous system produces both a sensory polyneuropathy and AIDS dementia complex (ADC) by a direct effect on the brain tissue. ADC gives progressive dementia, personality changes and cognitive impairment. CT scanning shows atrophic changes. CSF shows a raised protein count.

CMV virus tends to affect the nervous system by causing encephalitis. Symptoms are similar to ADC. However, the CSF examination shows a surprising increase in white cells, which are predominantly neutrophils.

Infection with **Herpes simplex type 2 virus** tends to come primarily from genital infection. In the immunocompromised host, infection can easily become disseminated. Encephalitis is a serious complication of primary infection. Symptoms include rapid onset of fitting, focal neurological signs and changes in personality. Examination of the CSF shows a moderately raised protein with a lymphocytosis. CT scanning often shows local inflammation within the temporal lobes.

BK virus is a polyomavirus frequently found in immunocompromised patients and has been linked with graft dysfunction in those with renal transplants.

328

Question on p.106.

Answer D
Warfarin

Atrial fibrillation is a risk factor for stroke. Independent risk depends on age, presence of risk factors for ischaemic heart disease, and presence or absence of heart failure. This gentleman has had a TIA probably secondary to AF. He has no other risk factors that we know about, which makes his annual risk about 6% (two previous episodes).

Warfarin has been shown to reduce the risk of having a further stroke in patients with AF. In one trial studying placebo versus warfarin, patients in the placebo arm suffered strokes at the rate of 6% (all ages), compared with 2% per annum in those taking warfarin.

The antiplatelet agents, **dipyridamole** and **aspirin**, both reduce incidence of TIAs and strokes in patients with vascular risks. However, there is minimal evidence that these drugs alter outcome in young patients with AF.

There is no need for **digoxin**, as this gentleman is already rate controlled.

Disopyramide is a sodium channel-blocker, class IA antiarrhythmic. It is not indicated in this situation.

329 Question on p.106.

Answer D
Stop unfractionated heparin

Whilst on unfractionated heparin for treatment of his DVT, this gentleman has acquired thrombocytopenia and an arterial thrombosis. This must be treated as heparin-induced thrombocytopenia syndrome (HITS) until proved otherwise. Clinically important thrombocytopenia occurs between day 6 and 10 of treatment and is immune mediated. It occurs in around 1% of patients receiving heparin for more than 5 days.

Paradoxically this syndrome may be complicated by thrombosis. Platelet aggregation and destruction occurs, which leads to severe arterial and venous thrombosis. Regular platelet counts for patients receiving heparin (including low-molecular-weight) are recommended if treatment is expected to exceed 5 days. **Heparin should be discontinued** if patients develop thrombocytopenia or if there is a drop in the platelet count of greater than 50%. Heparin should always be avoided in these patients in future.

Patients who have developed HITS still require anticoagulation and so an alternative should be used, such as lepirudin, or a heparinoid, such as danaparoid. **Low-molecular-weight heparin** should not be used, as HITS occurs with both low-molecular-weight and unfractionated heparin.

Low-molecular-weight heparins are best avoided in patients receiving dialysis as they precipitate the risk of bleeding. Unfractionated heparin is used preferentially as, unlike low-molecular-weight heparin, it does not accumulate in renal disease.

A surgical opinion should be sought in relation to perform an arterial **embolectomy**.

330 Question on p.107.

Answer C
CT brain

This man has a subdural haematoma until proved otherwise. He does have other factors that could be responsible for his condition; however, best medical practice is to rule out the most life-threatening diagnosis first. His risk factors for having a subdural haematoma include the following: ➤

of alcohol abuse:
 ˥lect
 ͻd clotting
 ͻed GCS
 ˌ˛eurology
 ˌgmus
 ͻry of epilepsy
 ˌf recently diagnosed, it could it be secondary to a bleed.

Subdural haematomas describe the accumulation of blood in the subdural space. They can be acute, subacute or chronic. **Acutely** they follow head injury and are associated with damage to the underlying brain tissue. Prognosis is poor. **Subacute** bleeds have fluctuating symptoms over the course of a few weeks. Headaches, drowsiness and confusion are common and often the initial injury cannot be remembered. **Chronic** bleeds have variable presentation. They are more common in the elderly and are frequently misdiagnosed as a stroke. As a rule, anyone presenting with progressive confusion and signs should have a CT scan to rule out a chronic bleed, having a low threshold in the elderly and alcoholics.

Skull X-rays are of no benefit in picking up subdurals because they do not alter your management at all. If a fracture is present, a scan is needed and, if no fracture is seen, it provides no reassurance to the absence of a bleed.

If the **CT scan** is normal, other diagnoses need to be considered:
Wernicke–Korsakoff's syndrome should be considered and **thiamine** prescribed whilst awaiting the scan.

Since **phenytoin** is metabolized by zero-order kinetics, toxicity occurs frequently in overdose and can have a similar presentation. One of the first things that should be checked is his blood glucose to rule out hypoglycaemia. However, dextrose administration without first giving thiamine can precipitate Wernicke–Korsakoff's syndrome.

A **lumbar puncture** should not be carried out before a CT scan because of the high risk of tentorial herniation.

331

Question on p.107.

Answer E
Uranium

Beryllium copper alloy is highly resistant to corrosion. It is used in industries such as electronics, aerospace and atomic reactors. Despite being inhaled through the lungs the disease it causes is a systemic one, similar to that of sarcoidosis. It can lead to pulmonary fibrosis if levels are uncontrolled in the normal working environment. Fortunately, there have been improvements in working conditions and now berrylliosis is very uncommon.

Pneumoconiosis is a disease caused by **coal dust** particles that are trapped in the small airways of the lungs. The greater the exposure to coal dust, the greater the incidence of disease. There are two forms: simple pneumoconiosis and progressive massive fibrosis.

Simple pneumoconiosis is a disease caused simply by the deposition of coal dust in the lungs. There are three grades and these are differentiated on X-ray appearance:

1. a few small round opacities
2. numerous small round opacities but with some normal lung markings
3. numerous small round opacities with few normal lung markings (30% of patients with grade 3 progress to progressive massive fibrosis).

Progressive massive fibrosis tends to affect the apices particularly where there is destruction of normal lung parenchyma and round fibrotic masses with occasional central necrotic areas. This often gives symptoms of severe dyspnoea. Prognosis is poor, as most patients develop respiratory failure.

Silica exposure occurs among stone masons, those involved in foundries, potters and ceramic industries. Silica and its dust are potentially exceedingly fibrotic. A small amount of silica can produce a large inflammatory reaction. The chest X-ray has a typical 'eggshell' calcification pattern.

Byssinosis is a disease occurring in those exposed to **cotton dust**. The exact nature of the disease is unclear but thought to be secondary to exposure to endotoxins present in bacteria in the cotton. Symptoms are similar to occupational asthma, dyspnoea and cough occurring on return to work. There are no X-ray changes.

Uranium has been found to increase the risk of lung cancer significantly. Miners of uranium suffering from lung ailments were first noticed as far back as 1540. However, it was not until this century that a firm connection was made. The quantum of risk is still not known because, as with mesothelioma, there is a considerable time lag between exposure and onset.

| 332 | Question on p. 107. |

Answer D
Severe alcohol poisoning

The blood gas picture shows a metabolic acidosis with an increased anion gap. The anion gap is calculated as below:

$$\text{Anion gap} = [(Na^+) + (K^+)] - [(HCO_3^-) + (Cl^-)]$$
$$\text{Normal range} = 13 - 19$$

In this case,

$$\text{Anion gap} = [(144) + (5.4)] - [(12) + (106)]$$
$$= 31.4$$

➤

If the anion gap is increased, it is assumed that there is an unmeasured anion present, which is either exogenous, e.g. salicylate or endogenous, e.g. lactate.

Causes of a metabolic acidosis with a raised anion gap are listed below.

- **Renal disease** – retention of H^+ along with SO_4^- and PO_4^-
- **Ketoacidosis:**
  – diabetic ketoacidosis
  – alcohol overdose
- **Exogenous acid**
  – salicylate
- **Lactic acidosis:**
  –Type A (lack of tissue O_2 and hence anaerobic metabolism), e.g. sepsis, hypotension
  –Type B (abnormal cell metabolism), e.g. metformin accumulation.

The patient in question has a normal BM and so **diabetic ketoacidosis** is unlikely. Severe **paracetamol overdose** can lead to drowsiness and metabolic acidosis in the later stages as the patient's liver decompensates. This is usually several days after the overdose and is usually accompanied by hypoglycaemia and deterioration in renal biochemistry, making this a less likely explanation.

Renal tubular acidosis is one of the few causes of a normal anion gap metabolic acidosis and is not the answer.

Salicylate overdose will initially cause a metabolic acidosis along with tinnitus, deafness, sweating and vasodilation. Coma is very rare and is usually accompanied by a centrally mediated compensatory respiratory alkalosis.

This leaves **severe alcohol poisoning**, which can explain the biochemical disturbance and clinical picture. Also common things are common and alcohol poisoning is one of the commonest non-trauma-related causes of young males presenting to casualty.

Causes of a normal anion gap metabolic acidosis
- Renal tubular acidosis
- Bicarbonate losing pancreatic fistula
- Uretosigmoid diversion
- Severe diarrhoea, e.g. cholera
- Acetazolamide

Answer A
Sjögren's syndrome

Coeliac disease is associated with many disorders. Of most importance is the increased incidence of malignancies of the upper GI tract in patients with untreated coeliac disease. These include small bowel lymphoma (relative risk 7:240), small bowel adenocarcinoma (relative risk 60:876) and oesophageal adenocarcinoma. Following treatment the risk of developing these malignancies decreases and, after 5 years of treatment, the risk is probably no greater than the average population risk.

Osteoporosis, iron-deficiency anaemia and vitamin B_{12} deficiency are all common in patients with coeliac disease. They are consequences of the enteropathy and usually respond to a gluten-free diet and appropriate replacement or drug therapy.

Conditions associated with coeliac disease

Condition	Incidence in coeliac disease	Coeliac disease incidence in patients with these conditions	Comments
Dermatitis herpetiformis	5%	70%	Treated with dapsone and gluten-free diet
Microscopic colitis		20%	
Sjögren's		15%	
Thyroid disease	25%	4%	
Diabetes mellitus		3%	Type 1 diabetes only
Pancreatic disease	30%	7%	Chronic pancreatic insufficiency
Down's syndrome		5%	
Turner's syndrome		2%	
Primary biliary cirrhosis	3%	4%	Liver does not improve with diet
Autoimmune hepatitis		3%	Liver does not improve with diet
Raised ALT	40%	9%	Normalizes with diet
Chronic juvenile arthritis		1%	
Idiopathic dilated cardiomyopathy		2%	
Alopecia areata		1%	

Answer B
Penicillamine

All the drugs mentioned in the question are used as disease-modifying drugs in patients with rheumatoid arthritis. Their mechanism of action is by modulating the immune system at various points including the inhibition of cytokine production. All have potentially serious side effects.

Gold is usually reserved for patients who are intolerant of or unresponsive to other therapies. It has to be used with great care, as immune reactions including angioneurotic oedema and exfoliative dermatitis are common. For this reason, a test dose is usually given. Other side effects include pulmonary fibrosis, cholestatic jaundice and glomerulonephritis. A total of 30% of patients have to stop the treatment because of side effects.

Penicillamine is also reserved for difficult cases. It has no effect on the disease for at least 3 months. Side effects include thrombocytopenia, rash, loss of taste and proteinuria. A number of patients develop drug-induced lupus, which resolves after stopping the drug.

Sulphasalazine is the most commonly used disease-modifying agent used in the treatment of rheumatoid arthritis. The reason for this is that it is effective (in 50%) and side effects are less than with the other agents. Common side effects include rash and macrocytosis. Rarely bone marrow suppression occurs.

Methotrexate is also effective and generally well tolerated in patients with rheumatoid arthritis. It can cause marrow suppression and a dose-related hepatic fibrosis (at a cumulative dose greater than 5 g). It is usually given with folic acid.

Hydroxychloroquine is used in mild to moderate disease with a response rate of approximately 50% at 4 weeks. Its main side effect is a retinopathy, which appears dose related. It is rare, even after protracted treatment. Patients should have careful visual field monitoring before starting and at 6 monthly intervals whilst receiving this drug.

Answer D
Phenoxybenzamine

This patient needs both α- and β-blockade prior to surgery. The α-blockade controls the blood pressure by reducing peripheral vasoconstriction. The β-blockade controls the tachycardia.

A β-blocker, e.g. **atenolol**, should never be given alone to a patient with a phaeochromocytoma. The reason for this is that, although the tachycardia may be controlled, β-blockade will exacerbate the peripheral vasoconstriction caused by the now unopposed α action of adrenaline. This may result in a fatal hypertensive crisis.

The treatment of choice is initially an α blocker. **Phenoxybenzamine** is the drug most frequently used, as it is an irreversible α blocker that cannot be overcome by a catecholamine surge. Treatment should be started several weeks prior to surgery as this will allow the volume depletion which is always present, to be corrected.

β-Blockers are added in once the patient has been established on phenoxybenzamine. **Labetalol**, which is an α- and β-blocker, has been used successfully in this situation but is not the preferred treatment option.

Hydralazine and **nifedipine** have no place in the management of hypertension in patients with phaeochromocytoma.

During surgery major changes in blood pressure can occur, and only an experienced anaesthetist should take on such a case. When the surgeon handles the tumour, a massive rise in blood pressure can occur. This may require the administration of sodium nitroprusside. After the tumour is removed, and sometimes immediately following clamping of the adrenal vein, major sustained hypotension may occur. This may require the infusion of large volumes of fluid with or without intravenous α- and β-agonists.

---

336 Question on p.109.

Answer D
Normal pressure hydrocephalus

The most significant feature in the presentation is urinary incontinence, as few dementias have dementia as a presenting feature. A **frontal lobe tumour** may present with personality change and unsociable behaviour, such as urinating in inappropriate places. However, the history does not describe typical frontal behaviour and the downgoing plantar makes this less likely.

Fifty per cent of **Alzheimer's** patients develop urinary incontinence but it is a late feature.

Vascular dementia may also feature urinary incontinence but the presentation is rarely gradual. Normally the patient has exacerbations with a stepwise deterioration in function. Tone is usually increased and plantars are upgoing.

The gait is broad-based, bradykinetic and shuffling, making **Parkinson's disease** a differential. However, it does not have rigidity, tremor or response to standard Parkinson's drugs. The gait is not strictly speaking ataxic (having no weakness or ataxia) and is described as a gait apraxia.

The clinical features are highly suggestive of **normal pressure hydrocephalus**. Normal pressure hydrocephalus (NPH) is a clinical symptom complex characterized by abnormal gait, urinary incontinence and dementia. It is an important diagnosis since it is a reversible cause of dementia. The history of falls may be purely due to the abnormal gait but ➤

it is also possible that the patient had a fall, sustaining a head injury, which caused the NPH. Treatment involves drainage of CSF initially by lumbar puncture followed by CSF shunting by surgical intervention.

337

Question on p.109.

Answer D
δ cells

The pancreas has two main functional organs: the exocrine pancreas and endocrine pancreas. The islets of Langerhans make up the endocrine pancreas and consist of four main cell types:

- **α cells** that secrete glucagon
- **β cells** that secrete insulin
- **δ cells** that secrete somatostatin
- **PP cells** that secrete pancreatic polypeptide.

The exocrine pancreas is involved in the production and secretion of proteases, amylase and lipase. Pancreatic **acinar cells** synthesize and secrete these digestive enzymes. These drain via the accompanying ductile and interlobular ducts into the pancreatic duct. This then empties via the ampulla of Vater into the duodenum. The acinar cell is subject to the activity of several hormones and neurotransmitters including:

- vasoactive intestinal polypeptide (VIP)
- secretin
- cholecystokinin (CCK)
- acetylcholine
- gastrin-releasing peptide (GRP).

Pancreatic juice consists of the following:

- amylase
- lipases–lipase, phospholipase A, carboxylesterase
- proteases – trypsinogen, chymotrypsinogen, proelastase, procarboxypeptidase
- bicarbonate
- chloride.

338

Question on p.109.

Answer B
Acetazolamide

This patient has a bicarbonate of 13 mmol/L and an anion gap of 13.3 mmol/L. She, therefore, has a metabolic acidosis with a normal anion gap.

The causes of a normal anion gap metabolic acidosis are as follows.

- Loss of bicarbonate from the gut:
  - ileostomy
  - diarrhoea
  - uterosigmoidostomy.
- Loss of bicarbonate from the kidney:
  - acetazolamide
  - type 2 renal tubular acidosis
  - hyperparathyroidism
  - heavy metal poisoning.
- Reduced renal H^+ loss:
  - type 1 renal tubular acidosis
  - type 4 renal tubular acidosis

Acetazolamide inhibits carbonic anhydrase, which is found in the gastric mucosa, pancreas, eye and kidney. In patients taking this drug, the kidneys are less able to secrete H^+, so producing an acidosis. It is used to prevent mountain sickness. One of the mechanisms by which it does this is by producing a metabolic acidosis and so increasing respiratory drive.

| 339 | Question on p.110. |

Answer B
Meilioidosis

This patient has a fever with multiple abscesses in the liver and spleen after returning from rural eastern Thailand. There are very few conditions that can cause this particular combination and the most likely diagnosis is meilioidosis.

Meilioidosis is a condition caused by a Gram-negative rod that is closely related to *Pseudomonas* sp. It affects horses and asses as well as humans. The causative organism is *Burkholderia pseudomallei*, which is fairly ubiquitous and can be isolated from soil samples from a large number of underdeveloped countries. It is found in large concentrations in soil samples from certain countries, particularly in eastern Thailand, Laos and Vietnam, and in these countries the disease is common in rural communities. Meilioidosis is also seen in rural northern Australia around the Darwin area.

Meilioidosis first came to prominence when a number of US servicemen developed the disease whilst serving in the Vietnam War in the 1960s. It is thought that the mode of transmission in these cases was perhaps caused by the effect of the down-draught of the helicopter blades producing an aerosol of contaminated soil, infecting embarking or disembarking servicemen. The orofaecal route is likely to be a more common mode of transmission in endemic areas. Meilioidosis is a serious disease and carries a mortality rate of 50%. Patients usually present, as in this case, with multiple abscesses with the following sites being involved (see table). ➤

Site	Incidence
Lung	50%
Soft tissue	10%
Liver	6%
Urinary	5%
Spleen	4%
Generalized sepsis with no focus	12%

As in this case, more than one site can be involved. Diabetes (40%) and chronic renal disease (15%) are predisposing factors. In children the disease has a very different pattern, with up to 30% presenting with a parotid abscess. Meilioidosis is resistant to many antibiotics. Treatment is by intravenous ceftazidine or carbepenen, followed by a 24-week course of oral antibiotic therapy. The disease can recur up to 30 years later and follow-up should be lifelong.

Typhoid fever and **malaria** do not present with multiple abscesses in the spleen and liver. **Amoebic abscess** is the commonest cause of an abscess in the liver in this part of the world. They are always single and can be very large. The second commonest cause of liver abscess is *Streptococcus milleri*. This can cause single or multiple hepatic abscesses, but coexisting multiple splenic abscesses would be very unusual. Most patients with abscesses due to *Streptococcus milleri* have an underlying focus of infection within the abdomen, e.g. diverticular abscess, which has often been clinically silent. As a result, patients with this problem are often over the age of 50.

340
Question on p.110.

Answer C
Hypertrichosis

Patients on cyclosporin commonly get *hypertrichosis* not *hirsuitism*. **Hirsuitism** refers to the male pattern of hair growth seen in females and differs to **hypertrichosis**, the state of excessive hair growth at any site, which may occur in either sex.

Causes of hypertrichosis include the following.

General.
- Anorexia nervosa
- Malnutrition
- Porphyria cutanea tarda
- Underlying malignancy
- Drugs:
  - cyclosporin
  - minoxidil.

Local
- Spina bifida
- Pigmented naevus
- Lichen simplex.

Adverse effects of cyclosporin
- Hypertrichosis
- Hypertension
- Nephrotoxicity
- Liver dysfunction
- Burning hands and feet
- Gum hypertrophy
- Risk of malignancy
- Fluid retention
- Hyperkalaemia
- Neuropathy
- Myopathy

Although **neuropathy** and **myopathy** are recognized adverse effects, they are much less common that hypertrichosis.

---

341 Question on p.110.

Answer A
Metformin

Metformin reduces cardiovascular mortality by 39% when given to overweight patients with type 2 diabetes mellitus, compared to diet alone. It also reduces all-cause mortality by 36%, and diabetic-related deaths by 42%.

The main complication of metformin therapy is lactic acidosis, which has an estimated prevalence of 1 to 5 in 100 000. Lactic acidosis can be precipitated by hypoxia or renal failure. Metformin has a short half-life and is excreted solely through the kidneys. A new set of guidelines has recently been drawn up for the withdrawal of metformin therapy in patients at risk of lactic acidosis.

Withdrawal of metformin therapy in patients at risk of lactic acidosis
- Stop if serum creatinine > 150 µmol/L or ejection fraction < 35%
- Withdraw
  - During periods of tissue hypoxia, e.g. myocardial infarction
  - For 3 days after iodine-containing contrast media*
  - 2 days before general anaesthesia*

*Restart metformin after checking renal function is stable.

Question on p.111.

Answer A
Aspirin

Isosorbide mononitrate and **bendrofluazide** are useful in symptomatic relief of angina and heart failure but there is no evidence that they specifically improve prognosis post-infarction.

β-Blockers reduce myocardial workload and oxygen consumption by reducing the heart rate, blood pressure and contractility, and they increase the threshold for ventricular fibrillation. A meta-analysis of such treatment in patients who have had myocardial infarctions shows a 20% reduction in long-term mortality and a 34% reduction in sudden cardiac death.

Calcium channel blockers have been shown not to improve outcome, with nifedipine increasing the risk of mortality and reinfarction.

The patient is already on an **ACE inhibitor** and many clinical trials have evaluated them in patients with myocardial infarction. They have been shown to reduce mortality at 2 years by 25–30%. Patients with large myocardial infarctions, clinical signs of heart failure, or objective evidence of having a left ventricular ejection fraction < 40% benefit most, with significant reduction in mortality and risk of heart failure.

Aspirin's benefit in secondary prevention is well established. In 19 791 patients who had had myocardial infarctions reviewed by the Antiplatelet Therapy Trialists, aspirin led to a 12% reduction in death, a 31% reduction in reinfarction and a 42% reduction in non-fatal stroke. Low to medium doses (75–325 mg/day) are as effective as high doses (1200 mg/day), with fewer gastrointestinal side effects.

Although this question does not mention **statins**, it is important to be aware of the evidence for their use in the secondary prevention post-myocardial infarction. Meta-analysis of secondary prevention trials suggests that lipid-lowering agents produce a reduction in fatal and non-fatal myocardial infarctions and cardiovascular deaths. The Scandinavian simvastatin survival study randomized over 4000 patients with angina or myocardial infarction, and raised low-density lipoprotein cholesterol concentration to receive simvastatin or placebo. During the median follow-up period of 5.4 years all cause mortality for the patients given simvastatin was reduced by 30%, which was largely attributed to the 42% reduction in the incidence of fatal coronary events in this group. Treatment led to a 34% reduction in the risk of a major coronary event and a 37% decrease in the need for revascularization during the study. The cholesterol and recurrent events trial used pravastatin in a population of patients with myocardial infarction whose mean total cholesterol concentration (5.42 mmol/L) and low-density lipoprotein cholesterol (3.60 mmol/L) were essentially the average for a general population. After a mean follow-up of 5 years, patients assigned pravastatin had a 24% reduction in fatal coronary artery disease and non-fatal myocardial infarctions.

Answer B
Progressive supranuclear palsy

This lady has Parkinsonism, as diagnosed by bradykinesia, shuffling gait, monotonous speech and tremor. There is no mention of rigidity, but other characteristics are present here and indicate the diagnosis.

The addition of gaze palsy suggests one of the Parkinson's plus syndromes. These are a group of conditions that all have Parkinsonism as a basis plus other neurological signs and symptoms.

Parkinson's plus syndromes

Name	Parkinson's	Plus	Treatment	Prognosis
Progressive supranuclear palsy	Parkinsonism	Axial rigidity Dementia Vertical and lateral gaze palsy	Anti-Parkinson's	Death 5–10 years after diagnosis
Multiple system atrophy	Parkinsonism	Autonomic dysfunction, e.g. postural hypotension	Anti-Parkinson's α-Blockers Fludrocortisone	Death 7–10 years after diagnosis
Corticobasal degeneration	Parkinsonism	Dysarthria Dysphasia Myoclonus Dystonia	Clonazepam Anti-Parkinson's no help	Death 6–8 years after diagnosis
Lewy body dementia	Parkinsonism	Visual hallucinations Confusion Loss memory Fluctuating cognition	Atypical antipsychotics, e.g. Risperidone	Poor Death 5 years after diagnosis

Answer C
Amoxicillin and probenecid

This patient has gonorrhoea as demonstrated by the presence of intracellular Gram-negative diplococci or *Neisseria gonorrhoea*. It can be diagnosed in clinic by Gram staining; however, this must always be confirmed by culture, particularly in females. Treatment is offered immediately in clinic and comprises a single dose of **amoxicillin and probenecid** im. **Cefuroxime** is used in those allergic to penicillin. Penicillin-resistant gonorrhoea is treated with a single dose of ciprofloxacin or spectinomycin. Systemic disease (perihepatitis, bacteraemia and salpingitis) is treated with cefuroxime im or iv.

Metronidazole is used to treat bacterial vaginosis.

Doxycycline is used in the treatment of *Chlamydia*.
Benzylpenicillin im is the initial treatment of choice for primary and secondary syphilis.

345

Question on p.112.

Answer A
Oral slow-release morphine sulphate

This patient has end-stage chronic obstructive pulmonary disease. His life expectancy is very limited and is probably a few months at best. In this situation, patients often have very distressing breathlessness that can make them suicidal. This patient has no evidence of an infective cause for the exacerbation of his symptoms, which are due to the relentless progression of his disease.

Biphasic positive airway pressure (BIPAP) may well improve his oxygenation, but most patients find this therapy very distressing and, in this context, is not appropriate. **Intravenous aminophylline** may also have a marginal effect on his airways and improve his oxygenation, but is unlikely to have a major effect on his breathlessness. It is also extremely arrhythmogenic, particularly in patients who are hypokalaemic.

This patient is terminally ill and is clearly past the stage of potential **lung reduction surgery**. This technique can, however, considerably improve patients' symptoms and effort tolerance in selected cases.

This patient is already on oral corticosteroid therapy and it is, therefore, unlikely that **intravenous corticosteroids** will have a major impact on his airways, oxygenation or breathlessness.

A recent meta-analysis of several small trials and a large double-blind trial from Australia have shown that patients with end-stage chronic obstructive pulmonary disease with severe dyspnoea obtain significant improvement in their symptoms when treated with **oral slow-release morphine sulphate**. Most patients treated in this way tolerate this opiate very well. The most common side effect is constipation, which can be minimized by the co-prescription of a regular laxative. A small number of patients develop nausea. This is due to stimulation of μ-opioid receptors in the vomiting centre of the brain. This usually passes but is easily remedied by a small dose of nocturnal dopamine antagonist, such as haloperidol.

The WHO and the US National Institute of Health regard opioids as being contraindicated in the management of dyspnoea due to chronic obstructive pulmonary disease. The basis for this is the risk of respiratory depression and the subsequent removal of hypoxic drive, leading to CO_2 retention. It is likely that the views of these two institutions will change in the light of these most recent data.

The optimum starting dose of slow-release morphine sulphate for the treatment of dyspnoea in patients with chronic obstructive pulmonary disease is unknown. It is probably prudent to start with 10 mg bd and titrate the dose upwards, depending on clinical response and side effects.

Question on p.112.

Answer D
12%

Venous thromboembolism is up to four times more likely to develop within 2–4 weeks of a flight. This risk appears to be highest within the first 2 weeks of a flight. The incidence of venous pulmonary embolism is greater among passengers who travel more than 10 000 kilometres.

A recent study from Australia has shown that a single long-haul flight per year increases the annual risk of venous thromboembolism by 12%. This equates to an absolute rate of developing thromboembolism of between 7 and 30 cases per million flights, with longer flights conferring the greater risk.

The optimal method of reducing the risk of venous thromboembolism in patients travelling by air remains to be determined.

 Question on p.112.

Answer B
HLA B51

Behçet's disease is an uncommon vasculitis of unknown cause. The HLA B51 haplotype carries a relative risk of approximately ten for developing this disorder. It is more common in certain ethnic groups and, in particular, in patients of Turkish origin.

The diagnosis should be considered in a patient with recurrent oral ulceration, and two or more of the following:

- genital ulceration
- ophthalmic symptoms or signs
  - uveitis
  - retinal changes
- dermatological symptoms or signs
  - erythema nodosum
  - pseudofolliculitis
- a positive pathergy test.

A skin pathergy test is based on the observation that patients with Behçet's disease develop a papule or pustule at the site of a needle prick. This usually occurs within 1–2 days.

Behçet's disease can also affect the gut by producing a florid colitis, which may be difficult to distinguish from inflammatory bowel disease. Thirty per cent of patients show neurological involvement, which includes aseptic meningitis, transverse myelitis, encephalitis and thrombosis of the cerebral veins. Patients with Behçet's commonly have joint symptoms. These are usually due to a mild large joint monoarthropathy or oligoarthropathy.

Treatment consists of immunosuppressive therapy with corticosteroids or cyclosporin.

348   Question on p.112.

Answer B
Performance status 1

The World Health Organization Performance Status is commonly used in the assessment of patients when planning appropriate treatment. Since risks will need to be weighed against potential benefits, it can be useful in assessing whether someone would benefit from active or palliative treatment. Clearly someone with a poor performance status is less likely to be able to withstand radical aggressive treatment and a more palliative approach can be considered.

The classification is outlined below:

0	Normal, no restrictions
1	Strenuous activity restricted
	Ambulatory, can do light work
2	Up and about > 50% of waking hours
	Limited self-care
3	Confined to bed or chair > 50% of waking hours
	Limited self-care
4	Confined to bed or chair
	Nil self-care, completely disabled.

349   Question on p.113.

Answer E
Occipital cortex infarction

Retinal artery occlusion produces blindness in the eye affected.

A **pituitary macroadenoma** causes a bitemporal hemianopia. The upper parts of the visual fields are usually affected first, as the tumour tends to grow upwards and distort the optic chiasm from below. In contrast, a craniopharyngioma (which is the other common cause of bitemporal hemianopia) tends to grow downwards from above the chiasm and the lower visual fields are, therefore, affected first.

Temporal lobe infarction causes an upper quadrantic homonymous hemianopia. It is very rare for a full homonymous hemianopia to be produced by this lesion.

Parietal lobe infarction causes a lower quadrantic homonymous hemianopia. It is very rare for a full homonymous hemianopia to be produced by this lesion.

Occipital cortex infarction causes a homonymous hemianopia, usually with macular sparing. The common cause of this is an infarction in the territory of the posterior cerebral artery. The macula is usually spared as the macula area in the occipital cortex has a separate blood supply from the middle cerebral artery.

Question on p.113.

Answer E
Mallory–Weiss tear

This patient gives a typical history of a **Mallory–Weiss tear**, i.e. recurrent vomiting with a small fresh haematemesis on the final vomit. Mallory–Weiss tears are a common cause of haematemesis and are particularly common in the younger age group. They often follow overindulgence with alcohol and are caused by vomiting, which induces a small tear at the gastro-oesophageal junction.

In most cases, the bleeding is minor or self-limiting but occasionally the bleeding can be torrential. There is a saying that 'a Mallory–Weiss tear will always stop bleeding on its own'. Whilst this is nearly always the case, sometimes the tear needs to be treated endoscopically, e.g. injected with adrenaline or clipped, or, very rarely, by surgery.

The other diagnoses given in the question are all possible causes of a haematemesis. In a case like this, it is not good medicine to rely solely on the history to make a diagnosis. It is mandatory, therefore, that this patient has an upper gastrointestinal endoscopy to make an accurate diagnosis. Only when this has been done can an appropriate treatment plan be devised.

APPENDIX OF SUBJECT CATEGORIES
(BY QUESTION)

Basic science:
24 p.10, 35 p.14, 48 p.18, 75 p.26, 87 p.30, 117 p.40, 134 p.45, 153 p.51, 166 p.56, 186 p.62, 202 p.66, 256 p.84, 337 p.109

Cardiology:
3 p.4, 14 p.7, 49 p.18, 60 p.22, 79 p.28, 85 p.29, 105 p.35, 122 p.41, 127, p.43, 143, p.48, 162 p.54, 185 p.61, 198 p.65, 215 p. 70, 220 p.72, 244 p.80, 252 p.82, 276 p.90, 278 p.91, 281 p.91, 300 p.97, 302 p.97, 311 p.100, 316 p.102, 325 p.105, 342 p.110

Dermatology:
4 p.4, 15 p.8, 59 p.22, 68 p.24, 93 p.32, 104 p.35, 118 p.40, 133 p.45, 149 p.50, 181 p.60, 200 p.66, 204 p.67, 219 p.72, 243 p.80, 274 p.89, 307 p.99, 323 p.104

Endocrine:
5 p.4, 16 p.8, 25 p.10, 62 p.22, 67 p.24, 83 p.29, 96 p.33, 125 p.42, 142 p.48, 168 p.56, 183 p.61, 193 p.64, 210 p.69, 222 p.73, 239 p.78, 255 p.83, 266 p.87, 275 p.90, 291 p.94, 298 p.96, 320 p.103, 335 p.108, 341 p.110

Gastroenterology:
6 p.5, 26 p.11, 34 p.14, 36 p.14, 45 p.17, 61 p.22, 70 p.25, 90 p.31, 95 p.32, 123 p.42, 139 p.46, 144 p.48, 152 p.51, 164 p.55, 167 p.56, 174 p.58, 187 p.62, 211 p.69, 224 p.73, 234 p.77, 251 p.82, 282 p.92, 296 p.96, 306 p.99, 333 p.108, 350 p.113

General medicine:
37 p.15, 50 p.19, 58 p.21, 109 p.37, 199 p.65, 225 p.74, 237 p.78, 249 p.81, 267 p.87, 290 p.94, 294 p.95, 305 p.98, 332 p.107, 348 p.112

Genetics:
17 p.8, 73 p.26, 88 p.30, 111 p.38, 128 p.43, 146 p.49, 169 p.57, 179 p.59, 216 p.71, 257 p.84

Haematology:
31 p.12, 44 p.17, 47 p.18, 54 p.20, 91 p.31, 110 p.38, 116 p.40, 137 p.46, 156 p.52, 182 p.60, 192 p.63, 212 p.69, 227 p.74, 247 p.81, 272 p.89, 289 p.94, 304 p.98, 308 p.99, 329 p.106, 346 p.112

Infectious diseases:
7 p.5, 18 p.8, 33 p.13, 39 p.15, 40 p.15, 53 p.20, 76 p.27, 78 p.27, 81 p.28, 102 p.35, 113 p.39, 138 p.46, 145 p.49, 158 p.53, 171 p.57, 175 p.58, 190 p.63, 203 p.66, 221 p.72, 238 p.78, 253 p.82, 263 p.86, 268 p.88, 280 p.91, 287 p.93, 292 p.94, 313 p.101, 327 p.105, 339 p.110, 344 p.111

Neurology:
8 p.5, 19 p.9, 22 p.10, 23 p.10, 30 p.12, 51 p.19, 52 p.19, 69 p.24, 94 p.32, 97 p.33, 100 p.34, 121 p.41, 130 p.44, 150 p.50, 163 p.55, 176 p.59, 189 p.62, 191 p.63, 207 p.68, 218 p.71, 230 p.75, 242 p.79, 246 p.80, 262 p.85, 265 p.87, 269 p.88, 286 p.93, 293 p.95, 295 p.95, 309 p.100, 321 p.104, 328 p.106, 330 p.107, 343 p.111

Oncology:
29 p.12, 57 p.21, 99 p.34, 214 p.70, 241 p.79, 258 p.84, 314 p.101, 322 p.104

Ophthalmology:
98 p.33, 173 p.58, 232 p.76, 349 p.113

Pharmacology:
9 p.6, 20 p.9, 27 p.11, 38 p.15, 42 p.16, 56 p.21, 74 p.26, 77 p.27, 92 p.32, 108 p.37, 120 p.41, 126 p.43, 132 p.44, 141 p.47, 147 p.49, 157 p.53, 170 p.57, 178 p.59, 206 p.67, 213 p.70, 226 p.74, 240 p.79, 254 p.83, 273 p.89, 279 p.91, 315 p.102, 324 p.104, 340 p.110

Psychiatry:
10 p.6, 43 p.16, 86 p.30, 106 p.36, 154 p.51, 160 p.54, 196 p.65, 260 p.85, 336 p.109

Renal:
1 p.3, 13 p.7, 21 p.9, 46 p.18, 55 p.29, 72 p.25, 80 p.28, 89 p.30, 103 p.35, 115 p.39, 119 p.40, 136 p.45, 140 p.47, 148 p.49, 161 p.54, 184 p.61, 201 p.66, 209 p.68, 223 p.73, 235 p.77, 261 p.85, 277 p.90, 288 p.93, 318 p.102, 319 p.103, 326 p.105, 338 p109

Respiratory:
2 p.3, 12 p.7, 64 p.23, 66 p.24, 71 p.25, 84 p.29, 107 p.36, 112 p.38, 124 p.42, 129 p.43, 135 p.45, 155 p.52, 165 p.55, 177 p.59, 188 p.62, 208 p.68, 217 p.71, 228 p.75, 245 p.80, 259 p.84, 264 p.86, 285 p.92, 297 p.96, 310 p.100, 331 p.107, 345 p.111

Rheumatology:
11 p.6, 28 p.12, 41 p.16, 63 p.23, 65 p.23, 82 p.28, 101 p.34, 114 p.39, 131 p.41, 151 p.50, 159 p.53, 172 p.57, 194 p.64, 195 p.64, 205 p.67, 229 p.75, 248 p.81, 250 p.82, 270 p.88, 284 p.92, 299 p.96, 312 p.101, 334 p.108, 347 p.112

Statistics:
32 p.13, 180 p.60, 197 p.65, 231 p.76, 233 p.77, 271 p.88, 283 p.92

INDEX